ELEMENTS OF MATHEMATICS

Springer
Berlin
Heidelberg
New York
Barcelona
Hong Kong
London
Milan
Paris
Tokyo

NICOLAS BOURBAKI

ELEMENTS OF MATHEMATICS

Lie Groups and Lie Algebras

Chapters 4–6

Springer

Originally published as
ÉLÉMENTS DE MATHÉMATIQUE,
GROUPES ET ALGÈBRES DE LIE 4, 5 et 6
© N. Bourbaki, 1968

Translator

Andrew Pressley
Department of Mathematics
King's College London
Strand, London WC2R 2LS
United Kingdom
andrew.pressley@kcl.ac.uk

First softcover printing of the 1st English edition of 2002

ISBN 978-3-540-69171-6

Library of Congress Control Number: 2008931305

Mathematics Subject Classification (2000): 22E10, 22E15, 22E60, 22-02

Cover-design: WMXDesign GmbH, Heidelberg

Printed on acid-free paper

9 8 7 6 5 4 3 2 1

springer.com

INTRODUCTION TO CHAPTERS IV, V AND VI

The study of semi-simple (analytic or algebraic) groups and their Lie algebras leads to the consideration of *root systems, Coxeter groups and Tits systems.* Chapters IV, V and VI are devoted to these structures.

To orient the reader, we give several examples below.

I. Let $\mathfrak{g}$ be a complex semi-simple Lie algebra and $\mathfrak{h}$ a Cartan subalgebra of $\mathfrak{g}$[1]. A *root* of $\mathfrak{g}$ with respect to $\mathfrak{h}$ is a non-zero linear form α on $\mathfrak{h}$ such that there exists a non-zero element x of $\mathfrak{g}$ with $[h, x] = \alpha(h)x$ for all $h \in \mathfrak{h}$. These roots form a reduced root system R in the vector space $\mathfrak{h}^*$ dual to $\mathfrak{h}$. Giving R determines $\mathfrak{g}$ up to isomorphism and every reduced root system is isomorphic to a root system obtained in this way. An automorphism of $\mathfrak{g}$ leaving $\mathfrak{h}$ stable defines an automorphism of $\mathfrak{h}^*$ leaving R invariant, and every automorphism of R is obtained in this way. The Weyl group of R consists of all the automorphisms of $\mathfrak{h}^*$ defined by the inner automorphisms of $\mathfrak{g}$ leaving $\mathfrak{h}$ stable; this is a Coxeter group.

Let G be a connected complex Lie group with Lie algebra $\mathfrak{g}$, and let Γ be the subgroup of G consisting of the elements h such that $\exp_G(2\pi i h) = 1$. Let $R^\vee$ be the root system in $\mathfrak{h}$ inverse to R, let $Q(R^\vee)$ be the subgroup of $\mathfrak{h}$ generated by $R^\vee$ and let $P(R^\vee)$ be the subgroup associated to the subgroup $Q(R)$ of $\mathfrak{h}^*$ generated by R (i.e. the set of $h \in \mathfrak{h}$ such that $\lambda(h)$ is an *integer* for all $\lambda \in Q(R)$). Then $P(R^\vee) \supset \Gamma \supset Q(R^\vee)$. Moreover, the centre of G is canonically isomorphic to $P(R^\vee)/\Gamma$ and the fundamental group of G to $\Gamma/Q(R^\vee)$. In particular, Γ is equal to $P(R^\vee)$ if G is the adjoint group and Γ is equal to $Q(R^\vee)$ if G is simply-connected. Finally, the weights of the finite-dimensional linear representations of G are the elements of the subgroup of $\mathfrak{h}^*$ associated to Γ.

II. Let G be a semi-simple connected compact real Lie group, and let $\mathfrak{g}$ be its Lie algebra. Let T be a maximal torus of G, with Lie algebra $\mathfrak{t}$, and let X be the group of characters of T. Let R be the set of non-zero elements α of X such that there exists a non-zero element x of $\mathfrak{g}$ with $(\operatorname{Ad} t).x = \alpha(t)x$ for all $t \in T$. Identify X with a lattice in the real vector space $V = X \otimes_{\mathbf{Z}} \mathbf{R}$; then R is a reduced root system in V. Let N be the normaliser of T in G; the action

[1] In this Introduction, we use freely the traditional terminology as well as the notions defined in Chapters IV, V and VI.

of N on T defines an isomorphism from the group N/T to the Weyl group of R. We have $P(R) \supset X \supset Q(R)$; moreover, $X = P(R)$ if G is simply-connected and $X = Q(R)$ if the centre of G reduces to the identity element.

The complexified Lie algebra $\mathfrak{g}_{(\mathbf{C})}$ of $\mathfrak{g}$ is semi-simple and $\mathfrak{t}_{(\mathbf{C})}$ is a Cartan subalgebra of it. There exists a canonical isomorphism from $V_{(\mathbf{C})}$ to the dual of $\mathfrak{t}_{(\mathbf{C})}$ that transforms R into the root system of $\mathfrak{g}_{(\mathbf{C})}$ with respect to $\mathfrak{t}_{(\mathbf{C})}$.

III. Let G be a connected semi-simple algebraic group over a commutative field k. Let T be a maximal element of the set of tori of G split over k and let X be the group of characters of T (the homomorphisms from T to the multiplicative group). We identify X with a lattice in the real vector space $V = X \otimes_{\mathbf{Z}} \mathbf{R}$. The roots of G with respect to T are the non-zero elements α of X such that there exists a non-zero element x of the Lie algebra $\mathfrak{g}$ of G with $(\mathrm{Ad}\, t).x = \alpha(t)x$ for all $t \in T$. This gives a root system R in V, which is not necessarily reduced. Let N be the normaliser and Z the centraliser of T in G and let $N(k)$ and $Z(k)$ be their groups of rational points over k. The action of $N(k)$ on T defines an isomorphism from $N(k)/Z(k)$ to the Weyl group of R.

Let U be a maximal element of the set of unipotent subgroups of G, defined over k and normalised by Z. Put $P = Z.U$. Then $P(k) = Z(k).U(k)$ and $P(k) \cap N(k) = Z(k)$. Moreover, there exists a basis $(\alpha_1, \ldots, \alpha_n)$ of R such that the weights of T in U are the positive roots of R for this basis; if S denotes the set of elements of $N(k)/Z(k)$ that correspond, via the isomorphism defined above, to the symmetries $s_{\alpha_i} \in W(R)$ associated to the roots α_i, the quadruple $(G(k), P(k), N(k), S)$ is a Tits system.

IV. In the theory of semi-simple algebraic groups over a local field, Tits systems are encountered whose Weyl group is the affine Weyl group of a root system. For example, let $G = \mathbf{SL}(n+1, \mathbf{Q}_p)$ (with $n \geq 1$). Let B be the group of matrices $(a_{ij}) \in \mathbf{SL}(n+1, \mathbf{Z}_p)$ such that $a_{ij} \in p\mathbf{Z}_p$ for $i < j$, and let N be the subgroup of G consisting of the matrices having only one non-zero element in each row and column. Then there exists a subset S of $N/(B \cap N)$ such that the quadruple (G, B, N, S) is a Tits system. The group $W = N/(B \cap N)$ is the affine Weyl group of a root system of type A_n; this is an infinite Coxeter group.

Numerous conversations with J. Tits have been of invaluable assistance to us in the preparation of these chapters. We thank him very cordially.

CONTENTS

CHAPTER V GROUPS GENERATED BY REFLECTIONS

CHAPTER VI ROOT SYSTEMS

CHAPTER IV
Coxeter Groups and Tits Systems

§ 1. COXETER GROUPS

In this section, W denotes a group written multiplicatively, with identity element 1, and S denotes a set of generators of W such that $\mathrm{S} = \mathrm{S}^{-1}$ and $1 \notin \mathrm{S}$. Every element of W is the product of a finite sequence of elements of S. From no. 3 onwards we assume that every element of S is of order 2.

1. LENGTH AND REDUCED DECOMPOSITIONS

DEFINITION 1. *Let $w \in \mathrm{W}$. The length of w (with respect to S), denoted by $l_{\mathrm{S}}(w)$ or simply by $l(w)$, is the smallest integer $q \geqslant 0$ such that w is the product of a sequence of q elements of* S. *A reduced decomposition of w (with respect to* S*) is any sequence $\mathbf{s} = (s_1, \ldots, s_q)$ of elements of* S *such that $w = s_1 \ldots s_q$ and $q = l(w)$.*

Thus 1 is the unique element of length 0 and S consists of the elements of length 1.

PROPOSITION 1. *Let w and w' be in* W. *We have the formulas:*

$$l(ww') \leqslant l(w) + l(w'), \tag{1}$$

$$l(w^{-1}) = l(w), \tag{2}$$

$$|l(w) - l(w')| \leqslant l(ww'^{-1}). \tag{3}$$

Let $(s_1, \ldots, s_p)$ and $(s'_1, \ldots, s'_q)$ be reduced decompositions of w and w' respectively. Thus $l(w) = p$ and $l(w') = q$. Since $ww' = s_1 \ldots s_p s'_1 \ldots s'_q$, we have $l(ww') \leqslant p + q$, proving (1). Since $\mathrm{S} = \mathrm{S}^{-1}$ and $w^{-1} = s_p^{-1} \ldots s_1^{-1}$, we have $l(w^{-1}) \leqslant p = l(w)$. Replacing w by w^{-1} gives the opposite inequality $l(w) \leqslant l(w^{-1})$, proving (2). Replacing w by ww'^{-1} in (1) and (2) gives the relations

$$l(w) - l(w') \leqslant l(ww'^{-1}), \tag{4}$$

$$l(ww'^{-1}) = l(w'w^{-1}). \tag{5}$$

Exchanging w and w' in (4) gives $l(w') - l(w) \leqslant l(ww'^{-1})$ by (5), proving (3).

COROLLARY. *Let* $\mathbf{s} = (s_1, \ldots, s_p)$ *and* $\mathbf{s}' = (s'_1, \ldots, s'_q)$ *be two sequences of elements of* S *such that* $w = s_1 \ldots s_p$ *and* $w' = s'_1 \ldots s'_q$*. If the sequence* $(s_1, \ldots, s_p, s'_1, \ldots, s'_q)$ *is a reduced decomposition of* ww'*, then* $\mathbf{s}$ *is a reduced decomposition of* w *and* $\mathbf{s}'$ *is one of* w'*.*

By hypothesis, $l(w) \leqslant p$, $l(w') \leqslant q$ and $l(ww') = p + q$. By (1), we must have $l(w) = p$ and $l(w') = q$, hence the corollary.

Remark In view of formulas (1) and (2), the formula $d(w, w') = l(ww'^{-1})$ defines a distance on W, invariant under right translations.

2. DIHEDRAL GROUPS

DEFINITION 2. *A dihedral group is a group generated by two distinct elements of order two.*

Example. Let M be the multiplicative group $\{1, -1\}$, and let m be an integer $\geqslant 2$ (resp. $m = \infty$). Then M acts on the group $\mathrm{Z}/m\mathrm{Z}$ (resp. on Z) by $(-1).x = -x$, and the corresponding semi-direct product of M by $\mathrm{Z}/m\mathrm{Z}$ (resp. of M by Z) is denoted by D_m. The elements of D_m are thus the pairs (ε, x) with $\varepsilon = \pm 1$ and $x \in \mathrm{Z}/m\mathrm{Z}$ (resp. $x \in \mathrm{Z}$); the group law on D_m is given by the formula

$$(\varepsilon, x).(\varepsilon', x') = (\varepsilon\varepsilon', \varepsilon' x + x'). \tag{6}$$

We denote by ι the class of 1 modulo m (resp. $\iota = 1$) and set

$$\rho = (-1, 0), \quad \rho' = (-1, \iota), \quad \pi = (1, \iota). \tag{7}$$

Then $\rho^2 = \rho'^2 = 1$ and $\pi = \rho\rho'$. The formulas

$$\pi^n = (1, n\iota), \quad \rho\pi^n = (-1, n\iota) \tag{8}$$

show that D_m is a dihedral group generated by $\{\rho, \rho'\}$.

PROPOSITION 2. *Assume that* S *consists of two distinct elements* s *and* s' *of order 2.*

(i) *The subgroup* P *of* W *generated by* $p = ss'$ *is normal, and* W *is the semi-direct product of the subgroup* $\mathrm{T} = \{1, s\}$ *and* P*. Moreover,* $(\mathrm{W} : \mathrm{P}) = 2$*.*

(ii) *Let* m *be the order (finite or infinite) of* p*. Then* $m \geqslant 2$ *and* W *is of order* $2m$*. There is a unique isomorphism* φ *from* D_m *to* W *such that* $\varphi(\rho) = s$ *and* $\varphi(\rho') = s'$*.*

(i) We have $sps^{-1} = sss's = s's = p^{-1}$, and hence

$$sp^n s^{-1} = p^{-n} \tag{9}$$

for every integer n. Since W is generated by $\{s, s'\}$, and hence by $\{s, p\}$, the subgroup P is normal. It follows that TP is a subgroup of W, and since TP contains s and $s' = sp$, we have $W = TP = P \cup sP$. To prove (i), it is therefore enough to show that $W \neq P$. If $W = P$, the group W would be commutative, so $p^2 = s^2 s'^2 = 1$. But then the only elements of $W = P$ would be 1 and p, contradicting the hypothesis that W contains at least three elements, namely 1, s and s'.

(ii) Since $s \neq s'$, we have $p \neq 1$ and so $m \geqslant 2$. Since P is of order m and $(W : P) = 2$, the order of W is $2m$. If m is finite (resp. infinite), there exists an isomorphism φ' from $\mathbf{Z}/m\mathbf{Z}$ (resp. $\mathbf{Z}$) to P taking π to p. Moreover, there exists an isomorphism φ'' from $M = \{1, -1\}$ to T taking -1 to s. The group W is the semi-direct product of T and P. In view of the formulas (9) and $\rho\pi^n\rho^{-1} = \pi^{-n}$, φ' and φ'' induce an isomorphism φ from D_m to W such that $\varphi(\rho) = s$ and $\varphi(\pi) = p$, and hence $\varphi(\rho') = s'$. The uniqueness of φ follows from the fact that D_m is generated by $\{\rho, \rho'\}$.

Remark. Consider a dihedral group W of order $2m$ generated by two distinct elements s and s' of order 2. Denote by $\mathbf{s}_q$ (resp. $\mathbf{s}'_q$) the sequence of length q whose odd (resp. even) numbered terms are equal to s and whose even (resp. odd) numbered terms are equal to s', and let w_q (resp. w'_q) be the product of the sequence $\mathbf{s}_q$ (resp. $\mathbf{s}'_q$). We have

$$w_{2k} = (ss')^k, \quad w_{2k+1} = (ss')^k s,$$
$$w'_{2k} = (s's)^k = (ss')^{-k}, \quad w'_{2k+1} = (s's)^k s' = (ss')^{-k-1} s.$$

If $\mathbf{s} = (s_1, \ldots, s_q)$ is a reduced decomposition (with respect to $\{s, s'\}$) of an element w of W, then clearly $s_i \neq s_{i+1}$ for $1 \leqslant i \leqslant q-1$. Hence, $\mathbf{s} = \mathbf{s}_q$ or $\mathbf{s} = \mathbf{s}'_q$.

If $m = \infty$, the elements $(ss')^n$ and $(ss')^n s$ for $n \in \mathbf{Z}$ are distinct. Hence, the elements w_q $(q \geqslant 0)$ and w'_q $(q > 0)$ are distinct, and if $\mathbf{s}$ is a reduced decomposition of w_q (resp. w'_q) we necessarily have $\mathbf{s} = \mathbf{s}_q$ (resp. $\mathbf{s} = \mathbf{s}'_q$). It follows from this that $l(w_q) = l(w'_q) = q$ and that *the set of reduced decompositions of the elements of* W *consists of the* $\mathbf{s}_q$ *and the* $\mathbf{s}'_q$. Moreover, every element of W has a unique reduced decomposition.

Suppose now that m is *finite*. If $q \geqslant 2m$, we have $w_q = w_{q-2m}$ and $w'_q = w'_{q-2m}$; if $m \leqslant q \leqslant 2m$, we have $w_q = w'_{2m-q}$, $w'_q = w_{2m-q}$. Hence, neither $\mathbf{s}_q$ nor $\mathbf{s}'_q$ are reduced decompositions if $q > m$. It follows that each of the $2m$ elements of W is one of the $2m$ elements $w_0 = w'_0$, w_q and w'_q for $1 \leqslant q \leqslant m-1$, and $w_m = w'_m$. These $2m$ elements are thus distinct and it follows as above that $l(w_q) = l(w'_q) = q$ for $q \leqslant m$ and that *the set of reduced decompositions of elements of* W *consists of the* $\mathbf{s}_q$ *and the* $\mathbf{s}'_q$ *for* $0 \leqslant q \leqslant m$. Every element of W except w_m has a unique reduced decomposition; w_m has two.

3. FIRST PROPERTIES OF COXETER GROUPS

Recall that from now on we assume that the elements of S are of order 2.

DEFINITION 3. (W, S) *is said to be a Coxeter system if it satisfies the following condition:*

(C) *For* s, s' *in* S, *let* $m(s, s')$ *be the order of* ss' *and let* I *be the set of pairs* (s, s') *such that* $m(s, s')$ *is finite. The generating set* S *and the relations* $(ss')^{m(s,s')} = 1$ *for* (s, s') *in* I *form a presentation*[1] *of the group* W.

When (W, S) is a Coxeter system, one also says, by abuse of language, that W is a *Coxeter group*.

Examples. 1) Let m be an integer $\geqslant 2$ or ∞ and let W be a group defined by a set of generators $S = \{s, s'\}$ and the relations $s^2 = s'^2 = 1$ when $m = \infty$, $s^2 = s'^2 = (ss')^m = 1$ when m is finite. Consider on the other hand the dihedral group D_m (no. 2, *Example*) and the elements ρ and ρ' of D_m defined by (7). Since $\rho^2 = \rho'^2 = 1$ and $(\rho\rho')^m = 1$ when m is finite, there exists a unique homomorphism f from W to D_m such that $f(s) = \rho$ and $f(s') = \rho'$. Since $\rho\rho'$ is of order m, it follows that ss' is itself of order m. Hence, (W, S) is a Coxeter system, W is a dihedral group of order $2m$ and f is an isomorphism (Prop. 2).

By transport of structure, it follows that every dihedral group is a Coxeter group.

2) Let $\mathfrak{S}_n$ be the symmetric group of degree n, with $n \geqslant 2$. Let s_i be the transposition of i and $i+1$ for $1 \leqslant i < n$, and let $S = \{s_1, \ldots, s_{n-1}\}$. One can show (§ 2, no.4, *Example* and § 1, Exerc. 4) that $(\mathfrak{S}_n, S)$ is a Coxeter system.

3) For the classification of finite Coxeter groups, cf. Chap. 4, § 4.

Remark. Suppose that (W, S) is a Coxeter system. There exists a homomorphism ε from W to the group $\{1, -1\}$ characterized by $\varepsilon(s) = -1$ for all $s \in S$. We call $\varepsilon(w)$ the signature of w; it is equal to $(-1)^{l(w)}$. The formula $\varepsilon(ww') = \varepsilon(w)\varepsilon(w')$ thus translates into $l(ww') \equiv l(w) + l(w') \bmod. 2$.

[1] This means that (W, S) has the following universal property: given a group G and a map f from S to G such that $(f(s)f(s'))^{m(s,s')} = 1$ for (s, s') in I, there exists a homomorphism g from W to G extending f. This homomorphism is unique because S generates W. An equivalent form of this definition is the following. Let $\overline{W}$ be a group, f a homomorphism from $\overline{W}$ to W and h a map from S to $\overline{W}$ such that $f(h(s)) = s$ and $(h(s)h(s'))^{m(s,s')} = 1$ for (s, s') in S and such that the $h(s)$ (for $s \in S$) generate $\overline{W}$. Then f is injective (and hence is an isomorphism from $\overline{W}$ to W).

PROPOSITION 3. *Assume that* (W, S) *is a Coxeter system. Then, two elements* s *and* s' *of* S *are conjugate*[2] *in* W *if and only if the following condition is satisfied:*

(I) *There exists a finite sequence* $(s_1, \ldots, s_q)$ *of elements of* S *such that* $s_1 = s, s_q = s'$ *and* $s_j s_{j+1}$ *is of finite* odd *order for* $1 \leqslant j < q$.

Let s and s' in S be such that $p = ss'$ is of finite order $2n+1$. By (9), $sp^{-n} = p^n s$ hence

$$p^n sp^{-n} = p^n p^n s = p^{-1} s = s'ss = s', \tag{10}$$

and s' is conjugate to s.

For all s in S, let A_s be the set of $s' \in S$ satisfying (I). With the hypotheses in (I), the elements s_j and s_{j+1} are conjugate for $1 \leqslant j < q$ by the above, hence every element s' of A_s is conjugate to s.

Let f be the map from S to $M = \{1, -1\}$ equal to 1 on A_s and to -1 on $S - A_s$. Let s' and s'' in S be such that $s's''$ is of finite order m. Then $f(s')f(s'') = 1$ if s' and s'' are both in A_s or both in $S - A_s$. In the other case, $f(s')f(s'') = -1$, but m is even. Thus $(f(s')f(s''))^m = 1$ in all cases. Since (W, S) is a Coxeter system, there exists a homomorphism g from W to M inducing f on S. Let s' be a conjugate of s. Since s belongs to the kernel of g, so does s', hence $f(s') = g(s') = 1$ and finally $s' \in A_s$. Q.E.D.

4. REDUCED DECOMPOSITIONS IN A COXETER GROUP

Suppose that (W, S) is a Coxeter system. Let T be the set of conjugates in W of elements of S. For any finite sequence $\mathbf{s} = (s_1, \ldots, s_q)$ of elements of S, denote by $\Phi(\mathbf{s})$ the sequence $(t_1, \ldots, t_q)$ of elements of T defined by

$$t_j = (s_1 \ldots s_{j-1}) s_j (s_1 \ldots s_{j-1})^{-1} \quad \text{for } 1 \leqslant j \leqslant q. \tag{11}$$

Then $t_1 = s_1$ and $s_1 \ldots s_q = t_q t_{q-1} \ldots t_1$. For any element $t \in T$, denote by $n(\mathbf{s}, t)$ the number of integers j such that $1 \leqslant j \leqslant q$ and $t_j = t$. Finally, put

$$R = \{1, -1\} \times T.$$

Lemma 1. (i) *Let* $w \in W$ *and* $t \in T$. *The number* $(-1)^{n(\mathbf{s},t)}$ *has the same value* $\eta(w, t)$ *for all sequences* $\mathbf{s} = (s_1, \ldots, s_q)$ *of elements of* S *such that* $w = s_1 \ldots s_q$.

(ii) *For* $w \in W$, *let* U_w *be the map from* R *to itself defined by*

$$U_w(\varepsilon, t) = (\varepsilon.\eta(w^{-1}, t), wtw^{-1}) \quad (\varepsilon = \pm 1, t \in T). \tag{12}$$

The map $w \mapsto U_w$ *is a homomorphism from* W *to the group of permutations of* R.

[2] Recall that two elements (resp. two subsets) of a group W are said to be *conjugate* if there exists an inner automorphism of W that transforms one into the other.

For $s \in \mathrm{S}$, define a map U_s from R to itself by

$$\mathrm{U}_s(\varepsilon, t) = (\varepsilon.(-1)^{\delta_{s,t}}, sts^{-1}) \quad (\varepsilon = \pm 1, t \in \mathrm{T}), \tag{13}$$

where $\delta_{s,t}$ is the Kronecker symbol. It is immediate that $\mathrm{U}_s^2 = \mathrm{Id}_\mathrm{R}$, which shows that U_s is a *permutation* of R.

Let $\mathbf{s} = (s_1, \dots, s_q)$ be a sequence of elements of S. Put $w = s_q \dots s_1$ and $\mathrm{U}_\mathbf{s} = \mathrm{U}_{s_q} \dots \mathrm{U}_{s_1}$. We shall show, by induction on q, that

$$\mathrm{U}_\mathbf{s}(\varepsilon, t) = (\varepsilon.(-1)^{n(\mathbf{s},t)}, wtw^{-1}). \tag{14}$$

This is clear for $q = 0, 1$. If $q > 1$, put $\mathbf{s}' = (s_1, \dots, s_{q-1})$ and

$$w' = s_{q-1} \dots s_1.$$

Using the induction hypothesis, we obtain

$$\begin{aligned}\mathrm{U}_\mathbf{s}(\varepsilon, t) &= \mathrm{U}_{s_q}(\varepsilon.(-1)^{n(\mathbf{s}',t)}, w'tw'^{-1}) \\ &= (\varepsilon.(-1)^{n(\mathbf{s}',t)+\delta_{s_q, w'tw'^{-1}}}, wtw^{-1}).\end{aligned}$$

But $\Phi(\mathbf{s}) = (\Phi(\mathbf{s}'), w'^{-1}s_qw')$ and $n(\mathbf{s}, t) = n(\mathbf{s}', t) + \delta_{w'^{-1}s_qw', t}$, proving formula (14).

Now let $s, s' \in \mathrm{S}$ be such that $p = ss'$ has finite order m. Let $\mathbf{s} = (s_1, \dots, s_{2m})$ be the sequence of elements of S defined by $s_j = s$ for j odd and $s_j = s'$ for j even. Then $s_{2m} \dots s_1 = p^{-m} = 1$ and formula (11) implies that

$$t_j = p^{j-1}s \quad \text{for } 1 \leqslant j \leqslant 2m. \tag{15}$$

Since p is of order m, the elements $t_1, \dots, t_m$ are distinct and $t_{j+m} = t_j$ for $1 \leqslant j \leqslant m$. For all $t \in \mathrm{T}$, the integer $n(\mathbf{s}, t)$ is thus equal to 0 or 2 and (14) shows that $\mathrm{U}_\mathbf{s} = \mathrm{Id}_\mathrm{R}$. In other words, $(\mathrm{U}_s\mathrm{U}_{s'})^m = \mathrm{Id}_\mathrm{R}$. Thus, by the definition of Coxeter systems, there exists a homomorphism $w \mapsto \mathrm{U}_w$ from W to the group of permutations of R such that U_s is given by the right-hand side of (13). Then $\mathrm{U}_w = \mathrm{U}_\mathbf{s}$ for every sequence $\mathbf{s} = (s_1, \dots, s_q)$ such that $w = s_q \dots s_1$ and Lemma 1 follows immediately from (14).

Lemma 2. Let $\mathbf{s} = (s_1, \dots, s_q)$, $\Phi(\mathbf{s}) = (t_1, \dots, t_q)$ *and* $w = s_1 \dots s_q$. *Let* T_w *be the set of elements of* T *such that* $\eta(w, t) = -1$. *Then* $\mathbf{s}$ *is a reduced decomposition of* w *if and only if the* t_i *are distinct, and in that case* $\mathrm{T}_w = \{t_1, \dots, t_q\}$ *and* $\mathrm{Card}(\mathrm{T}_w) = l(w)$.

Clearly $\mathrm{T}_w \subset \{t_1, \dots, t_q\}$. Taking $\mathbf{s}$ to be reduced, it follows that $\mathrm{Card}(\mathrm{T}_w) \leqslant l(w)$. Moreover, if the t_i are distinct, then $n(\mathbf{s}, t)$ is equal to 1 or 0 according to whether t does or does not belong to $\{t_1, \dots, t_q\}$. It follows that $\mathrm{T}_w = \{t_1, \dots, t_q\}$ and that $q = \mathrm{Card}(\mathrm{T}_w) \leqslant l(w)$, which implies that $\mathbf{s}$ is reduced. Suppose finally that $t_i = t_j$ with $i < j$. This gives $s_i = us_ju^{-1}$, with $u = s_{i+1} \dots s_{j-1}$, hence

$$w = s_1 \dots s_{i-1}s_{i+1} \dots s_{j-1}s_{j+1} \dots s_q.$$

This shows that $\mathbf{s}$ is not a reduced decomposition of w.

Lemma 3. Let $w \in \mathrm{W}$ and $s \in \mathrm{S}$ be such that $l(sw) \leqslant l(w)$. For any sequence $\mathbf{s} = (s_1, \dots, s_q)$ of elements of S *with $w = s_1 \dots s_q$, there exists an integer j such that $1 \leqslant j \leqslant q$ and*

$$ss_1 \dots s_{j-1} = s_1 \dots s_{j-1}s_j.$$

Let p be the length of w and $w' = sw$. By the *Remark* of no. 3, $l(w') \equiv l(w) + 1$ mod. 2. The hypothesis $l(w') \leqslant l(w)$ and the relation

$$|l(w) - l(w')| \leqslant l(ww'^{-1}) = l(s) = 1$$

thus leads to $l(w') = p - 1$. Choose a reduced decomposition

$$(s'_1, \dots, s'_{p-1})$$

of w' and put $\mathbf{s} = (s, s'_1, \dots, s'_{p-1})$ and $\Phi(\mathbf{s}') = (t'_1, \dots, t'_p)$. It is clear that $\mathbf{s}'$ is a reduced decomposition of w and that $t'_1 = s$. The elements $t'_1, \dots, t'_p$ being distinct by Lemma 2, we have $n(\mathbf{s}', s) = 1$. Since w is the product of the sequence $\mathbf{s}$, we have $n(\mathbf{s}, s) \equiv n(\mathbf{s}', s)$ mod. 2 by Lemma 1, hence $n(\mathbf{s}, s) \neq 0$. Consequently, s is equal to one of the elements t_j of the sequence $\Phi(\mathbf{s})$, hence the lemma.

Remark. The set T_w defined in Lemma 2 consists of the elements of the form $w''sw''^{-1}$ corresponding to the triples $(w', w'', s) \in \mathrm{W} \times \mathrm{W} \times \mathrm{S}$ such that $w = w''sw'$ and $l(w') + l(w'') + 1 = l(w)$.

5. THE EXCHANGE CONDITION

The "exchange condition" is the following assertion about (W, S):

(E) *Let $w \in \mathrm{W}$ and $s \in \mathrm{S}$ be such that $l(sw) \leqslant l(w)$. For any reduced decomposition $(s_1, \dots, s_q)$ of w, there exists an integer j such that $1 \leqslant j \leqslant q$ and*

$$ss_1 \dots s_{j-1} = s_1 \dots s_{j-1}s_j. \tag{16}$$

We assume in this number that (W, S) satisfies (E). By Lemma 3, this is so if (W, S) is a Coxeter system. The results of this number thus apply to Coxeter systems.

PROPOSITION 4. *Let $s \in \mathrm{S}$, $w \in \mathrm{W}$ and $\mathbf{s} = (s_1, \dots, s_q)$ be a reduced decomposition of w. Then one of the following must hold:*

a) $l(sw) = l(w) + 1$ and $(s, s_1, \dots, s_q)$ is a reduced decomposition of sw.

b) $l(sw) = l(w) - 1$ *and there exists an integer* j *such that* $1 \leqslant j \leqslant q$, $(s_1, \ldots, s_{j-1}, s_{j+1}, \ldots, s_q)$ *is a reduced decomposition of* sw *and* $(s, s_1, \ldots, s_{j-1}, s_{j+1}, \ldots, s_q)$ *is a reduced decomposition of* w.

Put $w' = sw$. By formula (3) of no. 1, we have

$$|l(w) - l(w')| \leqslant l(s) = 1.$$

We distinguish two cases:

a) $l(w') > l(w)$. Then $l(w') = q + 1$ and $w' = ss_1 \ldots s_q$, so

$$(s, s_1, \ldots, s_q)$$

is a reduced decomposition of w'.

b) $l(w') \leqslant l(w)$. By (E), there exists an integer j such that $1 \leqslant j \leqslant q$ and (16) is satisfied. Then $w = ss_1 \ldots s_{j-1}s_{j+1} \ldots s_q$ and hence

$$w' = s_1 \ldots s_{j-1}s_{j+1} \ldots s_q.$$

Since $q - 1 \leqslant l(w') \leqslant q$, it follows that $l(w') = q - 1$ and that $(s_1, \ldots, s_{j-1}, s_{j+1}, \ldots, s_q)$ is a reduced decomposition of w'.

Lemma 4. Let $w \in \mathrm{W}$ *have length* $q \geqslant 1$, *let* D *be the set of reduced decompositions of* w, *and let* F *be a map from* D *to a set* E. *Assume that* $\mathrm{F}(\mathbf{s}) = \mathrm{F}(\mathbf{s}')$ *if the elements* $\mathbf{s} = (s_1, \ldots, s_q)$, $\mathbf{s}' = (s'_1, \ldots, s'_q)$ *of* D *satisfy one of the following hypotheses:*

a) $s_1 = s'_1$ *or* $s_q = s'_q$.

b) There exist s *and* s' *in* S *such that* $s_j = s'_k = s$ *and* $s_k = s'_j = s'$ *for* j *odd and* k *even.*

Then F *is constant.*

A) Let $\mathbf{s}, \mathbf{s}' \in \mathrm{D}$ and put $\mathbf{t} = (s'_1, s_1, \ldots, s_{q-1})$. We are going to show that if $\mathrm{F}(\mathbf{s}) \neq \mathrm{F}(\mathbf{s}')$ then $\mathbf{t} \in \mathrm{D}$ and $\mathrm{F}(\mathbf{t}) \neq \mathrm{F}(\mathbf{s})$. Indeed, $w = s'_1 \ldots s'_q$ and hence $s'_1 w = s'_2 \ldots s'_q$ is of length $< q$. By Prop. 4, there exists an integer j such that $1 \leqslant j \leqslant q$ and the sequence $\mathbf{u} = (s'_1, s_1, \ldots, s_{j-1}, s_{j+1}, \ldots, s_q)$ belongs to D. We have $\mathrm{F}(\mathbf{u}) = \mathrm{F}(\mathbf{s}')$ by condition *a)*; if $j \neq q$ we would have $\mathrm{F}(\mathbf{s}) = \mathrm{F}(\mathbf{u})$ for the same reason, and hence $\mathrm{F}(\mathbf{s}) = \mathrm{F}(\mathbf{s}')$ contrary to our hypothesis. Thus $j = q$ and hence $\mathbf{t} = \mathbf{u} \in \mathrm{D}$ and $\mathrm{F}(\mathbf{t}) = \mathrm{F}(\mathbf{s}') \neq \mathrm{F}(\mathbf{s})$.

B) Let $\mathbf{s}$ and $\mathbf{s}'$ belong to D. For any integer j with $0 \leqslant j \leqslant q + 1$ define a sequence $\mathbf{s}_j$ of q elements of S as follows:

$$
\begin{aligned}
\mathbf{s}_0 &= (s'_1, \ldots, s'_q)\\
\mathbf{s}_1 &= (s_1, \ldots, s_q)\\
\mathbf{s}_{q+1-k} &= (s_1, s'_1, \ldots, s_1, s'_1, s_1, s_2, \ldots, s_k)\\
&\qquad \text{for } q - k \text{ even and } 0 \leqslant k \leqslant q\\
\mathbf{s}_{q+1-k} &= (s'_1, s_1, \ldots, s_1, s'_1, s_1, s_2, \ldots, s_k)\\
&\qquad \text{for } q - k \text{ odd and } 0 \leqslant k \leqslant q.
\end{aligned}
\tag{17}
$$

Denote by (H_j) the assertion "$\mathbf{s}_j \in \mathrm{D}, \mathbf{s}_{j+1} \in \mathrm{D}$ and $\mathrm{F}(\mathbf{s}_j) \neq \mathrm{F}(\mathbf{s}_{j+1})$". By A), $(\mathrm{H}_j) \Longrightarrow (\mathrm{H}_{j+1})$ for $0 \leqslant j < q$, and (H_q) is not satisfied by condition *b*). Hence, (H_0) is not satisfied. Since $\mathbf{s}_0 = \mathbf{s}'$ and $\mathbf{s}_1 = \mathbf{s}$, it follows that $\mathrm{F}(\mathbf{s}) = \mathrm{F}(\mathbf{s}')$.

PROPOSITION 5. *Let* M *be a monoid (with unit element* 1*) and* f *a map from* S *to* M. *For* $s, s' \in \mathrm{S}$, *let* $m(s, s')$ *be the order of* ss' *and put*

$$a(s,s') = \begin{cases} (f(s)f(s'))^l & \textit{if } m(s,s') = 2l,\ l \textit{ finite} \\ (f(s)f(s'))^l f(s) & \textit{if } m(s,s') = 2l+1,\ l \textit{ finite} \\ 1 & \textit{if } m(s,s') = \infty. \end{cases} \tag{18}$$

If $a(s, s') = a(s', s)$ *whenever* $s \neq s'$ *are in* S, *there exists a map* g *from* W *to* M *such that*

$$g(w) = f(s_1)\dots f(s_q) \tag{19}$$

for all $w \in \mathrm{W}$ *and any reduced decomposition* $(s_1, \dots, s_q)$ *of* w.

For any $w \in \mathrm{W}$, let D_w be the set of reduced decompositions of w and F_w the map from D_w to M defined by

$$\mathrm{F}_w(s_1, \dots, s_q) = f(s_1)\dots f(s_q).$$

We are going to prove by induction on the length of w that F_w is constant, which will establish Prop. 5. The cases $l(w) = 0, 1$ being trivial, we assume that $q \geqslant 2$ and that our assertion is proved for the elements w with $l(w) < q$. Let w be of length q and $\mathbf{s}, \mathbf{s}' \in \mathrm{D}_w$; by Lemma 4 it suffices to prove that $\mathrm{F}_w(\mathbf{s}) = \mathrm{F}_w(\mathbf{s}')$ in cases *a*) and *b*) of that lemma.

a) The formula

$$\mathrm{F}_w(s_1, \dots, s_q) = f(s_1)\mathrm{F}_{w''}(s_2, \dots, s_q) = \mathrm{F}_{w'}(s_1, \dots, s_{q-1})f(s_q)$$

for $w' = s_1 \dots s_{q-1}$ and $w'' = s_2 \dots s_q$ and the induction hypothesis show that $\mathrm{F}_w(\mathbf{s}) = \mathrm{F}_w(\mathbf{s}')$ if $s_1 = s'_1$ or $s_q = s'_q$.

b) Suppose that there exist two elements s and s' of S such that $s_j = s'_k = s$ and $s_k = s'_j = s'$ for j odd and k even. It suffices to treat the case $s \neq s'$. The sequences $\mathbf{s}$ and $\mathbf{s}'$ are then two distinct reduced decompositions of w in the dihedral group generated by s and s'. By the *Remark* in no. 2, the order m of ss' is necessarily finite and, in the notation of that remark, $\mathbf{s} = \mathbf{s}_m$ and $\mathbf{s}' = \mathbf{s}'_m$. Consequently, $\mathrm{F}_w(\mathbf{s}) = a(s, s')$ and $\mathrm{F}_w(\mathbf{s}') = a(s', s)$ and hence

$$\mathrm{F}_w(\mathbf{s}) = \mathrm{F}_w(\mathbf{s}').$$

6. CHARACTERISATION OF COXETER GROUPS

THEOREM 1. (W, S) *is a Coxeter system if and only if it satisfies the exchange condition* (E) *of no.* 5.

Lemma 3 of no. 4 shows that any Coxeter system satisfies (E).

Conversely, suppose that (E) is satisfied. Let G be a group and f a map from S to G such that $(f(s)f(s'))^m = 1$ whenever s and s' belong to S and ss' is of finite order m. By Prop. 5, there exists a map g from W to G such that

$$g(w) = f(s_1) \dots f(s_q) \tag{20}$$

whenever $w = s_1 \dots s_q$ is of length q. To prove that (W, S) is a Coxeter system, it suffices to prove that g is a homomorphism, which is a consequence of the formula

$$g(sw) = f(s)g(w) \quad \text{for } s \in \mathrm{S}, w \in \mathrm{W} \tag{21}$$

since S generates W. By Prop. 4 of no. 5, only two cases are possible:

a) $l(sw) = l(w) + 1$: if $(s_1, \dots, s_q)$ is a reduced decomposition of w, then $(s, s_1, \dots, s_q)$ is a reduced decomposition of sw, hence (21).

b) $l(sw) = l(w) - 1$: put $w' = sw$; then $w = sw'$ and $l(sw') = l(w') + 1$. By *a*), $g(w) = f(s)g(sw)$ and hence $f(s)g(w) = g(sw)$ since $(f(s))^2 = 1$.

7. FAMILIES OF PARTITIONS

Suppose that (W, S) is a Coxeter system. For any $s \in \mathrm{S}$, let P_s be the set of elements w in W such that $l(sw) > l(w)$. We have the following properties:

(A) $\bigcap_{s \in \mathrm{S}} \mathrm{P}_s = \{1\}$.

Indeed, let $w \neq 1$ be in W and let $(s_1, \dots, s_q)$ be a reduced decomposition of w. Then $q \geqslant 1$ and $(s_2, \dots, s_q)$ is a reduced decomposition of $s_2 w$, so $l(w) = q$ and $l(s_1 w) = q - 1$. Hence, $w \notin \mathrm{P}_{s_1}$.

(B) *For any s in* S, *the sets* P_s *and* $s\mathrm{P}_s$ *form a partition of* W.

Let $w \in \mathrm{W}$ and $s \in \mathrm{S}$. By Prop. 4 of no. 5, we must distinguish two cases:

a) $l(sw) = l(w) + 1$: then $w \in \mathrm{P}_s$.
b) $l(sw) = l(w) - 1$: put $w' = sw$ so $w = sw'$; then

$$l(w') < l(sw')$$

hence $w' \in \mathrm{P}_s$, that is $w \in s\mathrm{P}_s$.

(C) *Let s, s' be in* S *and let w be in* W. *If $w \in \mathrm{P}_s$ and $ws' \in \mathrm{P}_s$ then* $sw = ws'$.

Let q be the length of w. From $w \in \mathrm{P}_s$ it follows that $l(sw) = q + 1$; and from $ws' \in \mathrm{P}_s$ it follows that $l(sws') = l(ws') - 1 \leqslant q$. Since $l(sws') = l(sw) \pm 1$, we have finally that $l(ws') = q + 1$ and $l(sws') = q$.

Let $(s_1, \ldots, s_q)$ be a reduced decomposition of w and $s_{q+1} = s'$; then $(s_1, \ldots, s_q, s_{q+1})$ is a reduced decomposition of the element ws' of length $q+1$. By the exchange condition, there exists an integer j with $1 \leqslant j \leqslant q+1$ such that

$$ss_1 \ldots s_{j-1} = s_1 \ldots s_j. \tag{22}$$

If $1 \leqslant j \leqslant q$, we would have $sw = s_1 \ldots s_{j-1} s_{j+1} \ldots s_q$ contradicting the formula $l(sw) = q + 1$. Thus $j = q + 1$ and formula (22) can be written $sw = ws'$.

Conversely, we have the following result:

PROPOSITION 6. *Let* $(\mathrm{P}_s)_{s \in \mathrm{S}}$ *be a family of subsets of* W *satisfying* (C) *and the following conditions:*

(A′) $1 \in \mathrm{P}_s$ *for all* $s \in \mathrm{S}$.
(B′) *The sets* P_s *and* $s\mathrm{P}_s$ *are disjoint for all* $s \in \mathrm{S}$.

Then, (W, S) *is a Coxeter system and* P_s *consists of the elements* w *of* W *such that* $l(sw) > l(w)$.

Let $s \in \mathrm{S}$ and $w \in \mathrm{W}$. There are two possibilities:

a) $w \notin \mathrm{P}_s$. Let $(s_1, \ldots, s_q)$ be a reduced decomposition of w and

$$w_j = s_1 \ldots s_j$$

for $1 \leqslant j \leqslant q$; also put $w_0 = 1$. Since $w_0 \in \mathrm{P}_s$ by (A′) and since $w = w_q$ is not in P_s, there exists an integer j with $1 \leqslant j \leqslant q$ such that $w_{j-1} \in \mathrm{P}_s$ and $w_j = w_{j-1}s_j$ does not belong to P_s. By (C),

$$sw_{j-1} = w_{j-1}s_j.$$

We have thus proved the formula

$$ss_1 \ldots s_{j-1} = s_1 \ldots s_{j-1}s_j$$

which implies that $sw = s_1 \ldots s_{j-1}s_{j+1} \ldots s_q$ and $l(sw) < l(w)$.

b) $w \in \mathrm{P}_s$: put $w' = sw$, so that $w' \notin \mathrm{P}_s$ by (B′). By *a*), we then have $l(sw') < l(w')$, that is $l(w) < l(sw)$.

Comparison of *a*) and *b*) proves that P_s consists of those $w \in \mathrm{W}$ such that $l(sw) > l(w)$. The exchange condition follows from this as we have seen in *a*), hence (W, S) is a Coxeter system (Th. 1 of no. 6).

8. SUBGROUPS OF COXETER GROUPS

In this number, we assume that (W, S) is a Coxeter system. For any subset X of S, we denote by W_X the subgroup of W generated by X.

PROPOSITION 7. *Let w be in* W. *There exists a subset* S_w *of* S *such that* $\{s_1, \ldots, s_q\} = S_w$ *for any reduced decomposition* $(s_1, \ldots, s_q)$ *of* w.

Denote by M the monoid consisting of the subsets of S with the composition law $(A, B) \mapsto A \cup B$; the identity element of M is $\varnothing$. Put $f(s) = \{s\}$ for $s \in S$. We are going to apply Prop. 5 of no. 5 to M and f. We have $a(s, s') = \{s, s'\}$ for s, s' in S if $m(s, s')$ is finite, hence there exists a map $g : w \mapsto S_w$ from W to M such that $g(w) = f(s_1) \cup \cdots \cup f(s_q)$, that is $S_w = \{s_1, \ldots, s_q\}$ for any $w \in W$ and any reduced decomposition $(s_1, \ldots, s_q)$ of w.

COROLLARY 1. *For any subset* X *of* S, *the subgroup* W_X *of* W *consists of the elements* w *of* W *such that* $S_w \subset X$.

If $w = s_1 \ldots s_q$ with $s_1, \ldots, s_q$ in S, then $w^{-1} = s_q \ldots s_1$; hence

$$S_{w^{-1}} = S_w. \tag{23}$$

Prop. 4 of no. 5 shows that $S_{sw'} \subset \{s\} \cup S_{w'}$ for $s \in S$ and $w' \in W$, which implies the formula

$$S_{ww'} \subset S_w \cup S_{w'} \tag{24}$$

by induction on the length of w. By (23) and (24), the set U of $w \in W$ such that $S_w \subset X$ is a subgroup of W; we have $X \subset U \subset W_X$, hence $U = W_X$.

COROLLARY 2. *For any subset* X *of* S, *we have* $W_X \cap S = X$.

This follows from Cor. 1 and the formula $S_s = \{s\}$ for s in S.

COROLLARY 3. *The set* S *is a minimal generating set of* W.

If $X \subset S$ generates W, then $W = W_X$ and hence $X = S \cap W_X = S$ by Cor. 2.

COROLLARY 4. *For any subset* X *of* S *and any w in* W_X, *the length of w with respect to the generating set* X *of* W_X *is equal to* $l_S(w)$.

Let $(s_1, \ldots, s_q)$ be a reduced decomposition of w considered as an element of W. We have $w = s_1 \ldots s_q$ and $s_j \in X$ for $1 \leqslant j \leqslant q$ (Cor. 1); moreover, w cannot be a product of $q' < q$ elements of $X \subset S$ by definition of $q = l_S(w)$.

THEOREM 2. (i) *For any subset* X *of* S, *the pair* (W_X, X) *is a Coxeter system.*

(ii) *Let* $(X_i)_{i\in I}$ *be a family of subsets of* S. *If* $X = \bigcap_{i\in I} X_i$, *then* $W_X = \bigcap_{i\in I} W_{X_i}$.

(iii) *Let* X *and* X′ *be two subsets of* S. *Then* $W_X \subset W_{X'}$ *(resp.* $W_X = W_{X'}$*) if and only if* $X \subset X'$ *(resp.* $X = X'$*).*

Every element of X is of order 2 and X generates W_X. Let $x \in X$ and $w \in W_X$ with $l_X(xw) \leqslant l_X(w) = q$. By Cor. 4 of Prop. 7, we have

$$l_S(xw) \leqslant l_S(w) = q.$$

Let $x_1, \dots, x_q$ be elements of X such that $w = x_1 \dots x_q$. Since (W, S) satisfies the exchange condition (Th. 1 of no. 6), there exists an integer j such that $1 \leqslant j \leqslant q$ and $xx_1 \dots x_{j-1} = x_1 \dots x_{j-1}x_j$. Thus, (W_X, X) satisfies the exchange condition and is therefore a Coxeter system (Th. 1 of no. 6). This proves (i).

Assertions (ii) and (iii) follow immediately from Cor. 1 of Prop. 7.

9. COXETER MATRICES AND COXETER GRAPHS

DEFINITION 4. *Let* I *be a set. A Coxeter matrix of type* I *is a symmetric square matrix* $M = (m_{ij})_{i,j\in I}$ *whose entries are integers or* $+\infty$ *satisfying the relations*

$$m_{ii} = 1 \quad \text{for all } i \in I; \tag{25}$$

$$m_{ij} \geqslant 2 \quad \text{for } i, j \in I \text{ with } i \neq j. \tag{26}$$

A Coxeter graph of type I *is (by abuse of language) a pair consisting of a graph* Γ[3] *having* I *as its set of vertices and a map* f *from the set of edges of this graph to the set consisting of* $+\infty$ *and the set of integers* $\geqslant 3$. Γ *is called the underlying graph of the Coxeter graph* (Γ, f).

A Coxeter graph (Γ, f) is associated to any Coxeter matrix M of type I as follows:

the graph Γ has set of vertices I and set of edges the set pairs $\{i, j\}$ of elements of I such that $m_{ij} \geqslant 3$, and the map f associates to the edge $\{i, j\}$ the corresponding element m_{ij} of M.

It is clear that this gives rise to a *bijection* between the set of Coxeter matrices of type I and the set of Coxeter graphs of type I.

To assist the reader in following our arguments, we often represent a Coxeter graph of type I by the diagram used to represent its underlying graph, and write either next to or above each edge $\{i, j\}$ the number $f(\{i, j\})$. We generally omit these numbers if they are equal to 3.

[3] See the appendix for the definition and properties of *graphs* used here.

If (W, S) is a Coxeter system, the matrix $\mathrm{M} = (m(s, s'))_{s,s' \in \mathrm{S}}$, where $m(s, s')$ is the order of ss', is a Coxeter matrix of type S which is called the Coxeter matrix of (W, S): indeed, $m(s, s) = 1$ since $s^2 = 1$ for all $s \in \mathrm{S}$, and $m(s, s') = m(s', s) \geqslant 2$ if $s \neq s'$ since $ss' = (s's)^{-1}$ is then $\neq 1$. The Coxeter graph (Γ, f) associated to M is called the Coxeter graph of (W, S). We remark that two vertices s and s' of Γ are *joined* if and only if s and s' do not commute. For example, the Coxeter matrix of a dihedral group of order $2m$ is $\begin{pmatrix} 1 & m \\ m & 1 \end{pmatrix}$ and its Coxeter graph is represented by

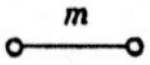

when $m \geqslant 3$ (or

if $m = 3$) and by

when $m = 2$. *The Coxeter graph of the symmetric group $\mathfrak{S}_n$ is represented by

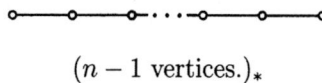

$(n - 1$ vertices.$)_*$

We show later (Chap. V, § 4) that, conversely, any Coxeter matrix is the matrix of a Coxeter system.

A Coxeter system (W, S) is said to be *irreducible* if the underlying graph of its Coxeter graph is *connected* (Appendix, no. 2) and *non-empty*. Equivalently, S is non-empty and there exists no partition of S into two distinct subsets S' and S'' of S such that every element of S' commutes with every element of S''. More generally, let $(\Gamma_i)_{i \in \mathrm{I}}$ be the family of connected components of Γ (Appendix, no. 2) and let S_i be the set of vertices of Γ_i. Let $\mathrm{W}_i = \mathrm{W}_{\mathrm{S}_i}$ be the subgroup of W generated by S_i (cf. no. 8). Then the $(\mathrm{W}_i, \mathrm{S}_i)$ are irreducible Coxeter systems (no. 8, Th. 2) called the *irreducible components of* (W, S). Moreover, the group W is the *restricted direct product*[4] of the subgroups W_i for $i \in \mathrm{I}$. Indeed, this follows from the following more general proposition:

[4] A group G is the *restricted direct product* of a family $(\mathrm{G}_i)_{i \in \mathrm{I}}$ of subgroups if, for any finite subset J of I, the subgroup G_J of G generated by the G_i for $i \in \mathrm{J}$ is the direct product of the G_i for $i \in \mathrm{J}$ and if G is the union of the G_J. Equivalently, every element of G_i commutes with every element of G_j for $i \neq j$ and every element of G can be written uniquely as a product $\prod_{i \in \mathrm{I}} g_i$ with $g_i \in \mathrm{G}_i$ and $g_i = 1$ for all but finitely many indices i. This last condition is equivalent to saying that G is generated by the union of the G_i and that $\mathrm{G}_i \cap \mathrm{G}_\mathrm{J} = \{1\}$ for all $i \in \mathrm{I}$ and all finite subsets J of I such that $i \notin \mathrm{J}$.

PROPOSITION 8. *Let* $(\mathrm{S}_i)_{i\in\mathrm{I}}$ *be a partition of* S *such that every element of* S_i *commutes with every element of* S_j *if* $i \neq j$. *For all* $i \in \mathrm{I}$, *let* W_i *be the subgroup generated by* S_i. *Then* W *is the restricted direct product of the family* $(\mathrm{W}_i)_{i\in\mathrm{I}}$.

It is clear that for all $i \in \mathrm{I}$ the subgroup W'_i generated by the union of the W_j for $j \neq i$ is also generated by $\mathrm{S}'_i = \bigcup_{i\neq j} \mathrm{S}_j$. Thus

$$\mathrm{W}_i \cap \mathrm{W}'_i = \mathrm{W}_\varnothing = \{1\}$$

by Th. 2 of no. 8. Since W is generated by the union of the W_i, this proves the proposition.

§ 2. TITS SYSTEMS

In this paragraph, the letters G, B, N, S, T, W *have the meaning indicated in no. 1 below.*

1. DEFINITIONS AND FIRST PROPERTIES

Let G be a group and B a subgroup of G. The group $\mathrm{B} \times \mathrm{B}$ acts on G by $(b, b').g = bgb'^{-1}$ for $b, b' \in \mathrm{B}$ and $g \in \mathrm{G}$. The orbits of $\mathrm{B} \times \mathrm{B}$ on G are the sets $\mathrm{B}g\mathrm{B}$ for $g \in \mathrm{G}$, and are called the *double cosets* of G with respect to B. They form a *partition* of G; the corresponding quotient is denoted by $\mathrm{B}\backslash\mathrm{G}/\mathrm{B}$. If C and C′ are double cosets, CC′ is a union of double cosets.

DEFINITION 1. *A Tits system is a quadruple* (G, B, N, S), *where* G *is a group,* B *and* N *are two subgroups of* G *and* S *is a subset of* $\mathrm{N}/(\mathrm{B} \cap \mathrm{N})$, *satisfying the following axioms:*

(T1) *The set* $\mathrm{B} \cup \mathrm{N}$ *generates* G *and* $\mathrm{B} \cap \mathrm{N}$ *is a normal subgroup of* N.
(T2) *The set* S *generates the group* $\mathrm{W} = \mathrm{N}/(\mathrm{B} \cap \mathrm{N})$ *and consists of elements of order* 2.
(T3) $s\mathrm{B}w \subset \mathrm{B}w\mathrm{B} \cup \mathrm{B}sw\mathrm{B}$ *for* $s \in \mathrm{S}$ *and* $w \in \mathrm{W}$. [5]
(T4) *For all* $s \in \mathrm{S}$, $s\mathrm{B}s \not\subset \mathrm{B}$.

The group $\mathrm{W} = \mathrm{N}/(\mathrm{B} \cap \mathrm{N})$ is sometimes called the *Weyl group* of the Tits system (G, B, N, S).

---

[5] Every element of W is a coset modulo $\mathrm{B} \cap \mathrm{N}$, and is thus a subset of G; hence products such as $\mathrm{B}w\mathrm{B}$ make sense. More generally, for any subset A of W, we denote by BAB the subset $\bigcup_{w\in\mathrm{A}} \mathrm{B}w\mathrm{B}$.

Remarks. 1) We shall see in no. 5 (Cor. of Th. 3) that, if (G, B, N) is given, there exists at most one subset S of $N/(B \cap N)$ such that (G, B, N, S) is a Tits system.

2) Let (G, B, N, S) be a Tits system, and let Z be a normal subgroup of G contained in B. Let $G' = G/Z, B' = B/Z, N' = N/(Z \cap N)$, and let S' be the image of S in $N'/(B' \cap N")$. Then one sees immediately that (G', B', N', S') is a Tits system.

Throughout this paragraph, with (G, B, N, S) *denoting a Tits system, we set* $T = B \cap N$ *and* $W = N/T$. *A double coset means a double coset of* G *with respect to* B. *For any* $w \in W$, *we set* $C(w) = BwB$; *this is a double coset.*

We are going to deduce several elementary consequences of the axioms (T1) to (T4). We denote by $w, w', \ldots$ elements of W and by $s, s', \ldots$ elements of S. The following relations are clear:

$$C(1) = B, \quad C(ww') \subset C(w).C(w'), \quad C(w^{-1}) = C(w)^{-1}. \tag{1}$$

Axiom (T3) can also be written in the form

$$C(s).C(w) \subset C(w) \cup C(sw). \tag{2}$$

Moreover, since $C(sw) \subset C(s).C(w)$ by (1) and since $C(s).C(w)$ is a union of double cosets, there are only two possibilities:

$$C(s).C(w) = \begin{cases} C(sw) & \text{if } C(w) \not\subset C(s).C(w) \\ C(w) \cup C(sw) & \text{if } C(w) \subset C(s).C(w). \end{cases} \tag{3}$$

By (T4), $B \neq C(s).C(s)$; putting $w = s$ in (3) and using the relation $s^2 = 1$, we obtain

$$C(s).C(s) = B \cup C(s). \tag{4}$$

This formula shows that $B \cup C(s)$ is a subgroup of G. Multiplying both sides of (4) *on the right* by $C(w)$, and using formula (3) and the relation

$$B.C(w) = C(w),$$

we obtain

$$C(s).C(s).C(w) = C(w) \cup C(sw). \tag{5}$$

Taking the inverses of the sets entering into formulas (2), (3) and (5) and then replacing w by w^{-1}, we obtain the formulas

$$C(w).C(s) \subset C(w) \cup C(ws) \tag{2'}$$

$$C(w).C(s) = \begin{cases} C(ws) & \text{if } C(w) \not\subset C(w).C(s) \\ C(w) \cup C(ws) & \text{if } C(w) \subset C(w).C(s) \end{cases} \tag{3'}$$

$$C(w).C(s).C(s) = C(w) \cup C(ws). \tag{5'}$$

Lemma 1. Let $s_1, \dots, s_q \in \mathrm{S}$ *and let* $w \in \mathrm{W}$. *We have*

$$\mathrm{C}(s_1 \dots s_q).\mathrm{C}(w) \subset \bigcup_{(i_1,\dots,i_p)} \mathrm{C}(s_{i_1} \dots s_{i_p} w),$$

where $(i_1, \dots, i_p)$ *denotes the set of strictly increasing sequences of integers in the interval* $[1, q]$.

We argue by induction on q, the case $q = 0$ being trivial. If $q \geqslant 1$, we have $\mathrm{C}(s_1 \dots s_q).\mathrm{C}(w) \subset \mathrm{C}(s_1).\mathrm{C}(s_2 \dots s_q).\mathrm{C}(w)$. By the induction hypothesis, $\mathrm{C}(s_2 \dots s_q).\mathrm{C}(w)$ is contained in the union of the $\mathrm{C}(s_{j_1} \dots s_{j_p} w)$, where

$$2 \leqslant j_1 < \dots < j_p \leqslant q.$$

By (T3), the set $\mathrm{C}(s_1).\mathrm{C}(s_{j_1} \dots s_{j_p} w)$ is contained in the union of the sets $\mathrm{C}(s_1 s_{j_1} \dots s_{j_p} w)$ and $\mathrm{C}(s_{j_1} \dots s_{j_p} w)$. This proves the lemma.

2. AN EXAMPLE

Let k be a field, n an integer $\geqslant 0$, and (e_i) the canonical basis of k^n. Let $\mathrm{G} = \mathbf{GL}(n, k)$, let B be the upper triangular subgroup of G, and let N be the subgroup of G consisting of the matrices having exactly one non-zero element in each row and column. An element of N permutes the lines ke_i; this gives rise to a surjective homomorphism $\mathrm{N} \to \mathfrak{S}_n$ whose kernel is the subgroup $\mathrm{T} = \mathrm{B} \cap \mathrm{N}$ of diagonal matrices, and allows us to identify $\mathrm{W} = \mathrm{N}/\mathrm{T}$ with $\mathfrak{S}_n$. We denote by s_j $(1 \leqslant j \leqslant n-1)$ the element of W corresponding to the transposition of j and $j+1$; let S be the set of s_j. *The quadruple* (G, B, N, S) *is a Tits system.* Indeed:

Axiom (T1) follows from Cor. 2 of Prop. 14 of *Algebra*, Chap. II, § 10, no. 13.

Axiom (T2) is proved in *Algebra*, Chap. I, Correction to p. 97.

Axiom (T4) is immediate.

It remains to verify axiom (T3), i.e.

$$s_j \mathrm{B} w \subset \mathrm{B} w \mathrm{B} \cup \mathrm{B} s_j w \mathrm{B} \quad \text{for } 1 \leqslant j \leqslant n-1, w \in \mathrm{W},$$

or equivalently,

$$s_j \mathrm{B} \subset \mathrm{B}\mathrm{B}' \cup \mathrm{B} s_j \mathrm{B}', \quad \text{with } \mathrm{B}' = w \mathrm{B} w^{-1}.$$

Let G_j be the subgroup of G consisting of the elements that fix the e_i for $i \neq j, j+1$ and stabilize the plane spanned by e_j and e_{j+1}; this group is isomorphic to $\mathbf{GL}(2, k)$. One checks that $\mathrm{G}_j \mathrm{B} = \mathrm{B} \mathrm{G}_j$. Since $s_j \in \mathrm{G}_j$, we have $s_j \mathrm{B} \subset \mathrm{B} \mathrm{G}_j$, and it suffices to prove that

$$\mathrm{G}_j \subset (\mathrm{B} \cap \mathrm{G}_j)(\mathrm{B}' \cap \mathrm{G}_j) \cup (\cap \mathrm{G}_j) s_j (\mathrm{B}' \cap \mathrm{G}_j).$$

Identify G_j with $\mathbf{GL}(2, k)$; the group $\mathrm{B} \cap \mathrm{G}_j$ is then identified with the upper triangular subgroup B_2 of $\mathbf{GL}(2, k)$, while the group $\mathrm{B}' \cap \mathrm{G}_j$ is identified with B_2 when $w(j) < w(j+1)$ and with the lower triangular subgroup B_2^- otherwise. In the first case, the formula to be proved can be written

$$\mathbf{GL}(2,k) = B_2 \cup B_2 s B_2 \quad \text{where } s = \begin{pmatrix} 0 & 1 \\ 1 & 0 \end{pmatrix};$$

this follows for example from the fact that B_2 is the stabilizer of a point for the action of $\mathbf{GL}(2,k)$ on the projective line $\mathbf{P}_1(k)$, and acts transitively on the complement of this point. In the second case, the formula to be proved can be written

$$\mathbf{GL}(2,k) = B_2 B_2^- \cup B_2 s B_2^-;$$

since $B_2^- = sB_2s$, this follows from the preceding formula by multiplying on the right by s.

3. DECOMPOSITION OF G INTO DOUBLE COSETS

THEOREM 1. *We have* $G = BWB$. *The map* $w \mapsto C(w)$ *is a bijection from* W *to the set* $B\backslash G/B$ *of double cosets of* G *with respect to* B.

It is clear that BWB is stable under $x \mapsto x^{-1}$, and Lemma 1 shows that it is stable under the product. Since it contains B and N, it is equal to G.

It remains to prove that $C(w) \neq C(w')$ if $w \neq w'$. For this, we shall prove by induction on the integer q the following assertion:

(A_q) If w and w' are distinct elements of W such that $l_S(w) \geqslant l_S(w') = q$, then $C(w) \neq C(w')$.

(For the definition of $l_S(w)$, see § 1, no. 1.)

This assertion is clear for $q = 0$, since then $w' = 1$ and $w \neq 1$, hence $C(w') = B$ and $C(w) \neq B$.

Assume that $q \geqslant 1$ and that w, w' satisfy the hypotheses of (A_q). There exists $s \in S$ such that sw' is of length $q-1$. We have

$$l_S(w) > l_S(sw') \tag{6}$$

hence $w \neq sw'$. Moreover, $sw \neq sw'$; by formula (3) of § 1, no. 1, we have

$$l_S(sw) \geqslant l_S(w) - 1 \geqslant l_S(sw') = q - 1. \tag{7}$$

By the induction hypothesis, $C(sw')$ is distinct from $C(w)$ and from $C(sw)$; from formula (2) it follows that

$$C(sw') \cap C(s).C(w) = \varnothing. \tag{8}$$

Since $C(sw') \subset C(s).C(w')$, we have finally that $C(w) \neq C(w')$.

Remark. Axiom (T4) was not used in the preceding proof.

4. RELATIONS WITH COXETER SYSTEMS

THEOREM 2. *The pair* (W, S) *is a Coxeter system. Moreover, for* $s \in \mathrm{S}$ *and* $w \in \mathrm{W}$, *the relations* $\mathrm{C}(sw) = \mathrm{C}(s).\mathrm{C}(w)$ *and* $l_{\mathrm{S}}(sw) > l_{\mathrm{S}}(w)$ *are equivalent.*

For any $s \in \mathrm{S}$, let P_s be the set of elements $w \in \mathrm{W}$ such that

$$\mathrm{C}(s).\mathrm{C}(w) = \mathrm{C}(sw).$$

We are going to verify that the P_s satisfy conditions (A′), (B′) and (C) of § 1, no. 7; the two assertions of the theorem will then follow from Prop. 6 of § 1, no. 7.

Condition (A′) is clear.

We verify (B′). If P_s and $s\mathrm{P}_s$ had an element w in common, we would have $w \in \mathrm{P}_s$ and $sw \in \mathrm{P}_s$, and hence

$$\mathrm{C}(s).\mathrm{C}(w) = \mathrm{C}(sw), \qquad \mathrm{C}(s).\mathrm{C}(sw) = \mathrm{C}(w).$$

It would follow that $\mathrm{C}(s).\mathrm{C}(s).\mathrm{C}(w) = \mathrm{C}(w)$ and, by formula (5), this would imply that $\mathrm{C}(w) = \mathrm{C}(sw)$, which would contradict Th. 1.

We verify (C). Let $s, s' \in \mathrm{S}$ and $w, w' \in \mathrm{W}$ with $w' = ws'$. The assumption that $w \in \mathrm{P}_s$ and $w' \notin \mathrm{P}_s$ implies that

$$\mathrm{C}(sw) = \mathrm{C}(s).\mathrm{C}(w) \tag{9}$$

$$\mathrm{C}(w') \subset \mathrm{C}(s).\mathrm{C}(w') \tag{10}$$

by (3).

From (9) and the relation $w = w's'$, it follows that

$$\mathrm{C}(s)w's'\mathrm{B} = \mathrm{C}(sw). \tag{11}$$

By formula (2′), $\mathrm{C}(w').\mathrm{C}(s') \subset \mathrm{C}(w') \cup \mathrm{C}(w's')$, which immediately implies that

$$\mathrm{C}(w')s'\mathrm{B} \subset \mathrm{C}(ws') \cup \mathrm{C}(w). \tag{12}$$

Since $\mathrm{C}(w')$ is a union of left cosets $g\mathrm{B}$ and since

$$\mathrm{C}(s).\mathrm{C}(w') = \mathrm{C}(s)w'\mathrm{B},$$

formula (10) shows that $\mathrm{C}(s)w'$ meets $\mathrm{C}(w')$ and *a fortiori* that $\mathrm{C}(s)w's'\mathrm{B}$ meets $\mathrm{C}(w')s'\mathrm{B}$. It follows from formulas (11) and (12) that the double coset $\mathrm{C}(sw)$ is equal to one of the double cosets $\mathrm{C}(ws')$ and $\mathrm{C}(w)$; since $sw \neq w$, Th. 1 allows us to conclude that $sw = ws'$.

COROLLARY 1. *Let* $w_1, \ldots, w_q \in \mathrm{W}$ *and let* $w = w_1 \ldots w_q$. *If*

$$l_{\mathrm{S}}(w) = l_{\mathrm{S}}(w_1) + \cdots + l_{\mathrm{S}}(w_q),$$

then

$$\mathrm{C}(w) = \mathrm{C}(w_1) \ldots \mathrm{C}(w_q).$$

On taking reduced decompositions of the w_i, one is reduced to the case of a reduced decomposition

$$w = s_1 \dots s_q, \qquad \text{with } s_i \in \mathrm{S}.$$

If $u = s_2 \dots s_q$, then $w = s_1 u$ and $l_{\mathrm{S}}(s_1 u) > l_{\mathrm{S}}(u)$, so $\mathrm{C}(w) = \mathrm{C}(s_1).\mathrm{C}(u)$ by the theorem. The required formula follows from this by induction on q.

COROLLARY 2. *Let $w \in \mathrm{W}$ and let T_w be the subset of* W *associated to w by the procedure of Lemma 2 of § 1, no. 4. If $t \in \mathrm{T}_w$, then*

$$\mathrm{C}(t) \subset \mathrm{C}(w).\mathrm{C}(w^{-1}).$$

If $t \in \mathrm{T}_w$, there exist by definition elements $w', w'' \in \mathrm{W}$ and $s \in \mathrm{S}$ such that

$$w = w'sw'', \quad l_{\mathrm{S}}(w) = l_{\mathrm{S}}(w') + l_{\mathrm{S}}(w'') + 1 \quad \text{and} \quad t = w'sw'^{-1}.$$

By Cor. 1,

$$\mathrm{C}(w).\mathrm{C}(w^{-1}) = \mathrm{C}(w').\mathrm{C}(s).\mathrm{C}(w'').\mathrm{C}(w''^{-1}).\mathrm{C}(s).\mathrm{C}(w'^{-1}).$$

Hence,

$$\mathrm{C}(w).\mathrm{C}(w^{-1}) \supset \mathrm{C}(w').\mathrm{C}(s).\mathrm{C}(s).\mathrm{C}(w'^{-1}).$$

By (4), $\mathrm{C}(s) \subset \mathrm{C}(s).\mathrm{C}(s)$. Hence,

$$\mathrm{C}(w).\mathrm{C}(w^{-1}) \supset \mathrm{C}(w').\mathrm{C}(s).\mathrm{C}(w'^{-1}) \supset \mathrm{C}(t).$$

COROLLARY 3. *Let $w \in \mathrm{W}$ and let H_w be the subgroup of* G *generated by* $\mathrm{C}(w).\mathrm{C}(w^{-1})$. *Then:*

a) For any reduced decomposition $(s_1, \dots, s_q)$ of w,

$$\mathrm{C}(s_j) \subset \mathrm{H}_w \quad \text{for } 1 \leqslant j \leqslant q.$$

b) The group H_w contains $\mathrm{C}(w)$ and is generated by $\mathrm{C}(w)$.

We prove *a*) by induction on j. Assume that $\mathrm{C}(s_k)$ is contained in H_w for $k < j$. Let

$$t = (s_1 \dots s_{j-1}) s_j (s_1 \dots s_{j-1})^{-1}.$$

The element t belongs to the subset T_w of W defined in Lemma 2 of § 1, no. 4. By Cor. 2, $\mathrm{C}(t) \subset \mathrm{H}_w$, and hence $\mathrm{C}(s_j) \subset \mathrm{H}_w$.

Since $\mathrm{C}(w) = \mathrm{C}(s_1) \dots \mathrm{C}(s_q)$, cf. Cor. 1, we have $\mathrm{C}(w) \subset \mathrm{H}_w$, and *b*) follows.

Example. Th. 2, applied to the Tits system described in no. 2, shows that *the symmetric group $\mathfrak{S}_n$*, with the set of transpositions of consecutive elements, *is a Coxeter group.*

5. SUBGROUPS OF G CONTAINING B

For any subset X of S, we denote by W_X the subgroup of W generated by X (cf. § 1, no. 8) and by G_X the union BW_XB of the double cosets $C(w)$, $w \in W_X$. We have $G_\varnothing = B$ and $G_S = G$.

THEOREM 3. *a) For any subset* X *of* S, *the set* G_X *is a subgroup of* G, *generated by* $\bigcup_{s \in X} C(s)$.

b) The map $X \mapsto G_X$ *is a bijection from* $\mathfrak{P}(S)$ *to the set of subgroups of* G *containing* B.

c) Let $(X_i)_{i \in I}$ *be a family of subsets of* X. *If* $X = \bigcap_{i \in I} X_i$, *then* $G_X = \bigcap_{i \in I} G_{X_i}$.

d) Let X *and* Y *be two subsets of* S. *Then* $G_X \subset G_Y$ *(resp.* $G_X = G_Y$*) if and only if* $X \subset Y$ *(resp.* $X = Y$*).*

It is clear that $G_X = (G_X)^{-1}$; Lemma 1 of no. 1 shows that $G_X.G_X \subset G_X$; and hence *a*) follows, taking into account Cor. 1 of Th. 2.

The injectivity of $X \mapsto G_X$ follows from that of $X \mapsto W_X$ (§ 1, no. 8, Th. 2). Conversely, let H be a subgroup of G containing B. Let U be the set of $w \in W$ such that $C(w) \subset H$. We have $H = BUB$ since H is a union of double cosets. Let $X = U \cap S$; we show that $H = G_X$. Clearly, $G_X \subset H$. On the other hand, let $u \in U$ and let $(s_1, \ldots, s_q)$ be a reduced decomposition of u. Cor. 3 of Th. 2 implies that $C(s_j) \subset H$, and hence that $s_j \in X$ for $1 \leqslant j \leqslant q$. Thus, $u \in W_X$, and since H is the union of the $C(u)$ for $u \in U$, we have $H \subset G_X$, which proves *b*).

Assertions *c*) and *d*) follow from analogous properties of W_X (§ 1, no. 8, Th. 2).

COROLLARY. *The set* S *consists of the elements* $w \in W$ *such that* $w \neq 1$ *and* $B \cup C(w)$ *is a subgroup of* G.

The elements $w \in W$ such that $B \cup C(w)$ is a subgroup of G are those for which there exists $X \subset S$ with $W_X = \{1, w\}$. Moreover, if $w \neq 1$, we necessarily have $\mathrm{Card}(X) = 1$, i.e. $w \in S$.

Remark. 1) The above corollary shows that S is determined by (G, B, N); for this reason, we sometimes allow ourselves to say that (G, B, N) is a Tits system, or that (B, N) is a *Tits system in* G.

PROPOSITION 1. *Let* X *be a subset of* S *and* N′ *a subgroup of* N *whose image in* W *is equal to* W_X. *Then,* (G_X, B, N', X) *is a Tits system.*

We have $G_X = BW_XB = BN'B$, which shows that G_X is generated by $B \cup N'$. The verification of the axioms (T1) to (T4) is now immediate.

PROPOSITION 2. *Let* $X, Y \subset S$ *and* $w \in W$. *We have*

$$G_X w G_Y = BW_X w W_Y B.$$

Let $s_1, \ldots, s_q \in \mathrm{X}$ and $t_1, \ldots, t_q \in \mathrm{Y}$. Lemma 1 shows that

$$\mathrm{C}(s_1 \ldots s_q).\mathrm{C}(w).\mathrm{C}(t_1 \ldots t_q) \subset \mathrm{BW_X}w\mathrm{W_Y B},$$

and hence that

$$\mathrm{G_X}w\mathrm{G_Y} \subset \mathrm{BW_X}w\mathrm{W_Y B}.$$

The opposite inclusion is obvious.

Remark. 2) Denote by $\mathrm{G_X}\backslash\mathrm{G}/\mathrm{G_Y}$ the set of subsets of G of the form $\mathrm{G_X}g\mathrm{G_Y}$, $g \in \mathrm{G}$; and define $\mathrm{W_X}\backslash\mathrm{W}/\mathrm{W_Y}$ analogously. The preceding proposition shows that the canonical bijection $w \mapsto \mathrm{C}(w)$ from W to $\mathrm{B}\backslash\mathrm{G}/\mathrm{B}$ defines by passage to the quotient a *bijection* $\mathrm{W_X}\backslash\mathrm{W}/\mathrm{W_Y} \to \mathrm{G_X}\backslash\mathrm{G}/\mathrm{G_Y}$.

PROPOSITION 3. *Let* $\mathrm{X} \subset \mathrm{S}$ *and* $g \in \mathrm{G}$. *The relation* $g\mathrm{B}g^{-1} \subset \mathrm{G_X}$ *implies that* $g \in \mathrm{G_X}$.

Let $w \in \mathrm{W}$ be such that $g \in \mathrm{C}(w)$. Since B is a subgroup of $\mathrm{G_X}$, the hypothesis $g\mathrm{B}g^{-1} \subset \mathrm{G_X}$ implies that $\mathrm{C}(w).\mathrm{C}(w^{-1}) \subset \mathrm{G_X}$, and hence that $\mathrm{C}(w) \subset \mathrm{G_X}$ by Cor. 3 of Th. 2, so g belongs to $\mathrm{G_X}$.

6. PARABOLIC SUBGROUPS

DEFINITION 2. *A subgroup of* G *is said to be parabolic if it contains a conjugate of* B.

It is clear that every subgroup that contains a parabolic subgroup is parabolic.

PROPOSITION 4. *Let* P *be a subgroup of* G.

a) P *is parabolic if and only if there exists a subset* X *of* S *such that* P *is conjugate to* $\mathrm{G_X}$ *(cf. no. 5 for the definition of* $\mathrm{G_X}$*).*

b) Let $\mathrm{X}, \mathrm{X}' \subset \mathrm{S}$ *and* $g, g' \in \mathrm{G}$ *be such that* $\mathrm{P} = g\mathrm{G_X}g^{-1} = g'\mathrm{G_{X'}}g'^{-1}$. *Then,* $\mathrm{X} = \mathrm{X}'$ *and* $g'g^{-1} \in \mathrm{P}$.

Assertion *a*) follows from Th. 3, *b*).

Under the hypotheses of *b*), we have

$$g^{-1}g'\mathrm{B}g'^{-1}g \subset g^{-1}g'\mathrm{G_{X'}}g'^{-1} = \mathrm{G_X},$$

and Prop. 3 shows that $g^{-1}g' \in \mathrm{G_X}$. Hence, $\mathrm{G_{X'}} = \mathrm{G_X}$ and $\mathrm{X}' = \mathrm{X}$ by Th. 3, *b*). Finally,

$$g'g^{-1} = g.g^{-1}g'.g^{-1} \in g\mathrm{G_X}g^{-1},$$

which proves *b*).

If the parabolic subgroup P is conjugate to $\mathrm{G_X}$, where $\mathrm{X} \subset \mathrm{S}$, then P is said to be of *type* X.

THEOREM 4. (i) *Let* P_1 *and* P_2 *be two parabolic subgroups of* G *whose intersection is parabolic and let* $g \in G$ *be such that* $gP_1g^{-1} \subset P_2$. *Then* $g \in P_2$ *and* $P_1 \subset P_2$.

(ii) *Two parabolic subgroups whose intersection is parabolic are not conjugate.*

(iii) *Let* Q_1 *and* Q_2 *be two parabolic subgroups of* G *contained in a subgroup* Q *of* G. *Then any* $g \in G$ *such that* $gQ_1g^{-1} = Q_2$ *belongs to* Q.

(iv) *Every parabolic subgroup is its own normaliser*[6].

Assertion (i) follows from Props. 3 and 4, and implies (ii). Under the hypotheses of (iii), we have $gQ_1g^{-1} \subset Q$, which implies that $g \in Q$ by (i). Finally, (iv) follows from (iii) by taking $Q_1 = Q_2 = Q$.

PROPOSITION 5. *Let* P_1 *and* P_2 *be two parabolic subgroups of* G. *Then* $P_1 \cap P_2$ *contains a conjugate of* T.

By first transforming P_1 and P_2 by an inner automorphism of G, we may assume that $B \subset P_1$. Let $g \in G$ be such that $gBg^{-1} \subset P_2$. By Th. 1, there exist $n \in N$ and $b, b' \in B$ such that $g = bnb'$. Since T is normal in N,

$$P_2 \supset gBg^{-1} = bnBn^{-1}b^{-1} \supset bnTn^{-1}b^{-1} = bTb^{-1}$$

and

$$P_1 \supset B \supset bTb^{-1},$$

which proves the proposition.

7. SIMPLICITY THEOREMS

Lemma 2. Let H *be a normal subgroup of* G. *There exists a subset* X *of* S *such that* $BH = G_X$ *and such that every element of* X *commutes with every element of* $S - X$.

Since BH is a subgroup of G containing B, there exists a unique subset X of S such that $BH = G_X$ (Th. 3).

Let $s_1 \in X$ and $s_2 \in S - X$; let n_1 and n_2 be representatives in N of s_1 and s_2, respectively. Then $n_1 \in G_X = BH$ and there exists $b \in B$ such that $bn_1 \in H$. Since H is normal in G, the element $h = n_2bn_1n_2^{-1}$ of G belongs to H. This means that

$$h \in C(s_2).C(s_1).C(s_2).$$

If the length of $s_2s_1s_2$ is equal to 3, Cor. 1 of Th. 2 implies that

$$C(s_2).C(s_1).C(s_2) = C(s_2s_1s_2),$$

[6] If H is a subgroup of a group G, the normaliser of H in G is the subgroup $\mathfrak{N}(H)$ consisting of the elements g of G such that $gHg^{-1} = H$. A subgroup H′ is said to normalise H if $H' \subset \mathfrak{N}(H)$, in which case $HH' = H'H$ is a subgroup of G in which H is normal.

and hence that $h \in \mathrm{H} \cap \mathrm{C}(s_2 s_1 s_2)$. Since $\mathrm{H} \cap \mathrm{C}(s_2 s_1 s_2)$ is non-empty, $s_2 s_1 s_2 \in \mathrm{W_X}$. As (s_2, s_1, s_2) is a reduced decomposition, it follows that $s_2 \in \mathrm{X}$, contrary to our assumption.

Thus $l_\mathrm{S}(s_2 s_1 s_2) \leqslant 2$; if $l_\mathrm{S}(s_2 s_1 s_2) = 1$, then $s_1 s_2 \in \mathrm{S}$ and so $(s_1 s_2)^2 = 1$, or $s_1 s_2 = s_2 s_1$. If $l_\mathrm{S}(s_2 s_1 s_2) = 2$, property (E) of § 1, no. 5 implies that $s_2 s_1 = s_1 s_2$, since $s_1 \neq s_2$. Q.E.D.

The following property of a group U enters into Th. 5 below:

(R) *For any normal subgroup* V *of* U *distinct from* U, *the commutator subgroup* (cf. *Algebra,* Chap. I, § 6, no. 8) *of* U/V *is distinct from* U/V.

Every soluble group satisfies (R); in particular, every abelian group satisfies (R). It can be shown that the symmetric group $\mathfrak{S}_n$ satisfies (R) (cf. Exerc. 29).

THEOREM 5. *Let* Z *be the intersection of the conjugates of* B, *let* U *be a subgroup of* B *and let* G_1 *be the subgroup generated by the conjugates of* U *in* G. *We make the following assumptions:*

(1) U *is normal in* B *and* B = UT.
(2) U *has property (*R*).*
(3) G_1 *is equal to its commutator subgroup.*
(4) *The Coxeter system* (W, S) *is irreducible* (cf. § 1, no. 9).

Then every subgroup H *of* G *normalised by* G_1 *is either contained in* Z *or contains* G_1.

First we show that $\mathrm{G} = \mathrm{G}_1\mathrm{T}$. The group $\mathrm{G}_1\mathrm{T}$ contains B and hence is its own normaliser (Th. 4); but as N normalises G_1 and T, it also normalises $\mathrm{G}_1\mathrm{T}$, so $\mathrm{N} \subset \mathrm{G}_1\mathrm{T}$. Since G is generated by B and N, it follows that $\mathrm{G} = \mathrm{G}_1\mathrm{T}$.

Next, set

$$\mathrm{G}' = \mathrm{G}_1\mathrm{H}, \quad \mathrm{B}' = \mathrm{B} \cap \mathrm{G}', \quad \mathrm{N}' = \mathrm{N} \cap \mathrm{G}',$$
$$\mathrm{T}' = \mathrm{T} \cap \mathrm{G}' = \mathrm{B}' \cap \mathrm{N}' \quad \text{and} \quad \mathrm{W}' = \mathrm{N}'/\mathrm{T}'.$$

We have $\mathrm{G} = \mathrm{G}'\mathrm{T}$ since G' contains G_1, and hence $\mathrm{N} = \mathrm{N}'\mathrm{T}$. The inclusion of N' into N thus defines, on passing to the quotient, an isomorphism $\alpha : \mathrm{W}' \to \mathrm{W}$. Let $\mathrm{S}' = \alpha^{-1}(\mathrm{S})$.

We now show that $(\mathrm{G}', \mathrm{B}', \mathrm{N}', \mathrm{S}')$ *is a Tits system.* Since G = BNB and B = TU = UT, we have G = UNU. Since U is a subgroup of G', it follows that $\mathrm{G}' = \mathrm{U}\mathrm{N}'\mathrm{U}$; since $\mathrm{U} \subset \mathrm{B}'$, this proves (T1). Axiom (T2) is satisfied since α is an isomorphism. Let $w \in \mathrm{W}$ and let $w' = \alpha^{-1}(w)$ be the corresponding element of W'. We have

$$\mathrm{B}w\mathrm{B} = \mathrm{B}w\mathrm{B}' = \mathrm{B}w'\mathrm{B}', \qquad \text{since } \mathrm{B} = \mathrm{B}'\mathrm{T}.$$

From this we conclude that $\mathrm{G}' \cap \mathrm{B}w\mathrm{B} = \mathrm{B}'w'\mathrm{B}'$, which means that the inclusion of G' into G defines on passing to the quotient a bijection from

$B'\backslash G'/B'$ to $B\backslash G/B$. Axiom (T3) follows immediately. Axiom (T4) follows from $B = B'T$.

The subgroup H is normal in G'. By Lemma 2 applied to (G', B', N', S'), there exists a subset X' of S' such that $B'H = G'_{X'}$ and every element of $S' - X'$ commutes with every element of X'. In view of assumption (4), there are only two possibilities:

a) $X' = \varnothing$, i.e. $B'H = B'$, so $H \subset B' \subset B$. If $g \in G$, then $g = g_1 t$ with $g_1 \in G_1$, $t \in T$, and $H \subset g_1 B g_1^{-1}$ since G_1 normalises H. Thus $H \subset gBg^{-1}$, and since Z is the intersection of the gBg^{-1}, we have $H \subset Z$.

b) $X' = S'$, i.e. $B'H = G'$. Since $G = G'T$, we have

$$G = B'HT = HB'T = HB.$$

As B normalises U, every conjugate of U is of the form hUh^{-1} with $h \in H$. Such a subgroup is contained in the group UH, hence $G_1 \subset UH$ by the definition of G_1. Thus, we have the isomorphisms

$$U/(U \cap H) \cong UH/H = G_1H/H \cong G_1/(G_1 \cap H).$$

By assumption (3), $G_1/(G_1 \cap H)$ is equal to its commutator subgroup. Assumption (2) now shows that the group $U/(U \cap H)$, which is isomorphic to $G_1/(G_1 \cap H)$, reduces to the identity element. Hence $G_1 \cap H = G_1$ and $G_1 \subset H$, which completes the proof.

COROLLARY. *Under the assumptions of Th. 5, the group* $G_1/(G_1 \cap Z)$ *is either simple non-abelian or reduces to the identity element.*

Th. 5 shows that $G_1/(G_1 \cap Z)$ is simple or reduces to the identity element. On the other hand, assumption (3) implies that it is equal to its commutator subgroup. Hence the corollary.

Remarks. 1) Assumptions (2), (3), (4) were not used in the proof that (G', B', N', S') is a Tits system.

2) Suppose that $Z \cap U = \{1\}$. Since Z and U are normal in B, it follows that every element of Z commutes with every element of U, and hence with every element of G_1. In view of the preceding corollary, it follows that $G_1 \cap Z$ *is the centre of* G_1.

3) Assumption (3) is implied by the following condition:

(3') U is generated by the commutators $b^{-1}u^{-1}bu$ with $u \in U$ and $b \in B \cap G_1$.

Examples. 1) Let k be a field, n an integer $\geqslant 0$, $G = \mathbf{GL}(n, k)$, and let (G, B, N, S) be the Tits system described in no. 2. Let U be the strictly upper triangular subgroup of G, i.e. the subgroup of B consisting of the matrices whose diagonal entries are equal to 1. Condition (1) in Th. 5 is immediate, and so is (2) since U is soluble. Condition (4) is satisfied if $n \geqslant 2$. One can show (cf. *Algebra*, Chap. II, § 10, Exerc. 13) that (3) is satisfied if $n \geqslant 3$ and $\mathrm{Card}(k) \geqslant 4$. Under these conditions, we conclude that $G_1/(G_1 \cap Z)$ is *simple* and that $G_1 \cap Z$ is the centre of G_1 (cf. *Remark* 2).

When k is commutative, $G_1 = \mathbf{SL}(n, k)$ (cf. *Algebra*, Chap. III, § 8, no. 9).

2) Let $\mathfrak{g}$ be a simple Lie algebra over $\mathbf{C}$, and let G be the group of inner automorphisms of $\mathfrak{g}$ (cf. Chap. III, § 6, no. 2, Prop. 2). By using Th. 5, one can show that G is simple non-abelian.

APPENDIX
GRAPHS

1. DEFINITIONS

DEFINITION 1. *A* combinatorial graph *(or simply a graph, if there is no risk of confusion) is a pair* (A, S), *where* S *is a set and* A *is a subset of* $\mathfrak{P}(\mathrm{S})$ *consisting of sets with two elements.*

Let $\Gamma = (\mathrm{A}, \mathrm{S})$ be a graph. The elements of A are called the *edges* and those of S the *vertices* of Γ; two vertices are said to be *joined* if $\{x, y\}$ is an edge. A vertex is called *terminal* if it is joined to at most one vertex, and a *ramification point* if it is joined to at least three vertices.

In accordance with the general definitions (*Sets* R, § 8), an *isomorphism* from the graph Γ to a graph $\Gamma' = (\mathrm{A}', \mathrm{S}')$ is a bijection from S to S′ that takes A to A′. A graph $\Gamma' = (\mathrm{A}', \mathrm{S}')$ is called a *subgraph* of Γ if $\mathrm{S}' \subset \mathrm{S}$ and $\mathrm{A}' \subset \mathrm{A}$; Γ is called a *full* subgraph of Γ if $\mathrm{S}' \subset \mathrm{S}$ and $\mathrm{A}' = \mathrm{A} \cap \mathfrak{P}(\mathrm{S})$. It is clear that every subset of S is the set of vertices of exactly one full subgraph of Γ.

To make the arguments easier to follow, we represent a graph by a diagram having points corresponding to the vertices, two points being joined by a line if and only if the vertices they represent are joined in the graph. For example, the diagram

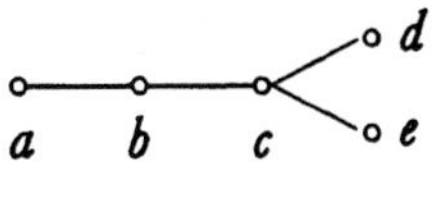

represents a graph whose vertices are a, b, c, d, e and whose edges are $\{a, b\}$, $\{b, c\}$, $\{c, d\}$ and $\{c, e\}$.

2. CONNECTED COMPONENTS OF A GRAPH

Let $\Gamma = (\mathrm{A}, \mathrm{S})$ be a graph. If a and b are two vertices, a *path* joining a and b is a sequence $(x_0, \ldots, x_n)$ of vertices of Γ with $x_0 = a, x_n = b$, the vertices x_i and x_{i+1} being joined for $0 \leqslant i < n$; the integer $n \geqslant 0$ is the *length* of the path. The path $(x_0, \ldots, x_n)$ is said to be injective if $x_i \neq x_j$ if $i \neq j$. If a path $(x_0, \ldots, x_n)$ joining a and b is of minimal length among such paths, it is necessarily injective; for if not, there would exist i and j with $0 \leqslant i < j \leqslant n$ and $x_i = x_j$ and then the sequence

$$(x_0, \ldots, x_i, x_{j+1}, \ldots, x_n)$$

would be a path of length $< n$ joining a and b.

The relation "there exists a path joining a and b" between two vertices a and b of Γ is an equivalence relation R on the set S of vertices. The equivalence classes of R are called the *connected components* of Γ; and Γ is said to be *connected* if S has at most one connected component, that is if any two vertices of Γ can be joined by at least one path.

PROPOSITION 1. *Let $\Gamma = (\mathrm{A}, \mathrm{S})$ be a graph and $(\mathrm{S}_\alpha)_{\alpha \in \mathrm{L}}$ its family of connected components. Denote by Γ_α the full subgraph of Γ having S_α as its set of vertices.*

(i) *For any α in L, the graph Γ_α is connected.*

(ii) *If $\Gamma' = (\mathrm{A}', \mathrm{S}')$ is a connected subgraph of Γ, there exists α in L such that $\Gamma' \subset \Gamma_\alpha$.*

(iii) *If $\alpha \neq \beta$, no element of S_α is joined in Γ to any element of S_β (equivalently, every edge of Γ is an edge of one of the Γ_α).*

(iv) *Let $(\mathrm{S}'_\lambda)_{\lambda \in \mathrm{M}}$ be a partition of S such that, if $\lambda \neq \mu$, no element of S'_λ is joined in Γ to any element of S'_μ; then each of the sets S'_λ is a union of connected components of Γ.*

(i) Let α be in L and a and b be in S_α. Then there exists a path $c = (x_0, \ldots, x_n)$ joining a and b in Γ. For any i with $0 \leqslant i \leqslant n$, the path $(x_0, \ldots, x_i)$ joins a to x_i in Γ, so $x_i \in \mathrm{S}_\alpha$. Thus, c is a path *in Γ_α* joining a and b. It follows that Γ_α is connected.

(ii) Let $\Gamma' = (\mathrm{A}', \mathrm{S}')$ be a non-empty connected subgraph of Γ, let a be an element of S' and let S_α be the connected component of S containing a. For any b in S', there exists a path c joining a and b in Γ', and *a fortiori* in Γ. It follows that $\mathrm{S}' \subset \mathrm{S}_\alpha$.

(iii) Given distinct elements α and β of L, and vertices $a \in \mathrm{S}_\alpha$ and $b \in \mathrm{S}_\beta$, there is no path joining a and b, and in particular no edge joining a and b.

(iv) Let a be in S'_λ and let S_α be the connected component of Γ containing a. Then, for any b in S_α, there exists a path $(x_0, \ldots, x_n)$ joining a and b in Γ. If i is an integer such that $0 \leqslant i < n$ and if $x_i \in \mathrm{S}'_\lambda$, then $x_{i+1} \in \mathrm{S}'_\lambda$ since x_i is joined to x_{i+1}. It follows by induction that $x_i \in \mathrm{S}'_\lambda$ for $0 \leqslant i \leqslant n$, and in particular that $b = x_n$ is in S'_λ. Thus, $\mathrm{S}_\alpha \subset \mathrm{S}'_\lambda$.

COROLLARY 1. *A graph $\Gamma = (\mathrm{A}, \mathrm{S})$ is connected if and only if there does not exist a partition $(\mathrm{S}', \mathrm{S}'')$ of S into two non-empty subsets such that no element of S' is joined in Γ to any element of S''.*

Suppose that Γ is not connected and let S' be one of its connected components. The set $\mathrm{S}'' = \mathrm{S} - \mathrm{S}'$ is non-empty by Prop. 1, (i) and no element of S' is joined to any element of S'' by Prop. 1, (iii).

Suppose now that Γ is connected and let (S', S'') be a partition with the stated property. By Prop. 1, (iv), the set S' contains at least one connected component, so $S' = S$ and $S'' = \varnothing$, a contradiction.

COROLLARY 2. *A subset* S' *of* S *is a union of connected components if and only if no vertex belonging to* S' *is joined to any vertex belonging to* $S - S'$.

The condition is sufficient by Prop. 1, (iv). It is necessary by Prop. 1, (iii).

3. FORESTS AND TREES

Let $\Gamma = (A, S)$ be a graph. A *circuit* of Γ is a sequence

$$(x_1, \ldots, x_n)$$

of distinct vertices of Γ such that $n \geqslant 3$, x_i is joined to x_{i+1} for $1 \leqslant i < n$ and x_n is joined to x_1. Γ is called a *forest* if there is no circuit in Γ; every subgraph of Γ is then also a forest. A connected forest is called a *tree*; the connected components of a forest are thus trees.

PROPOSITION 2. *Let* $\Gamma = (A, S)$ *be a forest having only a finite number of vertices.*

(i) *If* Γ *has at least one vertex, it has a terminal vertex.*

(ii) *If* Γ *has at least two vertices, there is a partition* (S', S'') *of its set of vertices into two non-empty subsets such that two distinct vertices that both belong to* S' *or both belong to* S'' *are never joined.*

Suppose that Γ has at least one vertex and let $(x_0, \ldots, x_n)$ be an injective path of maximal length in Γ. The vertex x_0 cannot be joined to a vertex y distinct from $x_0, x_1, \ldots, x_n$, since otherwise there would exist an injective path in Γ of length $n+1$, namely $(y, x_0, \ldots, x_n)$. The vertex x_0 is not joined to any vertex x_i with $2 \leqslant i \leqslant n$, since otherwise $(x_0, x_1, \ldots, x_i)$ would be a circuit in the forest Γ. Thus, x_0 is terminal.

We shall prove (ii) by induction of the number m of vertices of Γ, the case $m = 2$ being trivial. Suppose then that $m \geqslant 3$ and that assertion (ii) is proved for graphs with $m - 1$ vertices. Let a be a terminal vertex of Γ (cf. (i)). We apply the induction hypothesis to the full subgraph of Γ whose vertices are the vertices $x \neq a$ of Γ. Thus, there exist two non-empty disjoint subsets S'_1 and S''_1 of S with $S'_1 \cup S''_1 = S - \{a\}$, and such that two distinct vertices in S'_1 (resp. S''_1) are never joined. Since a is joined to at most one vertex of Γ, we can suppose for example that it is not joined to any vertex in S'_1. The partition $(S'_1, S''_1 \cup \{a\})$ then has the required property. Q.E.D.

For any integer $n \geqslant 1$, denote by A_n the graph whose vertices are the integers $1, 2, \ldots, n$ and whose edges are the pairs $\{i, j\}$ with $i - j = \pm 1$:

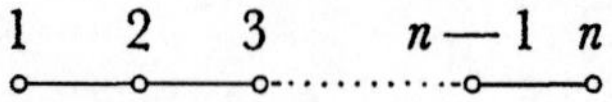

A graph Γ is said to be a *chain of length* $m \geqslant 0$ if it is isomorphic to A_{m+1}. This is equivalent to the existence in Γ of an injective path $(x_0, \ldots, x_m)$ containing all the vertices, the vertices x_i and x_j not being joined if $|i-j| > 1$.

PROPOSITION 3. *A graph is a chain if and only if its number of vertices is finite and non-zero and it is a tree with no ramification point.*

Suppose that the graph Γ is a chain $(x_0, \ldots, x_m)$ with the properties listed before the statement of Prop. 3. It is clear that any vertex of Γ is joined to at most two vertices. If $i < j$ the path $(x_i, \ldots, x_j)$ extracted from the path $(x_0, \ldots, x_m)$ joins x_i to x_j; thus, Γ is connected. Finally, let $(x_{p_1}, \ldots, x_{p_n})$ be a circuit in Γ, and let p_k be the smallest of the distinct integers $p_1, \ldots, p_n$. There exist distinct indices i and j such that x_{p_k} is joined to x_{p_i} and x_{p_j}: this follows from the definition of a circuit. Since $p_k < p_i$ and $p_k < p_j$, we necessarily have $p_i = p_j = p_k + 1$, which is a contradiction since $p_1, \ldots, p_n$ are distinct. Thus, there is no circuit in Γ.

Conversely, let Γ be a tree with no ramification point and with a finite non-zero number of vertices, and let $(x_0, \ldots, x_m)$ be an injective path of maximal length in Γ. Denote by T the set of vertices other than $x_0, \ldots, x_m$. A vertex $b \in \mathrm{T}$ cannot be joined to any vertex x_i, for we would have either

a) $i = 0$, but then $(b, x_0, \ldots, x_m)$ would be an injective path of length $m+1$ in Γ, or

b) $i = m$, but then $(x_0, \ldots, x_m, b)$ would be an injective path of length $m+1$ in Γ, or

c) $0 < i < m$, but then x_i would be joined to three distinct vertices x_{i-1}, x_{i+1} and b.

Since Γ is connected, T is empty by Cor. 1 of Prop. 1. Moreover, if there were i, j with $j - i > 1$ and x_i, x_j joined, there would be a circuit $(x_i, x_{i+1}, \ldots, x_j)$ in Γ. Thus, Γ is a chain. Q.E.D.

EXERCISES

§ 1

1) *a*) Let (W, S) be a Coxeter system and let $s_1, \dots, s_r$ be elements of S. Put $w = s_1 \dots s_r$. Show that if $l_S(w) < r$, there exist two integers p and q with $1 \leqslant p < q \leqslant r$ such that $w = s_1 \dots s_{p-1}s_{p+1} \dots s_{q-1}s_{q+1} \dots s_r$. Show that there is a strictly increasing sequence of integers $j(1), \dots, j(k)$ between 1 and r such that $(s_{j(1)}, \dots, s_{j(k)})$ is a reduced decomposition of w.

b) Let (W, S) be a Coxeter system and X, Y, Z three subsets of S. Show that

$$W_X \cap (W_Y.W_Z) = (W_X \cap W_Y).(W_X \cap W_Z)$$

(show that every element $w \in W_Y.W_Z$ has a reduced decomposition

$$(s_1, \dots, s_h, t_1, \dots, t_k)$$

such that $s_i \in Y$ and $t_j \in Z$ and use Cor. 1 of Prop. 7 of no. 8).

Show that

$$W_X.(W_Y \cap W_Z) = (W_X.W_Y) \cap (W_X.W_Z).$$

2) Let (W, S) be a Coxeter system and X a subset of S. Show that W_X is normal in W if and only if every element of X commutes with every element of S − X.

3) Let (W, S) be a Coxeter system and X, Y two subsets of S. Let $a \in W$. Show that there exists a unique element $w \in W_X a W_Y$ of minimal length and that every element

$$w' \in W_X a W_Y$$

can be written in the form $w' = xwy$, with $x \in W_X, y \in W_Y$ and $l(w') = l(x) + l(w) + l(y)$ (take an element of minimal length in $W_X a W_Y$ and use Exerc. 1). An element $w \in W$ is said to be (X, Y)-*reduced* if it is the element of minimal length in the double coset $W_X a W_Y$.

Show that if w is (X, ∅)-reduced then $l(xw) = l(x) + l(w)$ for all $x \in W_X$, and that every element of W can be written uniquely in the form xw where

$x \in W_X$ and w is $(X, \varnothing)$-reduced. Show that an element $w \in W$ is $(X, \varnothing)$-reduced if and only if $l(xw) > l(w)$ for all $x \in X$ (write w in the form yw', where $y \in W_X$ and w' is $(X, \varnothing)$-reduced).

Show that $w \in W$ is (X, Y)-reduced if and only if w is both $(X, \varnothing)$-reduced and $(\varnothing, Y)$-reduced.

4) Let n be an integer $\geqslant 2$. For any integer i with $1 \leqslant i \leqslant n-1$, denote by s_i the transposition of i and $i+1$ in the set $\{1, 2, \ldots, n\}$, and by H_i the set of $w \in \mathfrak{S}_n$ such that $w^{-1}(i) < w^{-1}(i+1)$; put $S = \{s_1, \ldots, s_{n-1}\}$. Show that $(\mathfrak{S}_n, S)$ is a Coxeter system and that H_i is the set of $w \in \mathfrak{S}_n$ such that $l(w) < l(s_i w)$ (use Prop. 6 of no. 7).

5) Let X be a non-empty set and W a set of permutations of X. Assume given a set $\mathfrak{R}$ of equivalence relations on X, an element $x_0 \in X$ and a map $\varphi : H \mapsto s_H$ from $\mathfrak{R}$ to W. Denote by $\mathfrak{R}_0$ the set of $H \in \mathfrak{R}$ such that $s_H(x_0) \equiv x_0$ mod. H' for all $H' \neq H$ in $\mathfrak{R}$, and by S_0 the set of s_H for H in $\mathfrak{R}_0$. We make the following assumptions:

(i) For any $H \in \mathfrak{R}$, there are two equivalence classes modulo H that are permuted by s_H and $s_H^2 = 1$.

(ii) For all $H \in \mathfrak{R}$ and all $w \in W$, the transform $w(H)$ of H by w is an equivalence relation belonging to $\mathfrak{R}$ and $s_{w(H)} = w s_H w^{-1}$.

(iii) For any $w \neq 1$ in W, the set of $H \in \mathfrak{R}$ such that $w(x_0) \not\equiv x_0$ mod. H is finite and meets $\mathfrak{R}_0$.

a) Prove that (W, S_0) is a Coxeter system (use Prop. 6 of no. 7).

b) Prove that the length $l_{S_0}(w)$ is equal to the number of elements $H \in \mathfrak{R}$ such that

$$w(x_0) \not\equiv x_0 \text{ mod. } H.$$

c) Let E be a finite set and X the set of total order relations on X. Denote by W the group of permutations of E, acting in the obvious way on E. Let i and j be distinct elements of E; say that two elements R and R′ of X are equivalent mod. H_{ij} if either $R(i,j)$ and $R'(i,j)$ or $R(j,i)$ and $R'(j,i)$; and denote the transposition of i and j by s_{ij}. Let $\mathfrak{R}$ be the set of equivalence relations of the form H_{ij} and φ the map from $\mathfrak{R}$ to W defined by $\varphi(H_{ij}) = s_{ij}$; finally let x_0 be an arbitrary element of X. Show that the objects thus defined satisfy assumptions (i) to (iii), and recover the results of Exerc. 4.

6) Let E be a set with 6 elements and F the set of structures of the projective line over the field $\mathbf{F}_5$ on E. Denote by $\mathfrak{S}_E$ the group of permutations of E; for any $\sigma \in \mathfrak{S}_E$ denote by $\tilde{\sigma}$ the permutation of F induced by σ by transport of structure. Show that there exists a bijection u from E to F, and that the map $\sigma \mapsto u^{-1}\tilde{\sigma}u$ is an outer automorphism of $\mathfrak{S}_E$ (if s is a transposition, $u^{-1}\tilde{s}u$ has three orbits of two elements).

7) Construct a group W and two subsets S and S′ of W such that (W, S) and (W, S′) are isomorphic Coxeter systems, but such that there exists no inner automorphism of W transforming S to S′ (use Exerc. 4 and Exerc. 6).

8) Construct a group W and two subsets S and S′ of W such that (W, S) and (W, S′) are non-isomorphic Coxeter systems, one of them being irreducible and the other not (for W take a dihedral group of order 12 generated by $\{s, s'\}$ where s and s' are of order 2 and $s \neq s'$, and put $S = \{s, s'\}$ and $S' = \{(ss')^3, s', s'(ss')^2\}$).

9) Let (W, S) be a Coxeter system with matrix $(m(s, s'))$, and let W^+ be the subgroup of W consisting of the elements of even length. Let $s_0 \in S$. Put $g_s = ss_0$. Show that the family $(g_s)_{s \in S - \{s_0\}}$ and the relations $g_s^{m(s,s_0)} = 1$ for $m(s, s_0) \neq \infty$ and $(g_s g_{s'}^{-1})^{m(s,s')} = 1$ for $s, s' \in S - \{s_0\}$ and $m(s, s') \neq \infty$, form a presentation of W^+. (Let H^+ be the group defined by the above presentation. Show that there exists an automorphism α of H^+, with square the identity, that transforms g_s to g_s^{-1} for all $s \in S - \{s_0\}$. If H_α is the semi-direct product of $\{1, -1\}$ and H^+, relative to α, define mutually inverse homomorphisms $H_\alpha \to W$ and $W \to H_\alpha$.) Show that if the elements of S are conjugate (cf. Prop. 3), the group W^+ is the *commutator subgroup* of W (remark that the elements g_s are then commutators).

10) Let $\mathfrak{A}_n$ be the alternating group consisting of the permutations $w \in \mathfrak{S}_n$ whose signature is equal to +1. Show that $\mathfrak{A}_n$ is the commutator subgroup of $\mathfrak{S}_n$ (use Exerc. 4 and 9). For any integer i with $1 \leqslant i \leqslant n-2$, put $u_i = s_i s_{i+1}$ (in the notation of Exerc. 4). Show that the family (u_i) and the relations $u_1^3 = 1$, $u_i^2 = 1$ for $i \geqslant 2$, $(u_i u_{i+1})^3 = 1$ for $1 \leqslant i \leqslant n-3$, and $u_i u_j = u_j u_i$ for $1 \leqslant i \leqslant n-4$ and $i+2 \leqslant j \leqslant n-2$, form a presentation of the group $\mathfrak{A}_n$ (use Exerc. 9).

*11) Let (W, S) be a Coxeter system. Let Γ_∞ be the graph whose set of vertices is S, two vertices s, s' being joined by an edge if and only if $m(s, s') \neq \infty$. Let S_α be the connected components of Γ_∞. Show that W can be identified with the *free product* of the W_{S_α}. In particular, every $w \in W$ can be written uniquely as a product $w_1 \dots w_h$ with $w_i \neq 1$, w_i belonging to $W_{S_{\alpha_i}}$, and $\alpha_i \neq \alpha_{i+1}$ for $1 \leqslant i \leqslant h-1$; show that the length of w is the sum of the lengths of the w_i.*

12) Let (W, S) be a Coxeter system such that $m(s, s')$ is even if $s \neq s'$ and let X be a subset of S. Show that there exists a unique homomorphism f_X from W to W_X such that $f_X(s) = s$ for $s \in X$ and $f_X(s) = 1$ for $s \in S - X$. Deduce that W is the semi-direct product of W_X and the kernel of f_X. Show that if $X \subset Y \subset S$, there exists a unique homomorphism $f_{X,Y}$ from W_Y to W_X such that $f_X = F_{X,Y} \circ f_Y$ and that W can be identified with a subgroup

of the projective system thus obtained from the W_X as X runs through the filtered set of finite subsets of S.

¶ 13) Let (W, S) be a Coxeter system. For $s, s' \in S$, define the sequence $\mathbf{a}(s, s')$ by means of the following rules:

(i) if ss' is of infinite order, $\mathbf{a}(s, s')$ is the empty sequence;
(ii) if ss' is of finite order m the sequence $\mathbf{a}(s, s')$ is of length m and its even (resp. odd) numbered terms are equal to s' (resp. s).

Denote by $a(s, s')$ the product of the sequence $\mathbf{a}(s, s')$.

a) Show that the generating set S and the relations $s^2 = 1$ and $\mathbf{a}(s, s') = \mathbf{a}(s', s)$ form a presentation of the group W.

b) Let q be an integer $\geqslant 1$. Let Σ_q be the set of sequences of q elements of S and let R_q be the smallest equivalence relation on Σ_q for which sequences of the form $(A, \mathbf{a}(s, s'), B)$ and $(A, \mathbf{a}(s', s), B)$ (where $s, s' \in S$ and A and B are sequences of elements of S) are equivalent. Let Σ_q^r be the set of sequences $\mathbf{s} = (s_1, \dots, s_q)$ such that $w(\mathbf{s}) = s_1 \dots s_q$ is of length q. Show that sequences $\mathbf{s}, \mathbf{s}' \in \Sigma_q^r$ are equivalent modulo R_q if and only if $w(\mathbf{s}) = w(\mathbf{s}')$ (argue by induction on q and apply Prop. 5 of no. 5).

c) Show that a sequence $\mathbf{s} \in \Sigma_q$ does not belong to Σ_q^r if and only if $\mathbf{s}$ is equivalent modulo R_q to a sequence in which two consecutive terms are equal. (Argue by induction on q and reduce to the case of a sequence $(s_1, \dots, s_q)$ which does not belong to Σ_q^r but which is such that $(s_1, \dots, s_{q-1})$ and $(s_2, \dots, s_q)$ belong to Σ_{q-1}^r; use Exerc. 1 to show that $s_1 \dots s_{q-1} = s_2 \dots s_q$ and apply *b*).)

*14) Let (W, S) be a Coxeter system and let (Γ, f) be its Coxeter graph. Let k be an integer $\geqslant 3$. If a is an edge of Γ, put $f_k(a) = f(a)$ if $f(a) \neq \infty$ and $f_k(a) = k$ if $f(a) = \infty$. Let (W_k, S) be a Coxeter system whose Coxeter graph is equal to (Γ, f_k) (Chap. V, § 4, no. 3, Cor. of Prop. 4). Show that there exists a unique homomorphism φ_k from W to W_k inducing the identity on S. Show that if k divides k', there exists a unique homomorphism $\varphi_{k,k'}$ from $W_{k'}$ to W_k such that $\varphi_k = \varphi_{k,k'} \circ \varphi_{k'}$. Show that the homomorphism (φ_k) from W to the projective limit of the W_k is injective (use Exerc. 13) *c*)), but in general not surjective (for example, in the case of the infinite dihedral group).*

15)[7] Let A be a set and $\mathfrak{C}$ a subset of $\mathfrak{P}(A)$. The elements of $\mathfrak{C}$ are called the *chambers* of A and a subset F of a chamber C is called a *facet*, the *codimension* of F in C being the cardinal of C − F. A facet F is said to be a *panel* of C if F is of codimension 1 in C. Two chambers C and C′ are said to be *adjoining*

[7] Exercises 15 to 24, as well as Exercises 3 to 17 of § 2, are hitherto unpublished and were communicated to us by J. Tits.

if they have a common panel F: then either $C = C'$ or $F = C \cap C'$. A *gallery* of length n is a sequence $\Gamma = (C_0, C_1, \ldots, C_n)$ of $n+1$ chambers such that C_i and C_{i+1} are adjoining for $0 \leqslant i \leqslant n-1$. Then C_0 and C_n are called the *ends* of Γ. The gallery Γ is called *injective* if $C_i \neq C_{i+1}$ for $0 \leqslant i \leqslant n-1$ and is called *minimal* if there is no gallery with the same ends and length $< n$.

The set A (together with $\mathfrak{C}$) is a *building* if every element of A belongs to at least one chamber and if any two chambers are the ends of a gallery. The *distance* between two chambers C and C′ is the length $d(C, C')$ of a minimal gallery with ends C and C′.

A *sub-building* of a building A is a subset D of A such that D together with $\mathfrak{C} \cap \mathfrak{P}(D)$ is a building.

a) Show that if A is a building, a facet has the same codimension in every chamber containing it; this allows us to speak of the codimension of a facet and of a panel of A without reference to a particular chamber. A *morphism* of a building B to A is a map f from B to A such that the restriction of f to every chamber C of B is a bijection from C to a chamber $f(C)$ of A. Show that the image under f of a facet of B is a facet of the same codimension.

b) A building is called an *apartment* if every panel is contained in exactly two chambers. Show that if A is an apartment, every automorphism of A (i.e. every permutation of A preserving $\mathfrak{C}$) that leaves fixed all the points of a chamber is the identity. More generally, let φ be an endomorphism of A and let C be a chamber of A such that $\varphi(a) = a$ for all $a \in C$. Let $(C, C_1, \ldots, C_n)$ be a gallery of A. Show that, either the gallery $(C, \varphi(C_1), \ldots, \varphi(C_n))$ is not injective, or $\varphi(a) = a$ for all a belonging to the union of the C_i.

16) Let (W, S) be a Coxeter system. For $s \in S$, denote by $W^{(s)}$ the subgroup $W_{S-\{s\}}$ of W, by A the set of subsets of W of the form $wW^{(s)}$ for $w \in W$ and $s \in S$, and by $\mathfrak{C}$ the set of subsets of A of the form $C_w = \{wW^{(s)} \mid s \in S\}$ for $w \in W$, which we call the chambers of A (Exerc. 15).

a) Show that the map $w \mapsto C_w$ is a bijection from W onto $\mathfrak{C}$.

b) Show that two distinct chambers C_w and $C_{w'}$ are adjoining if and only if there exists $s \in S$ such that $w' = ws$. Deduce that A (together with $\mathfrak{C}$) is an apartment (Exerc. 15), which we call the apartment of (W, S). Show that the length of a minimal gallery with ends C_w and $C_{w'}$ is equal to $l_S(w^{-1}w')$.

c) Let $\mathfrak{F}$ be the set of facets of A and let $F \in \mathfrak{F}$. Show that there exist a unique subset X of S and an element $w \in W$ such that $wW_X = \bigcap_{i \in F} i$. Then F is said to be of *type* X. Show that the codimension of F is equal to the cardinal of X. Show that the map $j : F \mapsto \bigcap_{i \in F} i$ is a *strictly decreasing bijection* (with respect to inclusion) from $\mathfrak{F}$ to the set of subsets of W of the form wW_X for $w \in W$ and $X \subset S$. Show that every facet of type X contains a unique facet of type Y for every Y such that $X \subset Y \subset S$.

d) Let W act on A be left translations and put $C = C_e$. Show that W acts simply-transitively[8] on $\mathfrak{C}$. Let $C_1, \ldots, C_n$ be chambers of A. Show that the following conditions are equivalent:

(i) the sequence $\Gamma = (C_0 = C, C_1, \ldots, C_n)$ is an injective gallery;

(ii) there exists a sequence $\mathbf{s} = (s_1, \ldots, s_n)$ of elements of S such that $C_j = t_j(C_{j-1})$ for $1 \leqslant j \leqslant n$, where t_j is the element of $\Phi(\mathbf{s})$ defined in no. 4, formula (11).

Show that if these conditions are satisfied, the sequence $\mathbf{s}$ is unique and $C_n = s_1 \ldots s_n(C)$. Show that the gallery Γ is minimal if and only if the sequence $\mathbf{s}(\Gamma) = \mathbf{s}$ is a reduced decomposition of $w = s_1 \ldots s_n$.

e) Let T be the union of the conjugates of S. For $t \in T$, the set L_t of points of A invariant under t is called the *wall* defined by t. Show that L_t is a union of panels and that a panel F is contained in L_t if and only if $j(F)$ is of the form $wW_{\{s\}}$ with $t = wsw^{-1}$. Deduce that, for any panel F, there is a unique element $t = t(F) \in T$ such that $F \subset L_t$: L_t is called the *support* of F.

Show that if $w(L_t) = L_t$ (for $w \in W$), then $w = 1$ or $w = t$.

f) Let $w', w'' \in W$. Put $C' = w'(C), C'' = w''(C)$ and let $\Gamma = (C_0 = C', C_1, \ldots, C_n = C'')$ be an injective gallery with ends C' and C''. Let t_j be the element of T defining the support wall of the panel $C_j \cap C_{j-1}$ (for $1 \leqslant j \leqslant n$). Show that the sequence $\Psi(T) = (w'^{-1} t_j w')_{1 \leqslant j \leqslant n}$ coincides with the sequence $\Phi(\mathbf{s}(w'^{-1}(\Gamma))$. For $t \in T$, let $n(\Gamma, t)$ be the number of times $w'^{-1} t w'$ appears in $\Psi(\Gamma)$. Deduce from Lemma 1 of no. 4 that the number $(-1)^{n(\Gamma,t)}$ depends only on C' and C'' and not on Γ: we denote it by $\eta(C', C'', t)$. Show that the relation $\eta(C', C'', t) = 1$ is an equivalence relation between C' and C'' that has two equivalence classes that are permuted by t. Denote by $\mathfrak{C}^+(t)$ the equivalence class containing C and by $\mathfrak{C}^-(t)$ the other.

Show that, for $w \in W$ and $s \in S$, the chamber $w(C)$ belongs to $\mathfrak{C}^+(s)$ if and only if $l(sw) > l(w)$.

g) Let $A^+(t)$ (resp. $A^-(t)$) be the union of the chambers belonging to $\mathfrak{C}^+(t)$ (resp. $\mathfrak{C}^-(t)$) (for $t \in T$). Show that $A^+(t) \cap A^-(t) = L_t$. (To show that $A^+(t) \cap A^-(t) \subset L_t$, reduce to the case $t \in S$. If $a \in A^+(t) \cap A^-(t)$, put $a = wW^{(s)}$ with $s \in S$ and w being $(\varnothing, S - \{s\})$-reduced (Exerc. 3). If $w(C) \in \mathfrak{T}^-(t)$, then $l(tw) < l(w)$ and $w = ts_1 \ldots, s_q$ with $s_j \in S$ and $l(w) = q + 1$. Since $a \in A^-(t)$, there exists $x \in W^{(s)}$ such that $wx(C) \in \mathfrak{C}^+(t)$. Then

$$l(twx) = 1 + l(wx) = 1 + l(w) + l(x),$$

but since $twx = s_1 \ldots s_q x$ this is a contradiction. Thus, $w(C) \in \mathfrak{C}^+(t)$ and $l(tw) = 1 + l(w)$. If $x \in W^{(s)}$ is such that $l(twx) < l(wx)$, deduce from Exerc. 1 that $twx = wx'$ with $x' \in W^{(s)}$, and hence that $ta = a$ and $a \in L_t$.)

---

[8] Let H be a group and E a non-empty set on which H acts. H is said to act *simply-transitively* on E if the map $h \mapsto h.x$ is a bijection from H onto E for all $x \in E$; then E is said to be a *principal homogeneous set* for H.

The subsets $A^+(t)$ and $A^-(t)$ are called the *halves* of A determined by the wall L_t. Two points of A are said to be on the same side (resp. strictly on opposite sides) of L_t if they belong (resp. do not both belong) to one of the two halves. Any facet is contained in one of the halves determined by L_t. If two facets are contained in different halves, they are said to be on opposite sides of L_t, or to be separated by L_t.

h) Let $w \in W$. Show that $l(w)$ is equal to the number of walls separating C and $w(C)$.

i) Show that the map φ that takes the half $A^+(t)$ (resp. $A^-(t)$) to $(1, t)$ (resp. $(-1, t)$) is a bijection from the set $\mathfrak{M}$ of halves of A onto the set $R = \{1, -1\} \times T$ (cf. no. 4). With the notation of Lemma 1 of no. 4, show that $\varphi(w(M)) = U_w(\varphi(M))$ for all $w \in W$ and $M \in \mathfrak{M}$.

17) We retain the notation of Exerc. 16 and assume that W is *finite*. Let $\mathfrak{H}$ be the set of walls of A. To any $H \in \mathfrak{H}$, we associate the half H^+ of A determined by H containing C. Show that the elements of $\mathfrak{H}$ can be numbered in such a way that the map $j \mapsto \bigcap_{i \leqslant j} H_i^+$ is strictly decreasing on the interval $[1, \mathrm{Card}(\mathfrak{H})]$. (Consider the family $\mathfrak{F}$ of intersections of the sets H^+ ordered by inclusion and consider a strictly decreasing sequence $(F_0, \dots, F_q)$ of elements of $\mathfrak{F}$ of maximal length. For any $H \in \mathfrak{H}$, there exists an i such that $H^+ \supset F_j$ for $j \geqslant i$ and $H^+ \not\supset F_{i-1}$: show that $F_i = H^+ \cap F_{i-1}$.)

18) Let A be an apartment (Exerc. 15). A *folding* of A is an endomorphism π of A such that $\pi^2 = \pi$ and such that every chamber of A is the image under π of 0 or 2 chambers.

a) Let π be a folding of A and C a chamber of A such that $\pi(C) = C$. For any neighbouring chamber C′ of C, either $\pi(C') = C'$ or $\pi(C') = C$; if $a \in C$ we have $\pi(a) = a$. Show that, if $(C_0 = C, C_1, \dots, C_n)$ is a gallery, either $\pi(C_i) = C_i$ for all i or $(C_0, \pi(C_1), \dots, \pi(C_n))$ is not minimal (and in fact has two consecutive equal chambers). Deduce that any minimal gallery whose extremities are invariant under π is invariant under π. If $(C = C_0, C_1, \dots, C_n)$ is a minimal gallery and if $\pi(C_n) \neq C_n$, there exists an index i with $0 \leqslant i < n$ such that $\pi(C_j) = C_j$ for $0 \leqslant j \leqslant i$ and $\pi(C_j) \neq C_j$ for $i < j \leqslant n$.

b) Let C_1 and C_2 be two distinct neighbouring chambers and π, π' two foldings of A. Assume that $\pi(C_0) = C_1$ and $\pi'(C_1) = C_0$. Let C be a chamber, and consider the following three conditions:

$$\pi(C) = C; \qquad (1)$$

$$d(C, C_1) < d(C, C_2); \qquad (2)$$

$$\pi'(C) \neq C. \qquad (3)$$

Show that (1) $\Longrightarrow$ (2) $\Longrightarrow$ (3) and deduce that the three conditions are equivalent. Show that π (resp. π') is the unique folding of A taking C_2 (resp.

C_1) to C_1 (resp. C_2) (assume that (2) is satisfied and let $(C_1, C'_2, \dots, C'_n = C)$ be a minimal gallery: show that $\pi'(C'_{j+1})$ is the unique chamber distinct from $\pi'(C'_j)$ and containing the panel $\pi'(C'_j \cap C'_{j+1})$). Show that $\pi(\mathfrak{C})$ and $\pi'(\mathfrak{T})$ form a partition of the set $\mathfrak{T}$ of chambers of A and that $\pi(a) = \pi'(a) = a$ for all $a \in \pi(A) \cap \pi'(A)$. Show that the map from A to itself that coincides with π' on $\pi(A)$ and with π on $\pi'(A)$ is an involutive automorphism of A. It is called the *reflection* with respect to the panel $C_1 \cap C_2$. Show that it is the only non-trivial automorphism of A leaving fixed all the points of $C_1 \cap C_2$ (use Exerc. 15 *b*)).

c) Suppose that A is the apartment associated to a Coxeter system (W, S) and retain the notation of Exerc. 16. Let C_1 and C_2 be two neighbouring chambers and let t be the element of T such that the wall L_t is the support of $C_1 \cap C_2$. Let M_j be the half of A determined by L_t and containing C_j (for $j = 1, 2$). Show that the map π defined by $\pi(a) = a$ if $a \in M_1$ and $\pi(a) = t(a)$ if $a \in M_2$ is a folding of A such that $\pi(C_2) = C_1$ and that the reflection with respect to the panel $C_1 \cap C_2$ is the map $a \mapsto t(a)$.

19) Let A be an apartment. Assume that, for any two distinct neighbouring chambers C_1 and C_2, there is a folding (Exerc. 18) of A taking C_1 to C_2. Let C be a chamber of A and $(C_i)_{i \in I}$ the family of chambers neighbouring C and distinct from C. Denote by s_i the reflection with respect to the panel $C \cap C_i$ (Exerc. 18 *b*)). Put $S = \{s_i \mid i \in I\}$ and denote by W the group of automorphisms of A generated by the s_i.

a) Show that, for any chamber C′, there exists $w \in W$ such that $C' = w(C)$ (argue by induction on $d(C, C')$).

b) Show that (W, S) is a Coxeter system (for $i \in I$, put

$$P_{s_i} = \{w \in W \mid w(C) \subset \pi_i(A)\},$$

where π_i is the folding taking C_i to C, and show that the assumptions of Prop. 6 are satisfied: to prove condition (C′), remark that if $w \in P_{s_i}$ and $ws_j \notin P_{s_i}$, then

$$w(C) \cap ws_j(C) \subset \pi_i(A) \cap s_i\pi_i(A).$$

Since $w(C)$ and $ws_j(C)$ are neighbouring, it follows that $s_i = ws_jw^{-1}$ (Exerc. 18 *b*)).)

c) Let F be a facet of the chamber C. Show that the stabilizer W_F of F in W is generated by the $s_i \in S$ such that $F \subset C \cap C_i$ (let $w \in W_F$ with $l_S(w) > 1$ and let $i \in I$ be such that $w = s_iw'$ with $l(w') = l(w) - 1$; by Prop. 6, $w' \in P_{s_i}$, hence $w(C) \subset s_i\pi_i(A)$, $F \subset \pi_i(A) \cap s_i\pi_i(A)$ and $s_i \in W_F$). In particular, $w(C) = C$ if and only if $w = 1$.

d) Show that the map $a \mapsto W_{\{a\}}$ is an isomorphism from the apartment A to the apartment associated to (W, S) (Exerc. 16), compatible with the action of W.

20) Let A be a building and S a set. Then A is said to be *numbered* by S if one is given a map f from A to S such that, for any chamber C of A, the restriction of f to C is a *bijection* from C to S. If F is a facet of A, $f(\mathrm{F})$ is called the *type* of F. Let A be a numbered building. An endomorphism φ of A is called *allowed* if a and $\varphi(a)$ are of the same type for all $a \in \mathrm{A}$.

a) Let φ be an endomorphism of A. Show that, if there exists a chamber C of A such that a and $\varphi(a)$ are of the same type for all $a \in \mathrm{C}$, then φ is allowed. Show that if A is an apartment and π is a folding of A (Exerc. 18), then π is an allowed endomorphism.

b) A subset D of A is called *convex* if, for all $a \in \mathrm{A} - \mathrm{D}$, there exists an allowed endomorphism φ of A such that $\varphi(x) = x$ for all $x \in \mathrm{D}$ and $\varphi(a) \neq a$. Show that any intersection of convex sets is convex and that, for any subset D of A, there exists a smallest convex subset containing D: this is called the *convex hull* of D and denoted by $\Gamma(\mathrm{D})$.

21) Let (W, S) be a Coxeter system and A the associated apartment (cf. Exerc. 16, of which we retain the notation).

a) Show that there exists a unique numbering of A (called the canonical numbering) for which the type of a facet F is that defined in Exerc. 16 *c*). We shall always consider A to be equipped with this numbering.

b) Show that the allowed automorphisms of A are the operations of W.

c) Let D be a subset of A containing at least one chamber. Show that the following conditions are equivalent:
(i) D is the intersection of the halves of A (Exerc. 16 *g*)) that contain D;
(ii) D is convex;
(iii) whenever two facets F_1 and F_2 are contained in D, the convex hull of $\mathrm{F}_1 \cup \mathrm{F}_2$ is contained in D;
(iv) whenever a chamber C_1 and a facet F are contained in D and $(\mathrm{C}_1, \ldots, \mathrm{C}_n)$ is a gallery of minimal length such that $\mathrm{F} \subset \mathrm{C}_n$, we have $\mathrm{C}_i \subset \mathrm{D}$ for $1 \leqslant i \leqslant n$.

(To show that (iii) $\Longrightarrow$ (iv), use Exerc. 15 *b*). To show that (iv) $\Longrightarrow$ (i), argue by contradiction. Let D′ be the intersection of the halves of A containing D; let $a \in \mathrm{D}' - \mathrm{D}$, let C_0 be a chamber contained in D and let $(\mathrm{C}_0, \mathrm{C}_1, \ldots, \mathrm{C}_n)$ be a gallery of minimal length such that $a \in \mathrm{C}_n$. Then $\mathrm{C}_j \subset \mathrm{D}'$ for all j. Show that there exists an integer j with $0 \leqslant j < n$ such that $\mathrm{C}_j \subset \mathrm{D}$ and $\mathrm{C}_{j+1} \not\subset \mathrm{D}$. Let M (resp. M′) be the half of A determined by the support wall of the panel $\mathrm{C}_j \cap \mathrm{C}_{j+1}$ and containing C_j (resp. C_{j+1}). Show that $\mathrm{D} \not\subset \mathrm{M}$. Let $b \in \mathrm{D} \cap (\mathrm{A} - \mathrm{M})$ and let $\Gamma = (\mathrm{C}_j, \mathrm{C}'_1, \ldots, \mathrm{C}'_p)$ be a gallery of smallest possible length such that $b \in \mathrm{C}'_p$. Then $\mathrm{C}'_k \subset \mathrm{D}$ for $1 \leqslant k \leqslant p$ and $\mathrm{C}'_p \subset \mathrm{M}'$. Let π be the folding of A with image M′ (Exerc. 18 *c*)): then $\pi(\mathrm{C}_j) = \mathrm{C}_{j+1}$ and the gallery $\pi(\Gamma)$ is not injective (Exerc. 18 *a*)). If $\Gamma' = (\mathrm{C}_{j+1}, \mathrm{C}'_2, \ldots, \mathrm{C}'_{p-2}, \mathrm{C}'_p)$

is the gallery obtained from $\pi(\Gamma)$ by suppressing one of the two equal consecutive chambers, the gallery $(C_j, C_{j+1}, C'_2, \ldots, C'_{p-2}, C'_p)$ is minimal by the definition of Γ. Deduce from (iv) that $C_{j+1} \subset D$. Contradiction.)

22) We retain the notation of Exerc. 16 and 21.

a) Let $t \in T$ and $w \in W$. Show that the chambers C and $w(C)$ are separated by the wall L_t if and only if $l(tw) < l(w)$ (use the folding determined by the half $A^+(t)$).

b) Let $w_0 \in W$. Show that the following conditions are equivalent:

$$l(ww_0) = l(w_0) - l(w) \qquad \text{for all } w \in W; \tag{i}$$

$$l(tw_0) < l(w_0) \qquad \text{for all } t \in T; \tag{ii}$$

whenever $t \in T$, the chambers C and $w_0(C)$ are separated by the wall L_t (iii)

(Use Exerc. 16 *h*) to show that (iii) $\Longrightarrow$ (i).)

Show that such an element w_0 is unique and exists if and only if W is *finite.* It is then the element of greatest length of W and is characterized by

$$l(sw_0) < l(w_0) \qquad \text{for all } s \in S. \tag{iv}$$

Moreover, $w_0^2 = 1, w_0Sw_0 = S$ and $l(w_0) = \mathrm{Card}(T)$.

(*c*) Assume that W is finite. Show that, for any chamber C_0, there exists a unique chamber $-C_0$ such that $C_0 \cup (-C_0)$ is not contained in any half of A. Show that there exists a unique involutive automorphism φ of A (not necessarily allowed such that $\varphi(C_0) = -C_0$ for any chamber C_0 and that $\varphi(L) = L$ for any wall L of A. We put $\varphi(a) = -a$ for $a \in A$. If F is a facet, the facet $-F = \varphi(F)$ will be said to be *opposed* to F.

d) Let C_0 be a chamber of A and F a partition of C_0. Show that the convex hull of $C_0 \cup (-F)$ is the half of A determined by the wall L that is the support of F and that contains C_0.

23) We retain the notation of Exerc. 16. Let Aut(A) be the group of automorphisms of the apartment A. Show that if $\varphi \in \mathrm{Aut}(A)$, then φ permutes the walls of A, and $\varphi t \varphi^{-1} \in T$ for all $t \in T$ (use Exerc. 18). Deduce that W (identified with a subgroup of Aut(A)) is normal and that Aut(A) is the semidirect product of the subgroup E of automorphisms preserving the chamber C by W. Show that the action of Aut(A) on W defines an isomorphism from E to the group of automorphisms of the Coxeter system (W, S), or to that of the Coxeter graph of (W, S) (cf. also Exerc. 19).

24) A *structured building* is a building I equipped with a set $\mathfrak{U}$ of sub-buildings satisfying the following conditions:

(SB 1) The sub-buildings $A \in \mathfrak{U}$ are apartments.

(SB 2) Any two chambers of I are contained in at least one element of $\mathfrak{U}$.
(SB 3) Whenever $A_1, A_2 \in \mathfrak{U}$ are such that $A_1 \cap A_2$ contains a chamber, there exists an isomorphism from A_1 to A_2 leaving fixed the points of $A_1 \cap A_2$.

Let $(I, \mathfrak{U})$ be a structured building. The elements of $\mathfrak{U}$ are called the apartments of $(I, \mathfrak{U})$, or simply those of I.

a) Show that any two apartments of I are isomorphic. Let C be a chamber of I and A an apartment of I containing C. Show that there exists a unique endomorphism ρ of I (called the *retraction with centre* C *of* I *onto* A) such that $\rho(a) = a$ for all $a \in A$ and that, for any apartment A′ containing C, the restriction of ρ to A′ is an isomorphism from A′ to A (remark that, by (SB 2) and Exerc. 15 *b*), for any apartment A′ containing C, there exists a unique isomorphism $\rho_{A'}$ of A′ leaving all the points of C fixed). Show that $\rho^2 = \rho$ and that $\rho^{-1}(C) = C$.

b) Let A be an apartment of I, C_0 a chamber and F a facet contained in A. Let $(C_0, C_1, \ldots, C_n)$ be a gallery of smallest possible length such that $F \subset C_n$. Show that $C_i \subset A$ for $1 \leqslant i \leqslant n$ (argue by contradiction: if $C_i \subset A$ and $C_{i+1} \not\subset A$, consider the retraction of I onto A with centre the chamber of A distinct from C_i and containing $C_i \cap C_{i+1}$).

c) Let A be an apartment of I, C a chamber of A, F a panel of C, C′ a chamber of I and $\Gamma = (C_0, \ldots, C_n = C')$ a gallery of smallest possible length such that $F \subset C_0$. Show that the retraction ρ of I onto A with centre C transforms Γ into a gallery

$$(C'_0, \ldots, C'_n = \rho(C'))$$

of smallest possible length such that $F \subset C'_0$ (consider an apartment A′ containing C′ and F and apply *b*) and the fact that the restriction of ρ to A′ is an isomorphism).

d) Let A be an apartment, C_1 and C_2 two distinct neighbouring chambers contained in A, C′ a chamber containing $C_1 \cap C_2$ and distinct from C_1 and C_2, and A'_i an apartment containing C_i and C′ (for $i = 1, 2$). Let φ_i (resp. ψ_i) be the retraction of I onto A (resp. A'_i) with centre C_i (resp. C′) and let ρ_i be the restriction of $\varphi_i \circ \psi_i$ to A. Let C be a chamber of A; show that if

$$d(C, C_1) \leqslant d(C, C_2),$$

then $\rho_1(a) = a$ for all $a \in C$ and $d(C, C_1) < d(C, C_2)$ (consider a minimal gallery Γ with extremities C and C_1 and apply *c*) to show that $\rho_1(\Gamma)$ is minimal; then use Exerc. 15 *b*)). Show that, if $d(C, C_2) < d(C, C_1)$, then $\rho_1(C) \neq C$ and $\rho_1^2(C) = \rho_1(C)$ (take a minimal gallery Γ with extremities C and C_2 and use *c*) to show that $\rho_1(\Gamma)$ is a gallery of smallest possible length having one extremity equal to $\rho_1(C)$ and the other containing $C_1 \cap C_2$; deduce that $d(C_1, \rho_1(C_1)) \leqslant d(C_2, \rho_1(C_1))$).

Show that ρ_i is a *folding* (Exerc. 19) of A (show that $A = \rho_1(A) \cup \rho_2(A)$ and define an involutive automorphism σ of A by putting $\sigma(a) = \rho_2(a)$ if $a \in \rho_1(A)$ and $\sigma(a) = \rho_1(a)$ if $a \in \rho_2(A)$; show that if C is a chamber contained in $\rho_1(A)$, then $\rho_1^{-1}(C) = \{C, \rho_2(C)\}$).

e) Let I be a *spacious* structured building, that is to say that every panel is contained in at least three chambers. Show that there exists a Coxeter system (W, S), unique up to isomorphism, such that the apartments of I are isomorphic to the apartment A_0 associated to (W, S) (use *d*) and Exerc. 19)). Let A be an apartment of I and φ an isomorphism from A_0 to A. Show that there exists a unique numbering of I, with values in S, such that the types of a and $\varphi(a)$ are equal for all $a \in A_0$ (choose a chamber C of A and show, by using *b*), that, if A′ and A″ are two apartments of I containing C, the numberings of A′ and A″ extending that determined on C coincide on $A' \cap A''$).

We shall say that the Coxeter system (W, S) and the numbering thus obtained are *adapted* to I.

Show that the retractions introduced in *a*) are allowed endomorphisms. Show that a subset of I contained in an apartment A of I is convex in I if and only if it is convex in A (Exerc. 20).

f) We retain the notation of *e*) and let $\mathfrak{A}$ be the set of allowed isomorphisms from A_0 to the various apartments of I. Show that, if $\varphi, \psi \in \mathfrak{A}$ and if C is a chamber and F a facet of I contained in $\varphi(A_0) \cap \psi(A_0)$, there exists an element $w \in W$ such that $\psi^{-1}(C) = w\varphi^{-1}(C)$ and $\psi^{-1}(F) = w\varphi^{-1}(F)$ (consider an isomorphism λ from $\varphi(A_0)$ to $\psi(A_0)$ leaving fixed the points of $\varphi(A_0) \cap \psi(A_0)$ and apply Exerc. 21 *b*) to the automorphism $\psi^{-1} \circ \lambda \circ \varphi^{-1}$ of A_0).

25) Let I be a set and let $\mathfrak{F}$ be the set of finite subsets of I. For any $A \in \mathfrak{F}$, put $\varepsilon(A) = (-1)^{\mathrm{Card}(A)}$. Let G be an abelian group written additively, and let φ and ψ be two maps from $\mathfrak{F}$ to G. Show that the following properties are equivalent:

$$\varphi(A) = \sum_{B \subset A} \psi(B) \quad \text{for all } A \in \mathfrak{F}; \tag{i}$$

$$\psi(A) = \sum_{B \subset A} \varepsilon(A - B)\varphi(B) \quad \text{for all } A \in \mathfrak{F}. \tag{ii}$$

26) Let (W, S) be a Coxeter system, with S finite. For any subset H of W, denote by H(t) the formal power series with integer coefficients defined by

$$H(t) = \sum_{w \in H} t^{l(w)}.$$

a) Assume that Card(S) = 2. Show that

$$W(t) = (1 + t - t^m - t^{m+1})/(1 - t) \quad \text{if W is of finite order } 2m,$$
$$W(t) = (1 + t)/(1 - t) \quad \text{if W is infinite.}$$

b) Assume that W is *finite*. Let w_0 be the element of W of greatest length (Exerc. 22) and let $m = l(w_0)$. Show that

$$W(t) = t^m W(t^{-1})$$

(use Exerc. 22).

c) Let X be a subset of S. Denote by A_X the set of $(X, \varnothing)$-reduced elements of W (Exerc. 3) and W_X the subgroup of W generated by X. We know (Exerc. 3) that an element $w \in W$ belongs to A_X if and only if $l(xw) = l(w) + 1$ for all $x \in X$, that every element $w \in W$ can be written uniquely in the form $w = uv$ with $u \in W_X$ and $v \in A_X$, and that in that case $l(w) = l(u) + l(v)$. Deduce the formula

$$W(t) = W_X(t).A_X(t).$$

d) Retain the above notation and denote by B_X the set of $w \in A_X$ such that $l(sw) = l(w) - 1$ for all $s \in S - X$. Show that

$$A_X(t) = \sum_{X \subset Y \subset S} B_Y(t).$$

Deduce that

$$B_X(t) = \sum_{X \subset Y \subset S} \varepsilon(Y - X) A_Y(t) \quad \text{with} \quad \varepsilon(Z) = (-1)^{\mathrm{Card}(Z)}$$

(use Exerc. 25).

e) Assume that W is *finite* and define m and w_0 as in *b*). Show that $B_\varnothing = \{w_0\}$ and that

$$t^m = \sum_{Y \subset S} \varepsilon(Y) \frac{W(t)}{W_Y(t)}$$

(use *c*) and *d*)).

f) Assume that W is *infinite*. Show that $B_\varnothing = \varnothing$ and that

$$0 = \sum_{Y \subset S} \frac{\varepsilon(Y)}{W_Y(t)}.$$

g) Show that the formal power series $W(t)$ is a rational function of t (use *f*) and argue by induction on Card(S)). Show that this rational function vanishes whenever t is a root of unity, and that $1/W(\infty)$ is an integer. Show that $\frac{1}{W(t^{-1})} \in \mathbf{Z}[[t]]$.

§ **2**

1) Let G be a group, B and N two subgroups of G and S a subset of $W = N/(B \cap N)$. For all $w \in W$, put $C(w) = BwB$. Assume that conditions (T1) and (T2) of Def. 1 of no. 1 are satisfied, that whenever $s \in S$ and $w \in W$ at least one of the two relations $C(s).C(w) = C(sw)$ and $C(s).C(sw) = C(w)$ is satisfied, and that $B \cup C(s)$ is a subgroup of G for all $s \in S$. Show that condition (T3) is satisfied. Moreover, if the index of B in $B \cup C(s)$ is $\geqslant 3$, then (G, B, N, S) is a Tits system.

2) Let G be a group, B and N two subgroups of G and S a subset of $W = N/(B \cap N)$. Let Z be a normal subgroup of G contained in B. Let B′ and N′ be the canonical images of B and N in $G' = G/Z$. Show that the canonical map from N to N′ defines an isomorphism from W to $W' = N'/(B' \cap N')$. Let S′ be the image of S under this isomorphism. Show that (G', B', N', S') is a Tits system if and only if (G, B, N, S) is one.

3) Let G be a group, B a subgroup of G and $(C(w))_{w \in W}$ the family of double cosets of G with respect to B. Then B is called a *Tits subgroup* of G if there exists a subset S of W such that the following conditions are satisfied:

(1) the union of the $C(s)$ for $s \in S$ generates G;
(2) for all $s \in S$, the set $B \cup C(s)$ is a subgroup of G and the index of B in $B \cup C(s)$ is $\geqslant 3$;
(3) for all $s \in S$ and all $w \in W$, there exists an element $w' \in W$ such that $C(s).C(w) \subset C(w) \cup C(w')$.

From now on we assume that B is a Tits subgroup of G and that we are given a subset S of W satisfying conditions (1), (2) and (3).

a) Show that $C(s)^{-1} = C(s)$ and that $C(s).C(s) = B \cup C(s)$ for all $s \in S$. Show that, for all $s \in S$ and all $w \in W$, there exists an element $w'' \in W$ such that $C(w).C(s) \subset C(w) \cup C(w'')$.

b) If $w \in W$, the *length* of w, denoted by $l(w)$, is the smallest integer $n \geqslant 0$ for which there exist $s_1, \ldots, s_n \in S$ with $C(w) \subset C(s_1) \ldots C(s_n)$. Show that $l(w)$ is finite for all $w \in W$.

Let $u, v \in W$ with $l(u) < l(v)$ and let $s \in S$. Show that, if $C(v) \subset C(u).C(s)$ (resp. $C(v) \subset C(s).C(u)$), then $C(v) = C(u).C(s)$ (resp, $C(v) = C(s).C(u)$) (argue by induction on the length of u. If $C(v) \neq C(u).C(s)$, then $C(u).C(s) = C(u) \cup C(v)$. By using the induction hypothesis, show that there exist $t \in S$ and $w \in W$ such that

$$C(u) = C(t).C(w) \quad \text{with} \quad l(w) = l(u) - 1.$$

From the relations $C(v) \subset C(u).C(s) = C(t).C(w).C(s)$ and $C(t).C(w) = C(u) \neq C(v)$, deduce the existence of an element $w' \neq w$ such that

$C(w') \subset C(w).C(s)$ and $C(v) \subset C(t).C(w')$, so $l(w') \geqslant l(v) - 1 > l(u) - 1 = l(w)$. The induction hypothesis now implies that

$$C(w') = C(w).C(s).$$

Moreover,

$$\begin{aligned} C(t).C(u).C(s) &= C(t).C(t).C(w).C(s) = C(t).C(w).C(s) \cup C(w).C(s) \\ &= C(u).C(s) \cup C(w') = C(u) \cup C(v) \cup C(w') \end{aligned}$$

and also

$$C(t).C(u).C(s) = C(t).(C(u) \cup C(v)) \supset C(t).C(t).C(w) \supset C(w),$$

which is a contradiction since $w \neq u, v, w'$.)

c) Show that, for all $w \in W$ and all $s \in S$, there exists a unique element, denoted by $s.w$ (resp, $w * s$), distinct from w and such that

$$C(s.w) \subset C(s).C(w) \subset C(w) \cup C(s.w)$$
$$(\text{resp. } C(w * s) \subset C(w).C(s) \subset C(w) \cup C(w * s)).$$

(Show by induction on $l(w)$ that $C(s).C(w) \neq C(w)$. For this, write

$$C(w) = C(u).C(t)$$

with $t \in S$, $u \in W$ and $l(w) = l(u) + 1$. If $C(s).C(w) = C(w)$, then

$$C(s).C(u).C(t) = C(u).C(t)$$

and multiplying on the right by $C(t)$, we obtain that $C(u) \cup C(w) = C(s).C(u) \cup C(w)$. Since $C(u) \neq C(s).C(u)$ by the induction hypothesis, we have, by *b*),

$$C(s).C(u) = C(w),$$

and hence

$$C(u) \subset C(s).C(s).C(u) = C(s).C(w) = C(w),$$

which is absurd).

d) Let $s \in S$. Show that the map $p_s : w \mapsto s.w$ (resp. $q_s : w \mapsto w * s$) is a permutation of W and that $p_s^2 = \mathrm{Id}$ (resp. $q_s^2 = \mathrm{Id}$). Show that $p_s \circ q_t = q_t \circ p_s$ for all $s, t \in S$ (study the product $C(s).C(w).C(t)$ for $w \in W$ and show that $(s.w) * t \in \{w, s.w, w * t, s.(w * t)\}$; show that $(s.w) * t \notin \{s.w, w * t\}$ and that if $(s.w) * t = w$ then $s.w = w * t$ and $w = s.(w * t)$).

e) Show that the group of permutations P (resp. Q) generated by the p_s (resp. q_s) for $s \in S$ acts simply-transitively on W (to show that P is transitive, use (2) and argue as in Lemma 1 of no. 1; to show that P is simply transitive, use *d*)). Deduce that W has a unique group structure such that the map $p \mapsto p(e)$

(where e denotes the element of W such that $\mathrm{B} = \mathrm{C}(e)$) is an isomorphism from P to W. The map $q \mapsto q(e)$ is then also an isomorphism; moreover, $s.w = w * s = sw$ for all $s \in \mathrm{S}$ and all $w \in \mathrm{W}$ and $\mathrm{C}(w)^{-1} = \mathrm{C}(w^{-1})$.

f) Show that the pair (W, S) is a Coxeter system and generalize the results of no. 4.

g) Let X be a subset of S and $\mathrm{W_X}$ the subgroup of W generated by X. Show that the union $\mathrm{G_X}$ of the $\mathrm{C}(w)$ for $w \in \mathrm{W_X}$ is a subgroup of G and that Th. 3 of no. 5 is still true. Show that B is a Tits subgroup of $\mathrm{G_X}$. Generalize Props. 2 and 3 of no. 5, and Def. 2, Prop. 4 and Th. 4 of no. 6. Show that S is the set of $w \in \mathrm{W}$ such that $\mathrm{B} \cup \mathrm{C}(w)$ is a subgroup of G distinct from B. The Coxeter system (W, S) and the group W (called the *Weyl group* of (G, B)) thus depend only on (G, B).

h) Let N be a subgroup of G such that $\mathrm{B} \cap \mathrm{N}$ is normal in N and such that the intersection with N of every double coset $\mathrm{C}(w)$ with respect to B is a double coset with respect to $\mathrm{B} \cap \mathrm{N}$. Show that the group $\mathrm{N}/(\mathrm{B} \cap \mathrm{N})$ can be identified with W and that (G, B, N, S) is a Tits system.

4) Let (G, B, N, S) and (G′, B′, N′, S′) be two Tits systems with $\mathrm{G} = \mathrm{G}'$ and $\mathrm{B} = \mathrm{B}'$, and with Weyl groups W and W′. Let j be the bijection from W to W′ defined by the relation

$$\mathrm{B}w\mathrm{B} = \mathrm{B}'j(w)\mathrm{B}'.$$

Show that j is a group isomorphism between W and W′ and that $j(\mathrm{S}) = \mathrm{S}'$.

5) Let $\Sigma = (\mathrm{G}, \mathrm{B}, \mathrm{N}, \mathrm{S})$ be a Tits system. Put $\mathrm{T} = \mathrm{B} \cap \mathrm{N}$ and let $\hat{\mathrm{N}}$ be the normaliser of N.

a) Let $b \in \mathrm{B} \cap \hat{\mathrm{N}}$. Show that $bnb^{-1}n^{-1} \in \mathrm{B} \cap \mathrm{N}$ for all $n \in \mathrm{N}$ (put $bn = n'b$ and use Th. 1) and that b belongs to the intersection $\tilde{\mathrm{T}}$ of the conjugates $n\mathrm{B}n^{-1}$ for $n \in \mathrm{N}$. Show that $\tilde{\mathrm{T}} \cap \mathrm{N} = \mathrm{T}$.

If $\tilde{\mathrm{T}} = \mathrm{T}$, Σ is said to be *saturated.*

b) Put $\tilde{\mathrm{N}} = \mathrm{N}.\tilde{\mathrm{T}}$. Show that $\tilde{\mathrm{N}}$ is a subgroup of G containing $\tilde{\mathrm{T}}$ as a normal subgroup and that $\tilde{\mathrm{N}} \cap \mathrm{B} = \tilde{\mathrm{T}}$. Show that the injection of N into $\tilde{\mathrm{N}}$ defines an isomorphism from the Weyl group W of Σ to $\tilde{\mathrm{N}}/\tilde{\mathrm{T}}$.

c) Show that $(\mathrm{G}, \mathrm{B}, \tilde{\mathrm{N}}, j(\mathrm{S}))$ is a saturated Tits system, which is said to be *associated* to Σ.

6) We use the notation of no. 2 and let $\mathrm{N_0}$ be the subgroup of N consisting of the matrices all of whose entries are equal to 0 or 1. Show that $\mathrm{B} \cap \mathrm{N_0} = \mathrm{T} \cap \mathrm{N_0} = \{1\}$ and that the canonical map j from $\mathrm{N_0}$ to $\mathrm{W} = \mathrm{N}/\mathrm{T}$ is an isomorphism. Put $\mathrm{S_0} = j^{-1}(\mathrm{S})$. Show that $(\mathrm{G}, \mathrm{B}, \mathrm{N_0}, \mathrm{S_0})$ is a Tits system and that (G, B, N, S) is the associated saturated Tits system.

7) Let G be a group acting on a set E. Then G is said to act *doubly-transitively* on E if, whenever $x, y, x', y' \in \mathrm{E}$ are such that $x \neq y$ and $x' \neq y'$, there exists an element $g \in \mathrm{G}$ such that $g.x = x'$ and $g.y = y'$.

a) Let (G, B, N, S) be a Tits system whose Weyl group W is of order 2. Show that G acts doubly-transitively on G/B.

b) Let G be a group acting doubly transitively on a set E. Assume that $\mathrm{Card(E)} \geqslant 3$. Let $e \in \mathrm{E}$ and let B be the stabilizer of e. Let $x \in \mathrm{E}$, with $x \neq e$, and let $n \in \mathrm{G}$ be such that $n(e) = x$ and $n(x) = e$. Let N be the subgroup of G generated by n. Let s be the canonical image of n in N/T. Show that $(\mathrm{G}, \mathrm{B}, \mathrm{N}, \{s\})$ is a Tits system whose Weyl group is of order 2.

8) Let (G, B, N, S) be a Tits system; put $\mathrm{T} = \mathrm{B} \cap \mathrm{N}$ and $\mathrm{W} = \mathrm{N}/\mathrm{T}$. Let $\tilde{\mathrm{G}}$ be a group containing G as a normal subgroup. Assume that for all $h \in \tilde{\mathrm{G}}$, there exists $g \in \mathrm{G}$ such that $h\mathrm{B}h^{-1} = g\mathrm{B}g^{-1}$ and $h\mathrm{N}h^{-1} = g\mathrm{N}g^{-1}$. Let $\hat{\mathrm{B}}$ (resp. $\hat{\mathrm{N}}$) be the normaliser of B (resp. N) in $\tilde{\mathrm{G}}$; put $\Gamma = \hat{\mathrm{B}} \cap \hat{\mathrm{N}}$, $\tilde{\mathrm{N}} = \Gamma.\mathrm{N}$ and $\tilde{\mathrm{T}} = \tilde{\mathrm{N}} \cap \mathrm{B}$.

a) Show that $\tilde{\mathrm{G}} = \Gamma.\mathrm{G}$, $\hat{\mathrm{B}} = \Gamma.\mathrm{B}$, $\Gamma \cap \mathrm{B} = \Gamma \cap \mathrm{G}$ and $\tilde{\mathrm{T}} = (\Gamma \cap \mathrm{B}).\mathrm{T}$. The groups $\Omega = \Gamma/(\Gamma \cap \mathrm{B})$, $\tilde{\mathrm{G}}/\mathrm{G}$ and $\hat{\mathrm{B}}/\mathrm{B}$ are thus canonically isomorphic. If $\Phi \subset \Omega$ and if H is a subgroup of G containing $\Gamma \cap \mathrm{B}$, we denote by $\Phi\mathrm{H}$ the union of the subsets $\varphi\mathrm{H}$ for $\varphi \in \Phi$.

b) Show that $\tilde{\mathrm{T}}$ is normal in $\tilde{\mathrm{N}}$ (to show that $n\gamma n^{-1} \in \tilde{\mathrm{N}}$ for $n \in \tilde{\mathrm{N}}$ and $\gamma \in \Gamma \cap \mathrm{B}$, use Exerc. 5 *a*)), that $\mathrm{N} \cap \tilde{\mathrm{T}} = \mathrm{T}$ and that $\Gamma \cap \tilde{\mathrm{T}} = \Gamma \cap \mathrm{B}$. The injection of N (resp. Γ) into $\tilde{\mathrm{N}}$ thus allows W (resp. Ω) to be identified with a subgroup of $\tilde{\mathrm{W}} = \tilde{\mathrm{N}}/\tilde{\mathrm{T}}$. Show that Ω normalises S and that $\tilde{\mathrm{W}}$ is the semi-direct product of Ω and W.

c) Show that, for all $s \in \mathrm{S}$ and all $u \in \tilde{\mathrm{W}}$,

$$\mathrm{B}s\mathrm{B}u\mathrm{B} \subset (\mathrm{B}u\mathrm{B}) \cup (\mathrm{B}su\mathrm{B}).$$

d) Show that the map $u \mapsto \mathrm{B}u\mathrm{B}$ is a bijection from $\tilde{\mathrm{W}}$ to $\mathrm{B}\backslash\tilde{\mathrm{G}}/\mathrm{B}$ (use Th. 1 and the fact that Γ normalises B).

e) Let $\mathfrak{B}$ be the set of pairs (Φ, X), where Φ is a subgroup of Ω and X is a subset of X normalised by Φ. Put $\mathrm{G}_{(\Phi,\mathrm{X})} = \Phi\mathrm{G}_\mathrm{X} = \mathrm{B}\Phi\mathrm{W}_\mathrm{X}\mathrm{B}$ (with the notation of no. 5). Show that the map $(\Phi, \mathrm{X}) \mapsto \mathrm{G}_{(\Phi,\mathrm{X})}$ is a bijection from $\mathfrak{B}$ to the set of subgroups of $\tilde{\mathrm{G}}$ containing B. Generalize assertions *b*) and *c*) of Th. 3 and Prop. 2 of no. 5.

Show that the normaliser of $\mathrm{G}_{(\Phi,\mathrm{X})}$ in $\tilde{\mathrm{G}}$ is the subgroup $\mathrm{G}_{(\Phi',\mathrm{X})}$, where Φ' is the set of elements of Ω normalizing both Φ and X.

f) Show that $\mathrm{G}_{(\Phi,\mathrm{X})}$ is a maximal subgroup of $\tilde{\mathrm{G}}$ if and only if one of the following two conditions is satisfied:

(i) $\mathrm{X} = \mathrm{S}$ and Φ is a maximal subgroup of Ω;

(ii) $\Phi = \Omega$ and Φ acts transitively on $S - X$ (which is non-empty).

Show that $G_{(\Phi,X)}$ is a maximal subgroup in the set of subgroups of $\tilde{G}$ not containing G if and only if

(iii) $X \neq S$, Φ is the normaliser of X in Ω and acts transitvely on $S - X$.

g) Let Φ be a normal subgroup of Ω and put $G' = \Phi G$, $B' = \Phi B$, $N' = \Phi N$ and $T' = B' \cap N'$. Show that $T' = \Phi\tilde{T}$ and that T' is normal in N' if and only if every element of Φ commutes with every element of W. Show that G' is then normal in $\tilde{G}$, that the injection of N into N' defines an isomorphism j from W to $W' = N'/T'$ and that (G', B', N', S') (with $S' = j(S)$) is a Tits system.

9) Let (G, B, N, S) be a Tits system and X, Y, Z three subsets of S. Show that

$$G_X \cap (G_Y.G_Z) = (G_X \cap G_Y).(G_X \cap G_Z)$$

(use Exerc. 1 of § 1 and Prop. 2 of no. 3).

10) Let G be a group and B a Tits subgroup of G. We use the notation of Exerc. 3. For $s \in S$, denote by $G^{(s)}$ the subgroup $G_{S-\{s\}}$ (Exerc. 3 *g*)). Let I be the set of subsets of G of the form $gG^{(s)}$ (for $g \in G$ and $s \in S$), and $\mathfrak{C}$ the set of subsets of I of the form $C_g = \{gG^{(s)} \mid s \in S\}$ for $g \in G$. The C_g are called the *chambers* of I (§ 1, Exerc. 15). Let G act on I by left translations.

a) Let $\mathfrak{F}$ be the set of facets of I (that is, the subsets of the chambers, cf. § 1, Exerc. 15). Let $F \in \mathfrak{F}$. Show that there exist a unique subset X of S and an element $g \in G$ such that $gG_X = \bigcap_{a \in F} a$; F is said to be *of type* X. Show that F is then the set of $gG^{(s)}$ for $s \in S - X$ and is of codimension Card(X) in any chamber containing it. Show that the map $j : F \mapsto \bigcap_{a \in F} a$ is a strictly decreasing bijection, compatible with left translations, from $\mathfrak{F}$ to the set of subsets of G of the form gG_X for $g \in G$ and $X \subset S$. Show that, if $X \subset Y \subset S$, every facet of type X contains a unique facet of type Y.

b) Show that G acts transitively on the set $\mathfrak{C}$ of chambers and that the stabilizer of the chamber C_g ($g \in G$) is equal to gBg^{-1}; the map $g \mapsto C_g$ thus defines a bijection from G/B to $\mathfrak{C}$.

c) Show that two chambers C_g and $C_{g'}$ ($g, g' \in G$) are *neighbouring* (§ 1, Exerc. 15) if and only if there exists $s \in S$ such that $g' \in g(B \cup BsB)$.

d) Let $C_1, \ldots, C_n$ be chambers of I and put $C_0 = C_e$. Show that the following conditions are equivalent:

(i) the sequence $\Gamma = (C_0, C_1, \ldots, C_n)$ is an injective gallery;
(ii) there exist a sequence $\mathbf{s} = (s_1, \ldots, s_n)$ of elements of S and a sequence $(b_1, \ldots, b_n)$ of elements of B such that $C_j = b_1\bar{s}_1b_2\bar{s}_2 \ldots b_j\bar{s}_j(C_0)$ (where $\bar{s}_j$ denotes a given element of the double coset Bs_jB) for $1 \leqslant j \leqslant n$.

Show that, if these conditions are satisfied, the sequence $\mathbf{s}$ is unique: it is then called the *type* of Γ and denoted by $\mathbf{s}(\Gamma)$. Show that an injective gallery is minimal if and only if its type is a reduced decomposition. Show that the following conditions are satisfied:

(WI 1) *For any two chambers* C *and* C′ *of* I, *there exists a unique element* $t(\mathrm{C}, \mathrm{C}')$ *of* W *such that the set of types of minimal galleries with extremities* C *and* C′ *is the set of reduced decompositions of* $t(\mathrm{C}, \mathrm{C}')$.

(WI 2) *For any chamber* C, *the map* $\mathrm{C}' \mapsto t(\mathrm{C}, \mathrm{C}')$ *from the set of chambers of* I *to* W *is surjective.*

e) Show that two minimal galleries of the same type and with the same extremities are identical. (Reduce to proving that, if $(s_1, \ldots, s_n)$ is a reduced decomposition and if $b_1, \ldots, b_n, b'_1, \ldots, b'_n$ are elements of B such that $b_1\bar{s}_1 \ldots b_n\bar{s}_n \in b'_1\bar{s}_1 \ldots b'_n\bar{s}_n\mathrm{B}$, then $b_1\bar{s}_1 \in b'_1\bar{s}_1\mathrm{B}$. For this, remark that if $\bar{s}_1^{-1}b_1^{-1}b'_1\bar{s}_1 \notin \mathrm{B}$, then this element would belong to $\mathrm{B}s_1\mathrm{B}$ and we would have $b_2\bar{s}_2 \ldots b_n\bar{s}_n \in b\bar{s}_1b'b'_2\bar{s}_2 \ldots b'_n\bar{s}_n\mathrm{B}$ with $b, b' \in \mathrm{B}$, contradicting Cor. 1 of Th. 2 of no. 4.)

f) Show that I equipped with $\mathfrak{C}$ is a *building*, said to be *associated* to the pair (G, B). Show that there exists a unique *numbering* (§ 1, Exerc. 20) of I for which the type of a facet is that defined in *a*).

g) Show that I is *spacious*, namely that every panel of I is contained in at least three chambers (cf. § 1, Exerc. 24). Show that the following condition is satisfied:

(G) G*iven a panel* F, *a chamber* C, *a gallery* $\Gamma = (\mathrm{C}_0, \ldots, \mathrm{C}_n)$ *such that* $\mathrm{F} \subset \mathrm{C}_n$ *and of smallest possible length, and chambers* C′ *and* C″ *containing* F *and distinct from* C_n, *there exists an element* $g \in \mathrm{G}$ *such that* $g(\mathrm{C}_i) = \mathrm{C}_i$ *for* $0 \leqslant i \leqslant n$ *and* $g(\mathrm{C}') = \mathrm{C}''$.

(Reduce to the case $\mathrm{C}_0 = \mathrm{C}$; let $u \in \mathrm{S}$ be such that F is of type $\mathrm{S} - \{u\}$ and let $\mathbf{s}$ be the type of Γ. Show that $(\mathbf{s}, u)$ is a reduced decomposition. Take $h \in \mathrm{G}$ such that $\mathrm{C}_n = h(\mathrm{C})$; there exist b' and $b'' \in \mathrm{B}$ such that $\mathrm{C}' = hb'u(\mathrm{C})$ and $\mathrm{C}'' = hb''u(\mathrm{C})$. Then use Cor. 1 of Th. 2 of no. 4 generalized to the case of a Tits subgroup (cf. Exerc. 3 *f*)) to show that there exists $b \in \mathrm{B}$ such that $bhb'u\mathrm{B} = hb''u\mathrm{B}$; then $b \in h\mathrm{B}u\mathrm{B}u^{-1}\mathrm{B}h^{-1} \subset (h\mathrm{B}h^{-1}) \cup (h\mathrm{B}u\mathrm{B}h^{-1})$. If $b \in h\mathrm{B}u\mathrm{B}h^{-1}$, we would have $\mathrm{B}h\mathrm{B} \subset \mathrm{B}h\mathrm{B}u\mathrm{B} = \mathrm{B}hu\mathrm{B}$ (*loc. cit.*), which is impossible. Hence $b(\mathrm{C}_n) = \mathrm{C}_n$ and *e*) implies that $b(\mathrm{C}_i) = \mathrm{C}_i$ for all *i*.)

11) Let (W, S) be a Coxeter system and I a building numbered by S (§ 1, Exerc. 20). If $\Gamma = (\mathrm{C}_0, \ldots, \mathrm{C}_n)$ is an injective gallery, the *type* of Γ, denoted by $\mathbf{s}(\Gamma)$, is the sequence $(s_1, \ldots, s_n)$ of elements of S such that the panel $\mathrm{C}_{i-1} \cap \mathrm{C}_i$ is of type $\mathrm{S} - \{s_i\}$ (for $1 \leqslant i \leqslant n$). If conditions (WI 1) and (WI 2) of Exerc. 10 are satisfied, I is called a (W, S)-*building.*

Let I be a spacious (W, S)-building (cf. Exerc. 10 *g*)) and let G be a group of allowed automorphisms of I satisfying the following condition:

(G_0) *Given three distinct chambers* C, C' *and* C'' *containing the same panel, there exists an element* $g \in G$ *such that* $g(C) = C$ *and* $g(C') = C''$.

Choose a chamber C of I and denote by B the stabilizer of C in G.

a) Show that G acts transitively on the set of chambers of I.

b) Let C' and C'' be two chambers. Show that $t(C, C') = t(C, C'')$ if and only if there exists $b \in B$ such that $C'' = b(C')$ (if $t(C, C') = t(C, C'') = w$, consider a reduced decomposition $\mathbf{s}$ of w and a minimal gallery Γ' (resp. Γ'') with extremities C and C' (resp. C'') and of type $\mathbf{s}$. Argue by induction on $l(w)$ using (G_0) and *a*)). Deduce that there exists a bijection $w \mapsto B(w)$ from W to $B\backslash G/B$.

c) Let F be the facet of C of type $S - \{s\}$. Show that the stabilizer of F in G is equal to $B \cup B(s)$ (if $g(F) = F$, then $t(C, g(C)) = 1$ or s). Show that $B \subset B(s)B(s)$ (use (G_0)).

d) Show that B is a Tits subgroup of G and that the Coxeter system of (G, B) is canonically isomorphic to (W, S). (Let $w \in W$ and $s \in S$ be such that $l_S(sw) = l_S(w) + 1$. Let $g \in B(w)$ and $u \in B(s)$; let $\mathbf{s} = (s_1, \dots, s_n)$ be a reduced decomposition of w, $(C = C_0, C_1, \dots, C_n = g(C))$ a minimal gallery of type $\mathbf{s}$ and choose an element $\bar{s}_i \in B(s_i)$; show, by using (G_0), that there exist elements $b_i \in B$ such that $C_i = b_1\bar{s}_1 \dots b_i\bar{s}_i(C)$. Put $C_i' = u(C_{i-1})$ and show that the gallery $(C, u(C), u(C_1), \dots, u(C_n))$ is of type $(s, \mathbf{s})$, and is therefore minimal. Deduce that $ug \in B(sw)$ and that $B(s)B(w) = B(sw)$. If now $l(sw) = l(w) - 1$, put $w' = sw$: then $B(s)B(w') = B(w)$ and hence

$$B(s)B(w) = B(s)B(s)B(w') \subset B(w') \cup (B(s)B(w')) = B(sw) \cup B(w);$$

finally, since $B \subset B(s)B(s)$, we also have $B(w') = B(sw) \subset B(s)B(w)$.)

e) Show that there exists a unique isomorphism from the building associated to (G, B) (Exerc. 10) to I, compatible with the action of G and taking the canonical chamber C_e to C.

12) Let (G, B, N, S) be a Tits system, $W = N/(B \cap N)$ its Weyl group, I the (W, S)-building associated to (G, B) (Exerc. 10) and $C = C_e$ the canonical chamber of I. Let A_0 be the apartment associated to the Coxeter system (W, S) (§ 1, Exerc. 16). For all $g \in G$, let φ_g be the map from A_0 to I that takes a point $wW^{(s)}$ of A_0 ($w \in W$, $s \in S$) to the point $gwG^{(s)}$ of I.

Show that, for all $g \in G$, the map φ_g is an isomorphism of numbered buildings from A_0 to a subset of I that is the union of chambers $gn(C_e)$ for $n \in N$. Show that I, equipped with the set $\mathfrak{U}$ of $\varphi_g(A_0)$ for $g \in G$, is a structured building (§ 1, Exerc. 24) (to prove (SB 2), remark that, if $g', g'' \in G$, there exist $b', b'' \in B$ and $n \in N$ such that $g'^{-1}g'' = b'nb''$; then put $g = g'b'n$ and show that $g'(C)$ and $g''(C)$ are contained in $\varphi_g(A_0)$. To prove (SB 3), reduce to the case of two apartments $A' = \varphi_e(A_0)$ and

$A'' = \varphi_b(A_0)$, with $b \in B$, and show that the map $a \mapsto b(a)$ leaves the points of $A' \cap A''$ fixed by using Prop. 2 of no. 5). Show that the Coxeter system (W, S) and the numbering of I are adapted to $(I, \mathfrak{U})$ (§ 1, Exerc. 24 *e*)) and that the set $\mathfrak{I}$ of allowed isomorphisms from A_0 to the various elements of $\mathfrak{U}$ is the set of φ_g for $g \in G$.

13) We use the notation of Exerc. 24 of § 1: $(I, \mathfrak{U})$ is a spacious structured building equipped with a Coxeter system (W, S) and an adapted numbering and $\mathfrak{I}$ is the set of allowed isomorphisms from the apartment A_0 associated to (W, S) to the various apartments of $(I, \mathfrak{U})$. Further, let G be a group of allowed automorphisms of I, preserving E: the group G then acts on $\mathfrak{I}$ and we assume that G acts *transitively* on $\mathfrak{I}$.

Denote by C a chamber of I, A an apartment of $\mathfrak{U}$ containing C, φ an allowed isomorphism from A_0 to A taking the canonical chamber C_e of A_0 to C, B the stabilizer of C in G and N the stabilizer of A in G.

a) Show that, if A' and A'' are two apartments belonging to $\mathfrak{U}$, and containing the same chamber, there exists $g \in G$ such that $g(A') = A''$ and that $g(a) = a$ for all $a \in A' \cap A''$. Show that G acts transitively on the set of pairs (A, C) where $A \in \mathfrak{U}$ and C is a chamber of A.

b) Show that the map $n \mapsto \varphi^{-1} \circ n \circ \varphi$ is a surjective homomorphism from N to W, with kernel $B \cap N$. We can thus identify $N/(B \cap N)$ with W.

c) Show that conditions (WI 1) and (WI 2) of Exerc. 10 *d*) are satisfied (use the following fact: if an apartment of I contains two chambers C' and C'', it contains every minimal gallery with extremities C' and C'' (§ 1, Exerc. 24 *b*))).

d) Show that condition (G) of Exerc. 10 *g*) (and *a fortiori* condition (G_0) of Exerc. 11) is satisfied (with the notation of (G), consider an apartment A' (resp. A'') of I containing C_0 and C' (resp. C''); show by using Exerc. 24 *b*) of § 1 that $\Gamma \subset A" \cap A''$ and use *a*)).

e) Show that (G, B, N, S) is a Tits system and that $(I, \mathfrak{U})$ is canonically isomorphic to the associated numbered structured building (Exerc. 12).

14) Let (G, B, N, S) be a Tits system and $(I, \mathfrak{U})$ the associated numbered structured building (Exerc. 12). Show that G, considered as a group of automorphisms of I, satisfies the conditions of Exerc. 13. With the notation of Exerc. 12, put $A = \varphi_e(A_0)$ and $C = \varphi_e(C_e)$; show that B is the stabilizer of C in G. Let $\tilde{N}$ be the stabilizer of A in G; show that $\tilde{N}/(B \cap \tilde{N})$ can be identified with W and that $(G, B, \tilde{N}, S)$ is the *saturated* Tits system associated to (G, B, N, S) (Exerc. 5).

15) We use the hypotheses and notation of Exerc. 10. Assume moreover that the Weyl group W of (G, B) is *finite* and denote by w_0 the longest element of W (§ 1, Exerc. 22). Two chambers C and C' are said to be *opposed* if $t(C, C') = w_0$.

a) Show that if C and C′ are opposed, so are C′ and C. Show that there exists a chamber opposed to any given chamber C. Show that the stabilizer of a chamber C in G acts transitively on the set of chambers opposed to C.

b) Let C and C′ be two opposed chambers. Show that for all $w \in W$, there exists a unique chamber C_w having the following property: if $(s_1, \dots, s_k)$ (resp. $(s'_1, \dots, s'_h)$) is a reduced decomposition of w (resp. of $w' = w_0 w^{-1}$), there exists a minimal gallery $(C_0 = C, C_1, \dots, C_n = C')$ of type $(s_1, \dots, s_k, s'_1, \dots, s'_h)$ (with $n = h + k$) such that $C_w = C_k$ (use Exerc. 22 of § 1 and Exerc. 10, *d*) and *e*)). Show that C_w and C_{ww_0} are opposed.

c) Let $\mathfrak{M}$ be the set of pairs of opposed chambers. For $m = (C, C') \in \mathfrak{M}$, let A_m be the union of the chambers C_w constructed above. Show that I equipped with the set $\mathfrak{U}$ of A_m for $m \in \mathfrak{M}$ is a structured building (§ 1, Exerc. 24) and that the Coxeter system (W, S) and the numbering of I are adapted to $(I, \mathfrak{U})$; define a canonical bijection from $\mathfrak{M}$ to the set denoted by $\mathfrak{J}$ in Exerc. 24 of § 1. We identify these two sets.

d) Let $m = (C, C') \in \mathfrak{M}$ with $C = C_e$, and let N be the stabilizer of A_m in G. Show that $N/(B \cap N)$ can be identified with W and that (G, B, N, S) is a saturated Tits system (use Exerc. 13).

16) We retain the hypotheses and notation of Exerc. 15.

a) Let C and C′ be two chambers. Show that there exists a chamber C″ opposed both to C and to C′ (take C″ opposed to C such that $t(C, C')$ is of greatest possible length; if $t(C', C'') \neq w_0$, there exists a neighbouring chamber C_1 of C″ such that $l(t(C', C_1)) > l(t(C', C''))$; show by using condition (G) of Exerc. 10 that we can assume that $C_1 \not\subset A_{(C,C'')}$ and that C_1 is then opposed to C).

b) Let $a \in \mathfrak{U}$; show that there exists a unique involutive automorphism j_A (not necessarily allowed) that takes every chamber of A to the opposed chamber (use Exerc. 22 *c*) of § 1). Let F and F′ be two facets of I; show that if $F' = j_A(F)$ for some $A \in \mathfrak{U}$ containing F and F′, then the same is true for all $A \in \mathfrak{U}$ containing F and F′ (if $F, F' \in A \cap A'$, with $A, A' \in \mathfrak{U}$, consider a chamber C (resp. C′) of A (resp. A′) containing F (resp. F′) and an $A'' \in \mathfrak{U}$ containing C and C′ and use (SB 3)). Then F and F′ are said to be *opposed.* Show that two facets have a common opposed facet if and only if they are of the same type T and that a facet opposed to a facet of type T is of type $w_0 T w_0^{-1}$.

c) Let A_0 be the apartment associated to a Coxeter system (W, S) (§ 1, Exerc. 16) and let $\mathfrak{J}$ be the set of allowed isomorphisms from A_0 to the various elements of $\mathfrak{U}$. If α is a half of A_0, with wall L (§ 1, Exerc. 16) and if $\varphi \in \mathfrak{J}$, we say that $\varphi(\alpha)$ is a *semi-apartment* of I, with *wall* $\varphi(L)$. Show that $\varphi(L)$ then depends only on $\varphi(\alpha)$ and not on the pair (φ, α). Let D_1 and D_2 be two distinct semi-apartments, with the same wall L: show that there exist $\varphi \in \mathfrak{J}$ and a wall L_0 of A_0 such that $L = \varphi(L_0)$ and that the D_i are the images under φ of the two halves of A_0 determined by L_0 (choose a panel F contained in L and two chambers C_1 and C_2, one contained in D_1 and the other in D_2 and such that C_1 contains F and C_2 contains the panel opposed to F in D_1 (which is also opposed to F in D_2) and consider the apartment of I containing C_1 and C_2).

17) We retain the hypotheses and notation of Exerc. 15 and 16. Choose an element $\varphi \in \mathfrak{I}$ taking the canonical chamber C of A_0 (§1, Exerc. 16) to the canonical chamber C_e of I and, as in Exerc. 15 *d*), denote by N the stabilizer of the apartment $\varphi(A_0) \in \mathfrak{U}$ in the group G. For any subset D of A_0, denote by B_D the subgroup of G leaving fixed all the points of $\varphi(D)$: we have $B = B_C$ and $B \cap N = B_{A_0}$.

a) Let α be a half of A_0 containing C. Show that B_α acts transitively on the semi-apartments of I distinct from $\varphi(\alpha)$ whose wall is the wall L of $\varphi(\alpha)$ (let X be such a semi-apartment, F a panel contained in L and C′ a chamber of $\varphi(\alpha)$ containing F; show, by using Exerc. 16 *c*) and Exerc. 13 *a*), that there exists $g \in G$ such that $g(X \cup \varphi(\alpha)) = \varphi(A_0)$ and $g(C') = C'$; show that $g(F) = F$ and deduce from Exerc. 22 *c*) of §1 that $g \in B_\alpha$). Deduce that B_L acts doubly transitively on the semi-apartments with wall L and that $(B_L, B_\alpha, B_L \cap N)$ is a Tits system whose Weyl group is of order 2 (cf. Exerc. 7).

b) Let D_1 and D_2 be two convex subsets of A_0 such that $C \subset D_1 \subset D_2$ and that there exists a unique half α of A_0 with $D_1 \subset \alpha$ and $D_2 \not\subset \alpha$: then $D_1 = D_2 \cap \alpha$ (§1, Exerc. 21 *c*)). Show that $B_{D_1} = B_\alpha B_{D_2}$ and that $B_\alpha \cap B_{D_2} = B \cap N$ (by considering a gallery of smallest possible length having one extremity equal to C and the other containing a point $a \in D_2 - D_1$, show that there exist two neighbouring chambers C'_1 and C'_2 of A_0 such that $C'_1 \subset D_1$, $C'_2 \subset D_2$, $C'_2 \not\subset D_1$ and $C'_1 \cap C'_2$ contained in the wall L′ of α. Put $C_i = \varphi(C'_i)$, $F = \varphi(C'_1 \cap C'_2)$ and $L = \varphi(L')$. Show that the convex hull of $D_1 \cup C'_2$ is equal to D_2. Let $b \in B_{D_1}$: then $b(C_1) = C_1$, so $b(F) = F$ and $b(C_2) \neq C_1$. Deduce that the convex hull of $b(C_2) \cup L$ is a semi-apartment X distinct from $\varphi(\alpha)$ and with wall L, and that there exists $b' \in B_\alpha$ such that

$$b'(\varphi(A_0)) = X \cup \varphi(\alpha).$$

Show that $b'b(a) = a$ for all $a \in \varphi(D_1 \cup C'_2)$ and that $b'b \in B_{D_2}$).

c) Let $(\alpha_i)_{1 \leqslant i \leqslant q}$ be the halves of A_0 containing C, numbered so that the map

$$j \mapsto \bigcap_{1 \leqslant i \leqslant j} \alpha_i$$

is strictly decreasing (cf. §1, Exerc. 17). Show that $B = B_{\alpha_1} \dots B_{\alpha_q}$ and that if $b_i, b'_i \in B_{\alpha_i}$ with $b_1 \dots b_q = b'_1 \dots b'_q$, then $b'_i \in b_i(B \cap N)$ for $1 \leqslant i \leqslant q$.

18) We use the hypotheses and notation of no. 2. Let V_i be the vector subspace of k^n generated by $e_1, \dots, e_i$ (for $1 \leqslant i \leqslant n-1$).

a) Show that, for any subset X of S, the subgroup G_X (no. 5) consists of the elements $g \in G$ such that $g(V_i) = V_i$ for all i such that $s_i \notin X$.

b) Let I be the building associated to a Tits system (G, B, N, S) (Exerc. 10 and 12). Show that the map j that associates to the point $gG^{(i)}$ of I (where $G^{(i)}$ denotes the subgroup $G_{S-\{s_i\}}$ of G, in other words the stabilizer of V_i) the vector subspace $g(V_i)$ is a *bijection* from I to the set $\mathfrak{B}$ of vector subspaces of k^n that are $\neq \{0\}$ and $\neq k^n$, compatible with the action of G.

c) If E is a vector space, a *flag* of E is a set of vector subspaces of E that is totally ordered by inclusion. Show that elements $a_1, \dots, a_k$ of I belong to the same facet of I if and only if $\{j(a_1), \dots, j(a_k)\}$ is a flag of k^n.

d) Show that G acts doubly-transitively on the set of 1-dimensional vector subspaces of k^n. Suppose that $n \geqslant 2$ and let N_1 be the subgroup of G generated by the element that interchanges e_1 and e_2 and leaves fixed the other e_i. Show that $(G, G^{(1)}, N_1)$ is a Tits system whose Weyl group is of order 2.

e) Assume that k is commutative. Set

$$G' = \mathbf{SL}(n,k), \quad B' = G' \cap B, \quad N' = G' \cap N \quad \text{and} \quad T' = N' \cap B' = T \cap G'.$$

Show that N'/T' can be identified with $\mathfrak{S}_n$ and that (G', B', N', S) is a Tits system (argue as in no. 2).

19) Let k be a commutative field of characteristic $\neq 2$ and let Q be the quadratic form $x_1x_3 + x_2^2$ on k^3. Show that the group $\mathbf{SO}(Q)$ acts doubly transitively on the set of isotropic lines in k^3. Compare the corresponding Tits system (Exerc. 7) with that obtained in no. 2 for $n = 2$ (cf. *Algebra* Chap. IX, § 9, Exerc. 15).

20) We use the notation of no. 2, and assume that k is commutative. Consider the following cases:

(B_l) $n = 2l + 1$ (with $l \geqslant 1$), k is of characteristic $\neq 2$ and k^n is equipped with the quadratic form $Q = x_1x_n + \dots + x_lx_{l+2} + x_{l+1}^2$;

(C_l) $n = 2l$ (with $l \geqslant 1$) and k^n is equipped with the alternating form Φ such that $\Phi(e_i, e_j) = 0$ for $1 \leqslant i \leqslant n$, $1 \leqslant j \leqslant n$ and $i \leqslant j$, except when $i \leqslant l$, $j = n + 1 - i$, when $\Phi(e_i, e_j) = 1$;

(D_l) $n = 2l$ (with $l \geqslant 2$), k is of characteristic $\neq 2$ and k^n is equipped with the quadratic form $Q = x_1x_n + \dots + x_lx_{l+1}$.

Denote by G_1 the special orthogonal group $\mathbf{SO}(Q)$ in cases (B_l) and (D_l), and the symplectic group $\mathbf{Sp}(\Phi)$ in case (C_l). Put

$$B_1 = G_1 \cap B, \quad N_1 = G_1 \cap N \quad \text{and} \quad T_1 = G_1 \cap T = B_1 \cap N_1.$$

a) Show that the action of N_1 on the set of lines ke_i defines a homomorphism from N_1, with kernel T_1, onto the subgroup W_1 of $\mathfrak{S}_n$, allowing us to identify W_1 with N_1/T_1. Show that W_1 is the subgroup of $\mathfrak{S}_n$ generated by

the $\sigma_j = s_j s_{n-j}$ for $1 \leqslant j < l$ and by $\sigma_l = s_{l-1} s_l s_{l-1}$ in case (B_l);
the $\sigma_j = s_j s_{n-j}$ for $1 \leqslant j < l$ and by $\sigma_l = s_l$ in case (C_l);
the $\sigma_j = s_j s_{n-j}$ for $1 \leqslant j < l$ and by $\sigma_l = s_{l-1} s_l s_{l-1} s_l s_{l+1} s_l$ in case (D_l).

b) Let S_1 be the set of σ_j for $1 \leqslant j \leqslant l$. Show that (G_1, B_1, N_1, S_1) is a Tits system (to prove that the subgroup H of G_1 generated by B_1 and N_1 is the whole of G_1, argue as in *Algebra*, Chap. II, § 10, no. 13), remarking that H contains the lower triangular subgroup of G_1 and that, for any $\xi_i \in k$ $(2 \leqslant i \leqslant n)$, there exists a matrix $b = (b_{ij}) \in B_1$ such that $b_{11} = 1$, $b_{1i} = \xi_i$ for $2 \leqslant i \leqslant n-1$ and $b_{1n} = \xi_n$ in case (C_l), and $b_{1n} = 0$ in cases (B_l) and (D_l). Then argue as in no. 2, introducing the subgroups $G_{1,j} = G_1 \cap (G_j, G_{n-j})$ for $1 \leqslant j < l$ and the subgroup $G_{1,l}$ of elements of G_1 leaving fixed

the e_i for $i \neq l, l+1, l+2$ and the subspace generated by e_l, e_{l+1} and e_{l+2} in case (B_l);

the e_i for $i \neq l, l+1$ and the plane generated by e_l and e_{l+1} in case (C_l);

the e_i for $i < l-1$ or $i > l+2$ and the two planes generated by e_{l-1} and e_{l+1} and by e_1 and e_{l+2} in case (D_l).

Show that $G_{1,j}$ can be identified, respectively, with $\mathbf{GL}(2, k)$, $\mathbf{SL}(2, k)$ or the special orthogonal group of Exerc. 19).

**c*) Show that the Coxeter graph of the group W_1 is of type (B_l), (C_l) or (D_l) in the three cases (Chap VI, § 4, no. 1).$_*$

d) Show that, for any subset X of S_1, the subgroup G_{1X} consists of the $g \in G_1$ such that $g(V_i) = V_i$ for all i such that $\sigma_i \notin X$, except in case (D_l) where the same assertion is valid provided that V_{r-1} denotes the subspace generated by $e_1, \ldots, e_{r-1}$ and e_{r+1}. Deduce, as in Exerc. 18 *b*), that there exists a bijection j from the building associated to (G_1, B_1) to the set of totally isotropic subspaces $\neq 0$ in cases (B_l) and (C_l), and to the set of totally isotropic subspaces of dimension $\neq 0$ and $\neq r-1$ in case (D_l). Show that points $a_1, \ldots, a_k$ of I belong to the same facet if and only if $\{j(a_1), \ldots, j(a_k)\}$ is a flag.

21) Let A be a discrete valuation ring (*Commutative Algebra*, Chap. VI, § 3, no. 6), $\mathfrak{m}$ its maximal ideal, γ a generator of $\mathfrak{m}$ and K the field of fractions of A. Let G be the group $\mathbf{SL}(2, K)$, B the subgroup of G consisting of the matrices $\begin{pmatrix} a & b \\ c & d \end{pmatrix}$ such that $a, b, d \in A$ and $c \in \mathfrak{m}$ (with $ad - bc = 1$) and N the subgroup consisting of the matrices belonging to G and having only one non-zero entry in each row and column.

a) Show that $T = B \cap N$ is normal in N and that $W = N/T$ is an infinite dihedral group generated by the classes s and s' of the matrices $\begin{pmatrix} 0 & 1 \\ -1 & 0 \end{pmatrix}$ and $\begin{pmatrix} 0 & \gamma \\ -\gamma^{-1} & 0 \end{pmatrix}$, respectively.

b) Show that (G, B, N, S) (with $S = \{s, s'\}$) is a Tits system.

c) Let $H = \mathbf{SL}(2, A)$ be the subgroup of G consisting of the matrices with coefficients in A. Show that $(H, B \cap H, N, \{s\})$ is a Tits system. Compare with Exerc. 18 *e*).

d) Let $\hat{A}$ be the completion of A and let $\hat{G}, \hat{B}, \hat{N}, \hat{T}$ be the groups defined as above but replacing A by $\hat{A}$. Show that the injection of G into $\hat{G}$ defines an isomorphism from the building I associated to (G, B) (Exerc. 10) to the building $\hat{I}$ associated to $(\hat{G}, \hat{B})$. Let $(I, \mathfrak{U})$ (resp. $(\hat{I}, \hat{\mathfrak{U}})$) be the *structured* building associated to (G, B, N) (resp. $(\hat{G}, \hat{B}, \hat{N})$) (Exerc. 12): show that $j(\mathfrak{U}) \subset \hat{\mathfrak{U}}$, but that $j(\mathfrak{U}) \neq \hat{\mathfrak{U}}$ if $A \neq \hat{A}$ (remark that the apartments $\hat{\mathfrak{U}}$ (resp. $\mathfrak{U}$) correspond bijectively to the conjugates of T (resp. $\hat{T}$) by G (resp. $\hat{G}$).

22) Let G be a group and B a subgroup of G.

a) Show that the following conditions are equivalent:

(i) $B \cap gBg^{-1}$ is of finite index in B for all $g \in G$;

(ii) every double coset BgB with respect to B is a finite union of left cosets with respect to B.

More precisely, show that, for all $g \in G$, the index q_g of $B \cap gBg^{-1}$ in B is equal to the number of left cosets with respect to B contained in the double coset BgB. Show that $q_{gh} \leqslant q_g q_h$ for all $g, h \in G$.

Assume from now on that conditions (i) and (ii) are satisfied and denote by k a commutative ring. For $t \in G/B$ (resp. $t \in B\backslash G/B$), denote by a_t the map from G to k defined by $a_t(g) = 0$ if $g \notin t$ and $a_t(g) = 1$ if $g \in t$. Let L (resp. H) be the k-module generated by the a_t for $t \in G/B$ (resp. $t \in B\backslash G/B$).

b) Show that there exists a unique linear form μ on L such that $\mu(a_t) = 1$ for all $t \in G/B$.

c) Let $\varphi \in L$ and $\psi \in H$. Show that, for all $x \in G$, the map

$$\theta_x : y \mapsto \varphi(y)\psi(y^{-1}x)$$

belongs to L and that the map $\varphi * \psi : x \mapsto \mu(\theta_x)$ belongs to L. Moreover, if $\varphi \in H$ then $\varphi * \psi \in H$. Show that the map $(\varphi, \psi) \mapsto \varphi * \psi$ makes H into an algebra over k, having a_B as its unit element, and makes L into a right H-module.

The algebra H is called the *Hecke algebra* of G with respect to H and is denoted by $H_k(G, B)$.

d) Show that, for $t, t' \in \mathrm{B}\backslash\mathrm{G}/\mathrm{B}$,

$$a_t * a_{t'} = \sum_{t''} m(t, t'; t'') a_{t''},$$

where $m(t, t'; t'')$ is the number of cosets with respect to B contained in $t \cap g t'^{-1}$ for all $g \in t''$.

e) Let G act on L by left translations. Show that the action of H on L defines an isomorphism from H to the commutant of the linear representation of G on L thus obtained.

**f*) Assume that G is *finite* and that the characteristic of k does not divide the order of G. Show that $\mathrm{H}_k(\mathrm{G}, \mathrm{B})$ is absolutely semi-simple over k (*Algebra*, Chap VIII, § 7, no. 5) (use Maschke's Theorem (Chap. V, Appendix) and Prop. 3 of *Algebra*, Chap. VIII, § 5, no. 1).$_*$

g) Assume that G is a topological group and that B is a compact open subgroup of G. Show that conditions (i) and (ii) are satisfied and that, when $k = \mathbf{R}$ or $\mathbf{C}$, the product $\varphi * \psi$ is simply the convolution product relative to the right Haar measure on G, normalised by the condition $\mu(\mathrm{B}) = 1$ (cf. *Integration*, Chap. VIII, § 4, no. 5).

23) Let (W, S) be a Coxeter system and k a commutative ring. Suppose that we are given, for all $s \in \mathrm{S}$, two elements λ_s and μ_s of k such that $\lambda_s = \lambda_{s'}$ and $\mu_s = \mu_{s'}$ whenever s and s' are conjugate in W. Put $\mathrm{E} = k^{(\mathrm{W})}$ and let $\{e_w\}$ be the canonical basis of E.

a) Show that E has a unique algebra structure such that, for $s \in \mathrm{S}$ and $w \in \mathrm{W}$,

$$e_s.e_w = \begin{cases} e_{sw} & \text{if } l(sw) > l(w) \\ \lambda_s e_w + \mu_s e_{sw} & \text{if } l(sw) < l(w) \end{cases}$$

(introduce the endomorphism P_s of E defined by the above formulas, where $e_s.e_w$ is replaced by $\mathrm{P}_s(w)$, and the endomorphism $\mathrm{Q}_s = j\mathrm{P}_s j^{-1}$, where j denotes the automorphism of E defined by $j(e_w) = e_{w^{-1}}$; show that $\mathrm{P}_s\mathrm{Q}_t = \mathrm{Q}_t\mathrm{P}_s$ for $s, t \in \mathrm{S}$ by remarking that the conditions $l(swt) = l(w)$ and $l(sw) = l(wt)$ imply that $sw = wt$; then argue as in Exerc. 3 *e*)). The module E, equipped with this algebra structure, will be denoted by $\mathrm{E}_k((\lambda_s), (\mu_s))$. Show that $\mathrm{E}((0), (1))$ is the group algebra $k[\mathrm{W}]$ of W (*Algebra*, Chap. III, § 2, no. 6).

b) Show that the family of generators $(e_s)_{s \in \mathrm{S}}$ and the relations

$$\begin{aligned} e_s^2 &= \lambda_s e_s + \mu_s \quad \text{for } s \in \mathrm{S} \\ (e_s e_t)^r &= (e_t e_s)^r \quad \text{for } s, t \in \mathrm{S} \text{ such that } st \text{ is of finite even order } 2r \\ (e_s e_t)^r e_s &= (e_t e_s)^r e_t \quad \text{for } s, t \in \mathrm{S} \text{ such that } st \text{ is of finite odd order } 2r+1 \end{aligned}$$

form a presentation of the algebra E (argue as in the proof of Th. 1 of no. 6 of § 1).

24) Let G be a group and B a Tits subgroup of G (Exerc. 3, of which we use the notation). Assume that, for all $s \in \mathrm{S}$, the double coset $\mathrm{C}(s)$ is the union of a finite number q_s of left cosets with respect to B. We use the notation of Exerc. 22 and put $a_w = a_{\mathrm{C}(w)}$ for all $w \in \mathrm{W}$.

a) Show that conditions (i) and (ii) of Exerc. 22 are satisfied. We can therefore speak of the Hecke algebra $\mathrm{H}_k(\mathrm{G}, \mathrm{B})$ (k being a commutative ring), of which $(a_w)_{w \in \mathrm{W}}$ is a basis.

b) Let $s \in \mathrm{S}$ and $w \in \mathrm{W}$. Show that $a_s * a_s = (q_s - 1)a_s + q_s$; show that if $l(sw) > l(w)$ then $a_s * a_w = a_{sw}$.

c) Show that the linear map from the algebra $\mathrm{E}_k((q_s - 1), (q_s))$ associated to the Coxeter system (W, S) (Exerc. 23) to $\mathrm{H}_k(\mathrm{G}, \mathrm{B})$ that sends e_w to a_w for all $w \in \mathrm{W}$ is an isomorphism of algebras.

25) We use the notation of Exerc. 8. Assume in addition that, for all $s \in \mathrm{S}$, the index q_s of $\mathrm{B} \cap g\mathrm{B}g^{-1}$ in B is finite for all $g \in \mathrm{B}s\mathrm{B}$.

a) Show that the pair $(\tilde{\mathrm{G}}, \mathrm{B})$ satisfies conditions (i) and (ii) of Exerc. 22.

b) Show that, for all $\gamma \in \Gamma$, the map $x \mapsto \gamma x \gamma^{-1}$ defines an automorphism σ of the Hecke algebra $\mathrm{H}_k(\mathrm{G}, \mathrm{B})$ and that σ depends only on the class ω of γ in $\Omega = \Gamma/(\Gamma \cap \mathrm{B})$.

c) Let $k[\Omega]$ be the group algebra of Ω and (e_ω) its canonical basis. Show that the linear map j from $k[\Omega] \otimes_k \mathrm{H}_k(\mathrm{G}, \mathrm{B})$ to $\mathrm{H}_k(\tilde{\mathrm{G}}, \mathrm{B})$ defined by $j(e_\omega \otimes a_{\mathrm{B}w\mathrm{B}}) = a_{\mathrm{B}\omega w\mathrm{B}}$ (in the notation of Exerc. 22), for $\omega \in \Omega$ and $w \in \mathrm{W}$, is bijective and that

$$j^{-1}(j(e_w \otimes x) j(e_{w'} \otimes y)) = e_{ww'} \otimes \sigma_\omega(x) y$$

for $\omega, \omega' \in \Omega$ and $x, y \in \mathrm{H}_k(\mathrm{G}, \mathrm{B})$.

¶ 26) If E is an absolutely semi-simple algebra of finite rank over a commutative field k, the *numerical invariant* of E is the sequence of integers $(n_1, \ldots, n_r)$ such that $n_1 \geqslant \cdots \geqslant n_r > 0$ and that $\bar{k} \otimes_k \mathrm{E}$ is isomorphic, for any algebraic closure $\bar{k}$ of k, to $\prod_i \mathbf{M}_{n_i}(\bar{k})$.

Let V be an integral ring, K its field of fractions, φ a homomorphism from V to a commutative field k, and E a V-algebra. Assume that E is a free V-module of finite rank and put $\mathrm{E}_0 = \mathrm{E} \otimes_{\mathrm{V}} k$ and $\mathrm{E}_1 = \mathrm{E} \otimes_{\mathrm{V}} \mathrm{K}$.

a) Assume that the bilinear form $(x, y) \mapsto \mathrm{Tr}_{\mathrm{E}_0/k}(xy)$ on E_0 is non-degenerate. Show that E_0 and E_1 are absolutely semi-simple (cf. *Algebra*, Chap IX, § 2, Exerc. 1).

b) Assume that E_0 and E_1 are absolutely semi-simple over k and K, respectively. Show that E_0 and E_1 have the same numerical invariant (reduce to the case where k and K are algebraically closed); let (e_i) be a basis of E over V and let (X_i) be indeterminates. Show that the characteristic polynomial of the element $\sum_i X_i e_i$ of $E_1 \otimes_K K[(X_i)]$ (resp. $E_0 \otimes_k k[(X_i)]$) is of the form $P = \prod_j P_j^{n_j}$ (resp. $Q = \prod_k Q_k^{m_k}$), where $(n_1, \ldots, n_r)$ (resp. $(m_1, \ldots, m_s)$) is the numerical invariant of E_1 (resp. E_0), with $\deg(P_j) = n_j$ (resp. $\deg(Q_k) = m_k$). Show that $P_j \in V[(X_i)]$ and that $Q = \varphi(P)$. Deduce that there exist integers $c_{jk} \geqslant 0$ such that

$$m_k = \sum_j c_{jk} n_j, \quad \text{and} \quad n_j = \sum_k c_{jk} m_k.)$$

*27) Let (G, B, N, S) be a Tits system and let k be a commutative field. Assume that G is *finite* and that the characteristic of k divides neither the order of G nor the order of the Weyl group $W = N/(B \cap N)$. Show that the algebras $H_k(G, B)$ (Exerc. 22) and $k[W]$ are absolutely semi-simple and have the same numerical invariant, and hence are isomorphic when k is algebraically closed (let q_s be the index of $B \cap gBg^{-1}$ in B for $g \in BsB$, $s \in S$. Consider the algebra $E_{k[X]}((X(q_s - 1)), (1 + X(q_s - 1)))$ constructed as in Exerc. 23 from the Coxeter system (W, S) and the polynomial ring $k[X]$ and use Exerc. 26 *a*) and *b*), remarking that, by Maschke's theorem (Chap. V, Appendix), the bilinear form $\mathrm{Tr}_{k[W]/k}(xy)$ is non-degenerate).*

28) Let G be a group, M a maximal subgroup of G and U a normal subgroup of M, satisfying condition (R) of no. 7. Assume that G is equal to its commutator subgroup, that it is generated by the union of the conjugates of U and that the intersection of the conjugates of M reduces to the unit element. Show that G is simple. (Consider a normal subgroup N of G distinct from $\{1\}$; show that $G = N.M$ and then that $G = N.U$.)

29) Let H be a simple non-abelian group. Let θ be an automorphism of H of prime order p and let U be the semi-direct product of $\mathbf{Z}/p\mathbf{Z}$ by H corresponding to θ. Show that, if θ is not an inner automorphism, the only normal subgroups of U are $\{1\}$, H and U. Deduce that U is not soluble, but that it satisfies condition (R) of no. 7. Apply this to show that the symmetric group $\mathfrak{S}_n$ satisfies condition (R).

CHAPTER V
Groups Generated by Reflections

§ 1. HYPERPLANES, CHAMBERS AND FACETS

In this section, E denotes a *real* affine space of finite dimension d and T the space of translations of E (cf. *Algebra*, Chap. II, § 9). If a and b are two points of E, $[ab]$ (resp. $]ab[$, resp. $]ab]$) will denote the closed segment (resp. open segment, resp. segment open at a and closed at b) with extremities a, b. The space T is provided with its unique separated topological vector space topology, cf. *Topological Vector Spaces*, Chap. I, § 2, no. 3; it is isomorphic to $\mathbf{R}^d$. The space E is provided with the unique topology such that, for all $e \in \mathrm{E}$, the map $t \mapsto e + t$ from T to E is a homeomorphism.

We denote by H a *locally finite* set of hyperplanes of E (*General Topology*, Chap. I, § 1, no. 5).

1. NOTATIONS

Let H be a hyperplane of E. Recall that E – H has two connected components, called the *open half-spaces* bounded by H. Their closures are called the *closed half-spaces* bounded by H. Let $x, y \in \mathrm{E}$. Then x and y are said to be *strictly on the same side* of H if they are contained in the same open half-space bounded by H, or equivalently, if the closed segment with extremities x and y does not meet H; x and y are said to be *on opposite sides* of H if x belongs to one of the open half-spaces bounded by H and y to the other. If $x \in \mathrm{E}$ and $t \in \mathrm{T}$, then x and t are said to be strictly on the same side of H if this is so for x and $h + t$ for all $h \in \mathrm{H}$.

Let A be a non-empty connected subset of E. For any hyperplane H of E that does not meet A, $\mathrm{D_H(A)}$ denotes the unique open half-space bounded by H that contains A. If $\mathfrak{N}$ is a set of hyperplanes of E, none of which meet A, put

$$\mathrm{D}_{\mathfrak{N}}(\mathrm{A}) = \bigcap_{\mathrm{H} \in \mathfrak{N}} \mathrm{D_H(A)}. \tag{1}$$

If A consists of a single point a, we write $\mathrm{D_H}(a)$ and $\mathrm{D}_{\mathfrak{N}}(a)$ instead of $\mathrm{D_H}(\{a\})$ and $\mathrm{D}_{\mathfrak{N}}(\{a\})$.

2. FACETS

The set of points of E that do not belong to any hyperplane H of the set $\mathfrak{H}$ is open since $\mathfrak{H}$ is locally finite. More precisely, we have the following result:

PROPOSITION 1. *Let a be a point of E. There exists a connected open neighbourhood of a that does not meet any hyperplane H that belongs to $\mathfrak{H}$ and does not pass through a. Moreover, there exist only finitely many hyperplanes that belong to $\mathfrak{H}$ and pass through a.*

The set $\mathfrak{N}$ of hyperplanes H such that $H \in \mathfrak{H}$ and $a \notin H$ is locally finite since it is contained in $\mathfrak{H}$. Hence, the set U of points of E that do not belong to any of the hyperplanes of the set $\mathfrak{N}$ is open. Since $a \in U$, there is a connected open neighbourhood of a contained in U. The remainder of the proposition is clear.

Given two points x and y of E, denote by $R\{x, y\}$ the relation

" For any hyperplane $H \in \mathfrak{H}$, either $x \in H$ and $y \in H$ or x and y are strictly on the same side of H."

Clearly, R is an equivalence relation on E.

DEFINITION 1. *A facet of E relative to $\mathfrak{H}$ is an equivalence class of the equivalence relation defined above.*

PROPOSITION 2. *The set of facets is locally finite.*

This is clear since $\mathfrak{H}$ is locally finite.

Let F be a facet and a a point of F. A hyperplane $H \in \mathfrak{H}$ contains F if and only if $a \in H$; the set $\mathfrak{F}$ of these hyperplanes is thus finite; their intersection is an affine subspace L of E, which we shall call the affine *support* of F; the dimension of L will be called the *dimension* of F.

If $\mathfrak{N}$ is the set of hyperplanes $H \in \mathfrak{H}$ not containing F, then

$$F = L \cap \bigcap_{H \in \mathfrak{N}} D_H(a). \tag{2}$$

We shall prove that the closure of F is given by

$$\overline{F} = L \cap \bigcap_{H \in \mathfrak{N}} \overline{D_H(a)}. \tag{3}$$

It is clear that the right-hand side contains the left-hand side. Conversely, let $x \in L \cap \bigcap_{H \in \mathfrak{N}} \overline{D_H(a)}$. The open segment with extremities a and x is contained in L and in each of the $D_H(a)$ for $H \in \mathfrak{N}$, and hence in F. It follows that x is in the closure of F, hence the formula.

PROPOSITION 3. *Let F be a facet and L its affine support.*

(i) *The set* F *is a convex open subset of the affine subspace* L *of* E.

(ii) *The closure of* F *is the union of* F *and facets of dimension strictly smaller than that of* F.

(iii) *In the topological space* L, *the set* F *is the interior of its closure.*

Since every open half-space and every hyperplane are convex subsets of E, formula (2) shows that F is the intersection of a family of convex subsets, and hence is convex. On the other hand, let a be in F, and let U be a convex open neighbourhood of a in E that does not meet any of the hyperplanes in the set $\mathfrak{N}$ of $\mathrm{H} \in \mathfrak{H}$ such that $a \notin \mathrm{H}$. For any $\mathrm{H} \in \mathfrak{N}$, we thus have $\mathrm{U} \subset \mathrm{D_H}(a)$, hence $\mathrm{L} \cap \mathrm{U} \subset \mathrm{F}$, so that F is open in the topological space L.

Let b be a point of $\overline{\mathrm{F}} - \mathrm{F}$, belonging to a facet F', and let $\mathfrak{N}'$ be the set of hyperplanes $\mathrm{H} \in \mathfrak{N}$ passing through b; put $\mathfrak{N}'' = \mathfrak{N} - \mathfrak{N}'$. For any H in $\mathfrak{N}''$, we have $b \notin \mathrm{H}$ and $b \in \overline{\mathrm{D_H}(a)}$, hence $b \in \mathrm{D_H}(a)$ and $\mathrm{D_H}(b) = \mathrm{D_H}(a)$; by the definition of a facet, we thus have

$$\mathrm{F}' = \mathrm{L} \cap \bigcap_{\mathrm{H} \in \mathfrak{N}'} \mathrm{H} \cap \bigcap_{\mathrm{H} \in \mathfrak{N}''} \mathrm{D_H}(a), \tag{4}$$

whereas (3) implies that

$$\overline{\mathrm{F}} = \mathrm{L} \cap \bigcap_{\mathrm{H} \in \mathfrak{N}'} \overline{\mathrm{D_H}(a)} \cap \bigcap_{\mathrm{H} \in \mathfrak{N}''} \overline{\mathrm{D_H}(a)}, \tag{5}$$

hence $\mathrm{F}' \subset \overline{\mathrm{F}}$. We cannot have $\mathfrak{N}' = \varnothing$, for this would imply that $\mathrm{F} = \mathrm{F}'$ by (2) and (4), contrary to the hypothesis that $b \notin \mathrm{F}$ and $b \in \mathrm{F}'$. The support of F' is the set $\mathrm{L}' = \mathrm{L} \cap \bigcap_{\mathrm{H} \in \mathfrak{N}'} \mathrm{H}$; we have $a \in \mathrm{L}$, but $a \notin \mathrm{H}$ for H in $\mathfrak{N}'$, so $\mathrm{L}' \neq \mathrm{L}$ and finally $\dim \mathrm{L}' < \dim \mathrm{L}$, that is $\dim \mathrm{F}' < \dim \mathrm{F}$. This proves (ii).

Let H be in $\mathfrak{N}'$ and let D be the open half-space bounded by H and distinct from $\mathrm{D_H}(a)$; we have $b \in \mathrm{H} \cap \mathrm{L}$, and it is immediate that $\mathrm{D} \cap \mathrm{L}$ is a half-space of L bounded by the hyperplane $\mathrm{H} \cap \mathrm{L}$ of L; consequently, every neighbourhood of b *in* L meets $\mathrm{D} \cap \mathrm{L}$, and since $\mathrm{D} \cap \mathrm{L}$ is disjoint from $\overline{\mathrm{F}}$ by (3), we see that the point b of $\overline{\mathrm{F}} - \mathrm{F}$ cannot be in the interior of $\overline{\mathrm{F}}$ in the topological space L. Since F is open in L, we have (iii). Q.E.D.

COROLLARY. *Let* F *and* F' *be two facets. If* $\overline{\mathrm{F}} = \overline{\mathrm{F}'}$, *the facets* F *and* F' *are equal.*

This follows from (iii).

PROPOSITION 4. *Let* F *be a facet, and let* L *be an affine subspace of* E *that is the intersection of hyperplanes belonging to* $\mathfrak{H}$; *denote by* $\mathfrak{N}$ *the set of hyperplanes* $\mathrm{H} \in \mathfrak{H}$ *that do not contain* L. *The following conditions are equivalent:*

(i) *There exists a facet* F' *with support* L *that meets* $\overline{\mathrm{F}}$.

(ii) *There exists a facet* F' *with support* L *contained in* $\overline{\mathrm{F}}$.

(iii) *There exists a point* x *in* $\mathrm{L} \cap \overline{\mathrm{F}}$ *that does not belong to any of the hyperplanes of* $\mathfrak{N}$.

If these conditions are satisfied, $L \cap D_{\mathfrak{N}}(F)$ *is the unique facet with support* L *contained in* $\overline{F}$.

(i) $\Longrightarrow$ (ii): Since $\overline{F}$ is a union of facets (Prop. 3, (ii)), every facet that meets $\overline{F}$ meets a facet contained in $\overline{F}$, and so is equal to it.

(ii) $\Longrightarrow$ (iii): Every point x of F' satisfies (iii) since every hyperplane of $\mathfrak{H}$ containing x contains F', and hence L.

(iii) $\Longrightarrow$ (i): Let x be a point satisfying (iii) and let F' be the facet containing x; it is clear that F' meets $\overline{F}$. Let $H \in \mathfrak{H}$; then $x \notin H$ if $H \in \mathfrak{N}$ and clearly $x \in H$ if $H \notin \mathfrak{N}$; consequently the support of F' is the intersection of the hyperplanes of $\mathfrak{H} - \mathfrak{N}$, and is equal to L.

Finally, let F' be a facet with support L contained in $\overline{F}$, and let x be a point of F'; since no hyperplane of $\mathfrak{N} \subset \mathfrak{H}$ passes through x, Prop. 1 shows that there exists a convex open neighbourhood U of x that does not meet any hyperplane of $\mathfrak{N}$. Since x is in the closure of F, $U \cap F \neq \varnothing$; now $\mathfrak{N}$ is the set of hyperplanes $H \in \mathfrak{H}$ that do not contain F', and for all H in $\mathfrak{N}$ we have $D_H(x) = D_H(U) = D_H(U \cap F) = D_H(F)$ and formula (2) implies that

$$F' = L \cap D_{\mathfrak{N}}(F). \qquad \text{Q.E.D.}$$

3. CHAMBERS

DEFINITION 2. *A* chamber of E relative to $\mathfrak{H}$ *(or simply a* chamber *if there is no ambiguity regarding* $\mathfrak{H}$*) is a facet of* E *relative to* $\mathfrak{H}$ *that is not contained in any hyperplane belonging to* $\mathfrak{H}$.

Let U be the open set in E consisting of the points that do not belong to any hyperplane of $\mathfrak{H}$; since a hyperplane of $\mathfrak{H}$ must contain any facet that it meets, the chambers are the facets contained in U; every chamber is a convex (hence connected) open subset of E by Prop. 3, (i); since the chambers form a partition of U, they are exactly the *connected components* of U. Every convex subset A of U is connected, and thus contained in a chamber, which is unique if A is non-empty. It is clear that the chambers are the facets with support E, and Prop. 3, (iii) shows that every chamber is the interior of its closure. Finally, let C be a chamber and A a non-empty subset of C; formulas (2) and (3) imply that

$$C = \bigcap_{H \in \mathfrak{H}} D_H(A) = D_{\mathfrak{H}}(A), \qquad \overline{C} = \bigcap_{H \in \mathfrak{H}} \overline{D_H(A)} \tag{6}$$

since $D_H(A) = D_H(a)$ for all $a \in A$.

PROPOSITION 5. *Let* C *be a non-empty subset of* E. *Assume that there exists a subset* $\mathfrak{H}'$ *of* $\mathfrak{H}$ *with the following properties:*

a) For any $H \in \mathfrak{H}'$, *there exists an open half-space* D_H *bounded by* H *such that* $C = \bigcap_{H \in \mathfrak{H}'} D_H$.

b) The set C *does not meet any hyperplane belonging to* $\mathfrak{H} - \mathfrak{H}'$.

Under these conditions, C *is a chamber defined by* $\mathfrak{H}$ *in* E, *and* $D_H = D_H(C)$ *for all* $H \in \mathfrak{H}$.

Properties *a*) and *b*) show that C is a convex subset of U; hence there is a chamber C′ with $C \subset C'$. Since $C \subset D_H$, we have $D_H = D_H(C)$ for all H in $\mathfrak{H}'$, hence $C = D_{\mathfrak{H}'}(C) \supset D_{\mathfrak{H}}(C)$ since $\mathfrak{H}' \subset \mathfrak{H}$; we have $D_{\mathfrak{H}}(C) = C'$ by (6), hence $C \supset C'$. Finally therefore, $C = C'$.

PROPOSITION 6. *Every point of* E *is in the closure of at least one chamber.*

If E reduces to a single point, this is clear. Otherwise, let $a \in E$ and let $H_1, \dots, H_m$ be the hyperplanes of $\mathfrak{H}$ containing a. Since $\mathfrak{H}$ is locally finite, there exists a neighbourhood V of a that does not meet any hyperplane of $\mathfrak{H}$ other than $H_1, \dots, H_m$. Let D be a straight line passing through a and not contained in any of the H_i; if $x \in D$, $x \neq a$, and x is sufficiently close to a, the open segment $]ax[$ is contained in V and does not meet any of the H_i. Then $]ax[\subset U$; since $]ax[$ is connected, it is contained in a chamber C, hence $a \in \overline{C}$.

PROPOSITION 7. *Let* L *be an affine subspace of* E *and* Ω *a non-empty open subset of* L.

(i) *There exists a point* a *in* Ω *that does not belong to any of the hyperplanes of* $\mathfrak{H}$ *that do not contain* L.

(ii) *If* L *is a hyperplane and* $L \notin \mathfrak{H}$, *there exists a chamber that meets* Ω.

(iii) *If* L *is a hyperplane and* $L \in \mathfrak{H}$, *there exists a point* a *in* Ω *that does not belong to any hyperplane* $H \neq L$ *of* $\mathfrak{H}$.

Denote by $\mathfrak{M}$ the set of hyperplanes H with $H \in \mathfrak{H}$ and $L \not\subset H$, and by $\mathfrak{L}$ the set of hyperplanes of *the affine space* L of the form $L \cap H$ with $H \in \mathfrak{M}$. It is clear that $\mathfrak{L}$ is a locally finite set of hyperplanes in L, and Prop. 6 shows that Ω meets a chamber Γ defined by $\mathfrak{L}$ in L. If a is a point of $\Gamma \cap \Omega$, then $a \notin H$ for all $H \in \mathfrak{M}$, hence (i).

Assume now that L is a hyperplane; any hyperplane containing L is then equal to it, so we may distinguish two cases:

a) $L \notin \mathfrak{H}$: then $\mathfrak{M} = \mathfrak{H}$, and we have $a \notin H$ for all $H \in \mathfrak{H}$; thus a belongs to a chamber defined by $\mathfrak{H}$ in E, hence (ii).

b) $L \in \mathfrak{H}$: then $\mathfrak{M} = \mathfrak{H} - \{L\}$, hence (iii).

4. WALLS AND FACES

DEFINITION 3. *Let* C *be a chamber of* E. *A face of* C *is a facet contained in the closure of* C *whose support is a hyperplane. A wall of* C *is a hyperplane that is the support of a face of* C.

Every wall of C belongs to $\mathfrak{H}$. Prop. 4 shows that a hyperplane $L \in \mathfrak{H}$ is a wall of C if and only if $C \neq D_{\mathfrak{H}-\{L\}}(C)$. Moreover, every wall of C is the support of a single face of C.

PROPOSITION 8. *Every hyperplane* H *belonging to* $\mathfrak{H}$ *is the wall of at least one chamber.*

By Prop. 7, (iii), there exists a point a of H that does not belong to any hyperplane $H' \neq H$ of $\mathfrak{H}$; by Prop. 6, there exists a chamber C such that $a \in \overline{C}$; Prop. 4 then shows that H is a wall of C.

PROPOSITION 9. *Let* C *be a chamber and* $\mathfrak{M}$ *the set of walls of* C. *Then* $C = D_{\mathfrak{M}}(C)$ *and every subset* $\mathfrak{L}$ *of* $\mathfrak{H}$ *such that* $C = D_{\mathfrak{L}}(C)$ *contains* $\mathfrak{M}$. *A subset* F *of* $\overline{C}$ *is a facet if and only if it is a facet of* E *relative to the family* $\mathfrak{M}$.

a) Let $\mathfrak{L}$ be a subset of $\mathfrak{H}$ such that $C = D_{\mathfrak{L}}(C)$. Consider a hyperplane L belonging to $\mathfrak{H}$ but not to $\mathfrak{L}$; let $\mathfrak{N}$ be the set of hyperplanes $H \neq L$ belonging to $\mathfrak{H}$. Then $\mathfrak{L} \subset \mathfrak{N}$, hence $C = D_{\mathfrak{N}}(C)$, and L does not meet $D_{\mathfrak{N}}(C)$. By the implication (i) $\Longrightarrow$ (iii) in Prop. 4, the hyperplane L is not a wall of C. Consequently, every wall of C belongs to $\mathfrak{L}$.

b) We assume that $C = D_{\mathfrak{L}}(C)$. Let H be a hyperplane belonging to $\mathfrak{L}$ that is not a wall of C, and put $\mathfrak{L}' = \mathfrak{L} - \{H\}$. By the implication (iii) $\Longrightarrow$ (i) in Prop. 4, the convex set $D_{\mathfrak{L}'}(C)$ does not meet H, so $D_{\mathfrak{L}'}(C) \subset D_H(C)$ and $C = D_{\mathfrak{L}'}(C)$. If $\mathfrak{F}$ is a finite subset of $\mathfrak{L}$ that does not contain any wall of C, we conclude by induction on the cardinal of $\mathfrak{F}$ that $C = D_{\mathfrak{L}-\mathfrak{F}}(C)$.

c) Let a be a point of C; clearly, $C \subset D_{\mathfrak{M}}(a)$. Let a' be a point of $D_{\mathfrak{M}}(a)$; since the closed segment $[aa']$ is compact, the set $\mathfrak{F}$ of hyperplanes $H \in \mathfrak{H}$ that meet $[aa']$ is finite. Since a and a' are strictly on the same side of every wall of C, no wall of C belongs to $\mathfrak{F}$; by *b*), we have $C = D_{\mathfrak{H}-\mathfrak{F}}(C)$. Since $a' \in D_{\mathfrak{H}-\mathfrak{F}}(a)$, we have $a' \in C$. We have therefore proved that $D_{\mathfrak{M}}(a) \subset C$, which establishes the first part of the proposition.

d) To prove the last assertion of the proposition, it clearly suffices to show that a subset F of $\overline{C}$ that is a facet of E relative to $\mathfrak{M}$ is a facet of E relative to $\mathfrak{H}$, or that every hyperplane $H \in \mathfrak{H}$ that meets F contains F. So let H be a hyperplane that meets F but does not contain it. Since F is open in its affine support, it is not completely on one side of H. It follows that $\overline{C}$ is not completely on one side of H and hence that the hyperplane H does not belong to $\mathfrak{H}$, which completes the proof.

Remarks. 1) It follows from formula (6) and Prop. 9 that the closure of a chamber C is the intersection of the closed half-spaces that are bounded by a wall of C and contain C.

2) Let F be a facet whose support is a hyperplane L; we shall show that F is a face of two chambers. Let $\mathfrak{N}$ be the set of hyperplanes $H \neq L$ belonging to $\mathfrak{H}$; put $A = D_{\mathfrak{N}}(F)$ and denote by D^+ and D^- the two open half-spaces bounded by L. The set A is open and contains $F \subset L$, and since every point of L is in the closure of D^+ and D^-, the sets $C^+ = A \cap D^+$ and $C^- = A \cap D^-$ are non-empty; these are chambers. Moreover, the hyperplane L meets $D_{\mathfrak{N}}(F) = D_{\mathfrak{N}}(C^+)$; Prop. 4 shows that L is a wall of C^+ and that

F, which meets $L \cap D_{\mathfrak{N}}(F)$, is a face of C^+; similarly, F is a face of C^-. Finally, let C be a chamber of which F is a face, and suppose for example that $D^+ = D_L(C)$; by Prop. 4, the set $D_{\mathfrak{N}}(C)$ meets F, and hence is equal to $D_{\mathfrak{N}}(F)$, and we have

$$C = D_{\mathfrak{H}}(C) = D_L(C) \cap D_{\mathfrak{N}}(C) = D^+ \cap D_{\mathfrak{N}}(F) = C^+.$$

5. INTERSECTING HYPERPLANES

Recall (*Algebra*, Chap. II, § 9, no. 3) that two affine subspaces P and P′ of E are said to be parallel if there exists a vector t in T such that $P' = t + P$. It is clear that the relation "P and P′ are parallel" is an equivalence relation on the set of affine subspaces of E.

Lemma 1. Any two non-parallel hyperplanes have non-empty intersection.

Let H and H′ be two non-parallel hyperplanes, $a \in H$ and $a' \in H'$; there exist two hyperplanes M and M′ of the vector space T such that $H = M + a$ and $H' = M' + a'$; since H and H′ are not parallel, we have $M \neq M'$ and hence $T = M + M'$; hence there exist $u \in M$ and $u' \in M'$ such that $a' - a = u - u'$, and the point $u + a = u' + a'$ belongs to $H \cap H'$.

Lemma 2. Let H *and* H′ *be two distinct hyperplanes of* E, *and* f, f' *two affine functions on* E *such that* H *(resp.* H′*) consists of the points* a *in* E *such that* $f(a) = 0$ *(resp.* $f'(a) = 0$*). Finally, let* L *be a hyperplane of* E. *Assume that one of the following hypotheses is satisfied:*

a) The hyperplanes H, H′ *and* L *are parallel.*

b) The hyperplanes H *and* H′ *are not parallel, and* $H \cap H' \subset L$.

Then there exist real numbers λ, λ', *not both zero, such that* L *consists of those points* $a \in E$ *at which the affine function* $g = \lambda.f + \lambda'.f'$ *vanishes.*

The lemma being trivial when $L = H$, we assume that there exists a point a in L with $a \notin H$. Put $\lambda = f'(a), \lambda' = -f(a)$ and

$$g = \lambda.f + \lambda'.f';$$

then $\lambda' \neq 0$ since $a \notin H$; moreover, since $H \neq H'$, there exists $b \in H$ such that $b \notin H'$, so that $f(b) = 0, f'(b) \neq 0$, and thus $g(b) = -f(a).f'(b)$ is non-zero. The set L_1 of points where the affine function $g \neq 0$ vanishes is then a hyperplane of E; we have $g(a) = 0$, so $a \in L_1$.

a) *Assume that* H *and* H′ *are parallel*: g and f both vanish at every point of $L_1 \cap H$, hence so does f' since $\lambda' \neq 0$; thus every point of $L_1 \cap H$ belongs to H′; but since H and H′ are parallel and distinct, they are disjoint, so $L_1 \cap H = \varnothing$, and Lemma 1 shows that L_1 is parallel to H. Since $a \in L$ and $a \in L_1$, we thus have $L = L_1$.

b) *Assume that* H *and* H′ *are not parallel*: by Lemma 1, there is a point c in $H \cap H'$; we give E the vector space structure obtained by taking c as the origin. Then $H \cap H'$ is a vector subspace of E of codimension 2, and since $a \notin H$, the vector subspace M of E generated by $H \cap H'$ and a is a hyperplane; since $H \cap H' \subset L \cap L_1$ and $a \in L \cap L_1$, we have $M \subset L \cap L_1$, hence $M = L = L_1$. Q.E.D.

PROPOSITION 10. *Let* C *be a chamber, let* H *and* H′ *be two walls of* C, *and let* L *be a hyperplane meeting* $D_H(C) \cap D_{H'}(C)$. *Assume that* H *is distinct from* H′ *and that one of the following conditions is satisfied:*

a) The hyperplanes H, H′ *and* L *are parallel.*

b) The hyperplanes H *and* H′ *are not parallel, and* $H \cap H' \subset L$.

Then, L *meets* C.

Let b (resp. b') be a point of the face of C with support H (resp. H′); it is immediate that every point of the segment $[bb']$ distinct from b and b' belongs to C.

Introduce an affine function f that vanishes at every point of H and is such that $f(x) > 0$ for x in $D_H(C)$; similarly, introduce an affine function f' having an analogous property with respect to H′. By applying Lemma 2, we can find numbers λ and λ' and an affine function g having the properties stated in the lemma. We have $(\lambda, \lambda') \neq (0,0)$, and for every point x of $L \cap D_H(C) \cap D_{H'}(C)$, we have $f(x) > 0$, $f'(x) > 0$ and $\lambda.f(x) + \lambda'.f'(x) = 0$, so $\lambda\lambda' < 0$. On the other hand, we have $g(b) = \lambda'.f'(b)$ and $g(b') = \lambda.f(b')$, and since $f(b') > 0$, $f'(b) > 0$, we have $g(b)g(b') < 0$. The points b and b' are thus strictly on opposite sides of the hyperplane L, hence there exists a point c of L which belongs to $[bb']$, and is distinct from b and b', hence that belongs to C.

6. EXAMPLES: SIMPLICIAL CONES AND SIMPLICES

a) Let a be a point of E, and $(e_1, \dots, e_d)$ a basis of T; every point of E can thus be written uniquely in the form

$$x = a + \xi_1.e_1 + \cdots + \xi_d.e_d \tag{7}$$

with $\xi_1, \dots, \xi_d$ being real numbers. Denote by e'_i the affine function on E which, at any $x \in E$, written in the form (7), takes the value ξ_i. Denote by H_i the hyperplane formed by those x such that $e'_i(x) = 0$, and by $\mathfrak{H}$ the set of hyperplanes $H_1, \dots, H_d$. For every subset J of the set $I = \{1, 2, \dots, d\}$, put $H_J = \bigcap_{i \in J} H_i$; for every sequence $(\varepsilon_1, \dots, \varepsilon_d)$ of numbers equal to 0, 1 or -1, denote by $F(\varepsilon_1, \dots, \varepsilon_d)$ the set of those $x \in E$ such that $e'_i(x)$ is of sign ε_i for all i in I (*General Topology*, Chap. 4, § 3, no. 2). It is immediate that the facets defined by $\mathfrak{H}$ in E are the sets $F(\varepsilon_1, \dots, \varepsilon_d)$ and that these sets are pairwise distinct; the support of $F(\varepsilon_1, \dots, \varepsilon_d)$ is equal to H_J if J is the set of $i \in I$ such that $\varepsilon_i = 0$; in particular, the chambers are the sets of the form $F(\varepsilon_1, \dots, \varepsilon_d)$ where each of the numbers ε_i is equal to 1 or -1.

The set $C = F(1, \dots, 1)$ formed by those x with $e'_i(x) > 0$ for all $i \in I$ is a chamber, called the *open simplicial cone with vertex* a *defined by the basis*

$(e_1, \ldots, e_d)$. Its closure consists of the points x such that $e'_i(x) \geqslant 0$ for all $i \in \mathrm{I}$ when $d \geqslant 1$; otherwise, its closure is empty. For every subset J of I, let $\mathrm{C_J}$ be the set of points x of E such that $e'_i(x) = 0$ for $i \in \mathrm{J}$ and $e'_i(x) > 0$ for $i \in \mathrm{I-J}$. Then $\mathrm{C_J}$ is a facet with support $\mathrm{H_J}$, and it is an open simplicial cone with vertex a in the affine space $\mathrm{H_J}$; moreover, $\overline{\mathrm{C}} = \bigcup_{\mathrm{J \subset I}} \mathrm{C_J}$. In particular, the walls of C are the hyperplanes H_i for $i \in \mathrm{I}$, and the face of C contained in H_i is equal to $\mathrm{C}_{\{i\}}$.

None of the sets $\mathrm{H}_i, \mathrm{H_J}, \mathrm{C}, \mathrm{C_J}$ and $\mathrm{F}(\varepsilon_1, \ldots, \varepsilon_d)$ change if we replace the basis $(e_1, \ldots, e_d)$ by a basis $(\lambda_1 e_1, \ldots, \lambda_d e_d)$ with $\lambda_i > 0$ for all i.

b) Suppose now that we are given an affinely free system of points of E, say $(a_0, a_1, \ldots, a_d)$. We know that every point of E can be written uniquely in the form $x = \xi_0.a_0 + \cdots + \xi_d.a_d$, where $\xi_0, \ldots, \xi_d$ are real numbers with $\xi_0 + \cdots + \xi_d = 1$ (*Algebra*, Chap. 2, § 9, no. 3). Define affine functions $f_0, \ldots, f_d$, the function f_i associating to the point x, written as above, the number ξ_i. Denote by H_i the hyperplane of E defined by $f_i(x) = 0$ and by $\mathfrak{H}$ the set of hyperplanes $\mathrm{H}_0, \mathrm{H}_1, \ldots, \mathrm{H}_d$; finally, put $\mathrm{I} = \{0, 1, \ldots, d\}$. The *open simplex with vertices* $a_0, \ldots, a_d$ is the set C of points x of E such that $f_i(x) > 0$ for all $i \in \mathrm{I}$; it is one of the chambers defined by $\mathfrak{H}$ in E. The closure of C is the set $\overline{\mathrm{C}}$ of points x such that $f_i(x) \geqslant 0$ for all $i \in \mathrm{I}$; it is the convex envelope of the finite set $\{a_0, \ldots, a_d\}$ and it is easy to see that the extreme points of $\overline{\mathrm{C}}$ are $a_0, \ldots, a_d$.

For any subset J of I distinct from I, put $\mathrm{H_J} = \bigcap_{i \in \mathrm{J}} \mathrm{H}_i$ and let $\mathrm{C_J}$ be the set of points x of E such that $f_i(x) = 0$ for $i \in \mathrm{J}$ and $f_i(x) > 0$ for $i \in \mathrm{I-J}$. The set $\mathrm{C_J}$ is an open simplex in the affine space $\mathrm{H_J}$ with vertices the points a_i for $i \in \mathrm{I-J}$; we have $\mathrm{C}_\varnothing = \mathrm{C}, \overline{\mathrm{C}} = \bigcup_{\mathrm{J \neq I}} \mathrm{C_J}$ and $\mathrm{C_J} \neq \mathrm{C_{J'}}$ if $\mathrm{J} \neq \mathrm{J'}$; moreover, $\mathrm{C_J}$ is a facet with support $\mathrm{H_J}$. In particular, the walls of C are $\mathrm{H}_0, \ldots, \mathrm{H}_d$ and $\mathrm{C}_{\{i\}}$ is the face contained in H_i.

For any non-empty subset K of I, let $\mathrm{B_K}$ be the set of points x of E such that $f_i(x) > 0$ for $i \in \mathrm{K}$ and $f_i(x) < 0$ for $i \in \mathrm{I-K}$. The sets $\mathrm{B_K}$ are the chambers defined by $\mathfrak{H}$ in E and we have $\mathrm{B_I} = \mathrm{C}$. It is easy to see that $\overline{\mathrm{C}}$ is compact; on the other hand, if K is a subset of I distinct from I, of cardinal p, the chamber $\mathrm{B_K}$ contains the sequence of points x_n defined for $n \geqslant 2$ by

$$f_i(x_n) = \begin{cases} n & \text{for } i \in \mathrm{K} \\ (1 - pn)/(d + 1 - p) & \text{for } i \in \mathrm{I-K} \end{cases}$$

showing that $\mathrm{B_K}$ is not relatively compact.

§ 2. REFLECTIONS

In this paragraph, K denotes a commutative field, assumed not to be a characteristic 2 from no. 2 onwards. We denote by V a vector space over K.

1. PSEUDO-REFLECTIONS

DEFINITION 1. *An endomorphism s of the vector space* V *is said to be a pseudo-reflection if* $1 - s$ *is of rank* 1.

Let s be a pseudo-reflection in V, and let D be the image of $1 - s$. By definition, D is of dimension 1; thus, given $a \neq 0$ in D, there exists a non-zero linear form a^* on V such that $x - s(x) = \langle x, a^* \rangle . a$ for all $x \in \mathrm{V}$.

Conversely, given $a \neq 0$ in V and a linear form $a^* \neq 0$ on V, the formula

$$s_{a,a^*}(x) = x - \langle x, a^* \rangle . a \quad (x \in \mathrm{V}) \tag{1}$$

defines a pseudo-reflection s_{a,a^*}; the image of $1 - s_{a,a^*}$ is generated by a and the kernel of $1 - s_{a,a^*}$ is the hyperplane of V consisting of those x such that $\langle x, a^* \rangle = 0$. If V^* is the dual of V, it is immediate that the transpose $s_{a^*,a}$ of s_{a,a^*} is the pseudo-reflection of V^* given by the formula

$$s_{a^*,a}(x^*) = x^* - \langle x^*, a \rangle . a^* \quad (x^* \in \mathrm{V}^*). \tag{2}$$

If a is a non-zero vector, a *pseudo-reflection with vector a* is any pseudo-reflection s such that a belongs to the image of $1 - s$. The *hyperplane of a pseudo-reflection s* is the kernel of $1 - s$, the set of vectors x such that $s(x) = x$.

PROPOSITION 1. *Let* G *be a group and ρ an irreducible linear representation of* G *on a vector space* V*; assume that there exists an element g of* G *such that $\rho(g)$ is a pseudo-reflection.*

(i) *Every endomorphism of* V *commuting with $\rho(\mathrm{G})$ is a homothety, and ρ is absolutely irreducible.*

(ii) *Assume that* V *is finite dimensional. Let* B *be a non-zero bilinear form on* V *invariant under $\rho(\mathrm{G})$. Then* B *is non-degenerate, either symmetric or skew-symmetric, and every bilinear form on* V *invariant under $\rho(\mathrm{G})$ is proportional to* B.

Let u be an endomorphism of V commuting with $\rho(\mathrm{G})$. Let g be an element of G such that $\rho(g)$ is a pseudo-reflection and let D be the image of $1 - \rho(g)$. Since D is of dimension 1 and $u(\mathrm{D}) \subset \mathrm{D}$, there exists α in K such that $u - \alpha.1$ vanishes on D; the kernel N of $u - \alpha.1$ is then a vector subspace of V invariant under $\rho(\mathrm{G})$ and is non-zero as it contains D; since ρ is irreducible, $\mathrm{N} = \mathrm{V}$ and $u = \alpha.1$. The second part of (i) follows from the first by *Algebra*, Chap. VIII, § 13, no. 4, Cor. of Prop. 5.

Let N (resp. N′) be the subspace of V consisting of those x such that $B(x,y)=0$ (resp. $B(y,x)=0$) for all y in V; since B is invariant under $\rho(G)$, the subspaces N and N′ of V are stable under $\rho(G)$ and distinct from V since $B \neq 0$. Since ρ is irreducible, $N = N' = 0$ and B is non-degenerate.

Since V is finite dimensional, every bilinear form on V is given by the formula

$$B'(x,y) = B(u(x),y) \tag{3}$$

for some endomorphism u of V. If B′ is invariant under $\rho(G)$, the endomorphism u commutes with $\rho(G)$. Indeed, let x, y be in V and let g be in G; since B and B′ are invariant under $\rho(G)$, we have

$$\begin{aligned} B(u(\rho(g)(x)),y) &= B'(\rho(g)(x),y) = B'(x,\rho(g^{-1})(y)) \\ &= B(u(x),\rho(g^{-1})(y)) = B(\rho(g)(u(x)),y), \end{aligned}$$

hence $u(\rho(g)(x)) = \rho(g)(u(x))$ since B is non-degenerate. By (i), there exists α in K with $u = \alpha.1$, so $B' = \alpha.B$.

In particular, we can apply this to the bilinear form $B'(x,y) = B(y,x)$; then $B(y,x) = \alpha.B(x,y) = \alpha^2.B(y,x)$ for all x, y in V, and since B is non-zero we have $\alpha^2 = 1$, hence $\alpha = 1$ or $\alpha = -1$. Thus, B is either symmetric or skew-symmetric.

2. REFLECTIONS

Recall that from now on, unless stated otherwise, the field K is assumed to be of characteristic different from 2. A *reflection* in V is a pseudo-reflection s such that $s^2 = 1$; if s is a reflection, we denote by V_s^+ the kernel of $s - 1$ and by V_s^- that of $s + 1$.

PROPOSITION 2. *Let s be an endomorphism of* V.

(i) *If s is a reflection,* V *is the direct sum of the hyperplane V_s^+ and the line V_s^-.*

(ii) *Conversely, assume that* V *is the direct sum of a hyperplane* H *and a line* D *such that $s(x) = x$ and $s(y) = -y$ for $x \in H$ and $y \in D$. Then s is a reflection and $H = V_s^+$, $D = V_s^-$. Finally,* D *is the image of $1 - s$.*

(i) If s is a reflection, V_s^+ is a hyperplane. If x belongs to $V_s^+ \cap V_s^-$, then $x = s(x) = -x$, so $x = 0$ since K is of characteristic $\neq 2$. Finally, for x in V, the vector $x' = s(x) + x$ (resp. $x'' = s(x) - x$) belongs to V_s^+ (resp. V_s^-) since $s^2 = 1$, and $2x = x' - x''$. Thus V is the direct sum of V_s^+ and V_s^-, and V_s^- is necessarily of dimension 1 since V_s^+ is a hyperplane.

(ii) Under the stated hypotheses, every element of V can be written uniquely in the form $v = x + y$ with $x \in H$ and $y \in D$ and we have $s(v) = x - y$; assertion (ii) follows immediately from this.

COROLLARY. *If* V *is finite dimensional, every reflection is of determinant* -1.

Let s be a reflection in V. Prop. 2, (i) shows that there exists a basis $(e_1, \dots, e_n)$ of V such that $s(e_1) = e_1, \dots, s(e_{n-1}) = e_{n-1}$ and $s(e_n) = -e_n$, hence $\det(s) = -1$.

PROPOSITION 3. *Let* s *be a reflection in* V.

(i) *A subspace* V' *of* V *is stable under* s *if and only if* $V_s^- \subset V'$ *or* $V' \subset V_s^+$.

(ii) *An endomorphism* u *of* V *commutes with* s *if and only if* V_s^+ *and* V_s^- *are stable under* u.

(i) If $V' \subset V_s^+$, then $s(x) = x$ for all x in V', so $s(V') \subset V'$. Assume that $V_s^- \subset V'$; then, for any x in V', $s(x) - x \in V_s^- \subset V'$, hence $s(x) \in V'$; thus $s(V') \subset V'$. Conversely, assume that $s(V') \subset V'$; if $V' \not\subset V_s^+$, there exists x in V' with $s(x) \neq x$; the non-zero vector $a = s(x) - x$ belongs to the line V_s^-, and hence generates this space; since $a \in V'$, we have $V_s^- \subset V'$.

(ii) Assume first that u commutes with s. If x is a vector such that $s(x) = \varepsilon.x$ (where $\varepsilon = \pm 1$), then $s(u(x)) = u(s(x)) = \varepsilon.u(x)$, so V_s^+ and V_s^- are stable under u. Conversely, assume that V_s^+ and V_s^- are stable under u; it is clear that $us - su$ vanishes on V_s^+ and on V_s^-, and since V is the direct sum of V_s^+ and V_s^-, we have $us - su = 0$.

COROLLARY. *Two distinct reflections* s *and* u *commute if and only if* $V_s^- \subset V_u^+$ *and* $V_u^- \subset V_s^+$.

If $V_s^- \subset V_u^+$ and $V_u^- \subset V_s^+$, Prop. 3, (i) shows that V_u^+ and V_u^- are stable under s, hence $su = us$ by Prop. 3, (ii).

Conversely, if $su = us$, the subspace V_s^- is stable under u by (ii); by (i), there are two possible cases:

a) We have $V_u^- \subset V_s^-$: since they are both of dimension 1, these spaces are therefore equal, hence $V_s^- \not\subset V_u^+$; since V_u^+ is stable under s, we have $V_u^+ \subset V_s^+$ and so these two hyperplanes are equal. But then $s = u$, contrary to our assumptions.

b) We have $V_s^- \subset V_u^+$: the image of $1-s$ is thus contained in the kernel of $1-u$, so $(1-u).(1-s) = 0$. Since s and u commute, we have $(1-s).(1-u) = 0$, in other words $V_u^- \subset V_s^+$.

Remark. Let $a \neq 0$ be in V and let a^* be a non-zero linear form on V: it follows from formula (1) that

$$s_{a,a^*}^2(x) = x + (\langle a, a^* \rangle - 2)\langle x, a^* \rangle.a$$

and hence that s_{a,a^*} *is a reflection if and only if* $\langle a, a^* \rangle = 2$. In this case, we have $s_{a,a^*}(a) = -a$.

3. ORTHOGONAL REFLECTIONS

Assume that V is finite dimensional. Let B be a non-degenerate bilinear form on V. By *Algebra*, Chap. IX, § 6, no. 3, Prop. 4, B is invariant under a reflection s in V if and only if the subspaces V_s^+ and V_s^- of V are orthogonal with respect to B; they are then non-isotropic. Moreover, for any non-isotropic hyperplane H in V, there is a unique reflection s that preserves B and induces the identity on H; this is the *symmetry with respect to* H, cf. *Algebra*, Chap. IX, §6, no. 3. If a is a non-zero vector orthogonal to H, we have $B(a,a) \neq 0$ and the reflection s is given by the formula

$$s(x) = x - 2\frac{B(x,a)}{B(a,a)}.a \quad \text{for any } x \in V, \tag{4}$$

by *Algebra*, Chap. IX, § 6, no. 4, formula (6). The reflection s is also called the *orthogonal reflection with respect to* H.

PROPOSITION 4. *Assume that* V *is finite dimensional. Let* B *be a non-degenerate symmetric bilinear form on* V, X *a subspace of* V *and* X^0 *the orthogonal complement of* X *with respect to* B; *finally, let* s *be the orthogonal reflection with respect to a non-isotropic hyperplane* H *of* V. *The following conditions are equivalent:*

(i) X *is stable under* s.
(ii) X^0 *is stable under* s.
(iii) H *contains* X *or* X^0.

We have $V_s^+ = H$, and by what we have said, V_s^- is the orthogonal complement H^0 of H with respect to B. By Prop. 3, X is stable under s if and only if $X \subset H$ or $H^0 \subset X$; but the relation $H^0 \subset X$ is equivalent to $X^0 \subset H$ by *Algebra*, Chap. IX, § 1, no. 6, Cor. 1 to Prop. 4. This proves the equivalence of (i) and (iii); that of (ii) and (iii) follows by interchanging the roles of X and X^0, since $(X^0)^0 = X$.

4. ORTHOGONAL REFLECTIONS IN A EUCLIDEAN AFFINE SPACE

We retain the notation of the preceding number, and let E be an affine space of which V is the space of translations. Giving the form B on V provides E with the structure of a *euclidean space* (*Algebra*, Chap. IX, § 6, no. 6).

Let H be a non-isotropic hyperplane of E. The symmetry with respect to H (*Algebra*, Chap. IX, § 6, no. 6) is also called the *orthogonal reflection with respect to* H; we often denote it by s_H. We have $s_H^2 = 1$ and s_H is the unique *displacement* (*loc. cit.*, Def. 3) of E, distinct from the identity and leaving fixed the elements of H. The automorphism of V associated to s_H is the orthogonal reflection with respect to the direction of H (which is a non-isotropic hyperplane of V).

Every x in E can be written uniquely in the form $x = h + v$, with $h \in \mathrm{H}$ and $v \in \mathrm{V}$ orthogonal to H; we have

$$s_{\mathrm{H}}(h + v) = h - v.$$

PROPOSITION 5. *Let* H *and* H′ *be two parallel, non-isotropic hyperplanes of* E. *There exists a unique vector* $v \in \mathrm{V}$ *orthogonal to* H *and such that* $\mathrm{H}' = \mathrm{H} + v$. *The displacement* $s_{\mathrm{H}'}s_{\mathrm{H}}$ *is the translation by the vector* $2v$.

The existence and uniqueness of v are immediate. The automorphism of V associated to $s_{\mathrm{H}'}s_{\mathrm{H}}$ is the identity; thus $s_{\mathrm{H}'}s_{\mathrm{H}}$ is a translation. On the other hand, let $a \in \mathrm{H}'$; then $a - v \in \mathrm{H}$ and

$$s_{\mathrm{H}'}s_{\mathrm{H}}(a - v) = s_{\mathrm{H}'}(a - v) = a + v = (a - v) + 2v,$$

showing that $s_{\mathrm{H}'}s_{\mathrm{H}}$ is the translation by the vector $2v$.

COROLLARY. *Let* H *and* H′ *be two distinct, parallel, non-isotropic hyperplanes. If* K *is of characteristic zero (resp.* $p > 0$, *with* $p \neq 2$*), the group of displacements of* E *generated by* s_{H} *and* $s_{\mathrm{H}'}$ *is an infinite dihedral group (resp. a dihedral group of order* $2p$*).*

Indeed, by Prop. 2 of Chap. IV, § 1, no. 2, it suffices to show that $s_{\mathrm{H}'}s_{\mathrm{H}}$ is of infinite order (resp. order $2p$), which is clear.

Remark. We retain the notation of Prop. 5 and assume in addition that $\mathrm{K} = \mathbf{R}$. Put $s = s_{\mathrm{H}}$ and $s' = s_{\mathrm{H}'}$. Let H_n be the hyperplane $\mathrm{H} + n.v$ and let C_n be the set of points of E of the form $a + \xi.v$ with $a \in \mathrm{H}$ and $n < \xi < n + 1$. The C_n are connected open sets forming a partition of $\mathrm{E} - \bigcup_n \mathrm{H}_n$. They are therefore the *chambers* defined by the system $\mathfrak{H} = (\mathrm{H}_n)_{n \in \mathbf{Z}}$ in E. The translation $(s's)^n$ transforms the chamber $\mathrm{C} = \mathrm{C}_0$ into the chamber C_{2n}, and since $s(\mathrm{C}_0) = \mathrm{C}_{-1}$, we have $(s's)^n s(\mathrm{C}) = \mathrm{C}_{2n-1}$. It follows that *the dihedral group* W *generated by* s *and* s' *permutes the chambers* C_n *simply-transitively*. Moreover, as we shall now show, *if the chambers* C *and* $w(\mathrm{C})$ *are on opposite sides of* H (for $w \in \mathrm{W}$), *we have* $l(sw) = l(w) - 1$ (the lengths being taken with respect to $\mathrm{S} = \{s, s'\}$ (Chap. IV, § 1, no. 1)). Indeed, we then have $w(\mathrm{C}) = \mathrm{C}_n$ for some $n < 0$. If $n = -2k$, then $w = (ss')^k$ and $sw = (s's)^{k-1}s'$, so $l(w) = 2k$ and $l(sw) = 2k - 1$ (Chap. IV, § 1, no. 2, *Remark*). If $n = -2k - 1$, then $w = (ss')^k s$ and $sw = (s's)^k$, so $l(w) = 2k + 1$ and $l(sw) = 2k$.

5. COMPLEMENTS ON PLANE ROTATIONS

In this no., V denotes a real vector space of dimension 2, provided with a *scalar product* (that is, a *non-degenerate*, positive, symmetric bilinear form) and an *orientation*. The measures of angles will be taken with respect to the base 2π; the principal measure of an angle between half-lines (resp. lines) is thus a real number θ such that $0 \leqslant \theta < 2\pi$ (resp. $0 \leqslant \theta < \pi$) (*General Topology*, Chap. VIII, § 2, no. 3 and no. 6). By abuse of language, for any real number θ, we shall use θ to denote an angle whose measure is θ and denote by ρ_θ the rotation with angle θ (*Algebra*, Chap. IX, § 10, no. 3).

PROPOSITION 6. *Let s be the orthogonal reflection with respect to a line* D *of* V. *If Δ and Δ' are two half-lines starting at the origin (resp. two lines passing through the origin) of* V, *we have*

$$(\widehat{s(\Delta), s(\Delta')}) \equiv -(\widehat{\Delta, \Delta'}) \quad (\text{mod. } 2\pi) \quad (\text{resp. } (\text{mod. } \pi)).$$

Let u be a rotation transforming Δ into Δ'. Since su is an orthogonal transformation of V of determinant -1, it is a reflection and thus $(su)^2 = 1$. Consequently, $u^{-1} = sus^{-1}$ transforms $s(\Delta)$ into $s(\Delta')$, hence the proposition.

COROLLARY. *Let* D *and* D′ *be two lines of* V *and let θ be a measure of the angle* $(\widehat{\mathrm{D}, \mathrm{D}'})$. *Then* $s_{\mathrm{D}'}s_{\mathrm{D}} = \rho_{2\theta}$.

We know that $s_{\mathrm{D}'}s_{\mathrm{D}}$ is a rotation since it is of determinant 1. Let Δ and Δ' be two half-lines starting at the origin carried by D and D′. We have

$$\begin{aligned}(\widehat{\Delta, s_{\mathrm{D}'}s_{\mathrm{D}}(\Delta)}) &\equiv (\widehat{\Delta, s_{\mathrm{D}'}(\Delta)}) \equiv (\widehat{\Delta, \Delta'}) + (\widehat{\Delta', s_{\mathrm{D}'}(\Delta)}) \\ &\equiv (\widehat{\Delta, \Delta'}) + (\widehat{s_{\mathrm{D}'}(\Delta'), s_{\mathrm{D}'}(\Delta)}) \\ &\equiv (\widehat{\Delta, \Delta'}) - (\widehat{\Delta', \Delta}) \equiv 2(\widehat{\Delta, \Delta'}) \quad (\text{mod. } 2\pi),\end{aligned}$$

hence the corollary.

Now let Δ and Δ' be two half-lines of V such that

$$\Delta \neq \Delta' \quad \text{and} \quad \Delta \neq -\Delta',$$

and let s and s' be the orthogonal reflections with respect to the lines D and D′ containing Δ and Δ'. Let θ be the principal measure of the angle $(\widehat{\mathrm{D}, \mathrm{D}'})$. If $\theta \in \pi\mathbf{Q}$, denote by m the smallest integer $\geqslant 1$ such that $m\theta \in \pi\mathbf{Z}$. If $\theta \notin \pi\mathbf{Q}$, put $m = \infty$. Let W be the group generated by s and s'.

PROPOSITION 7. *The group* W *is dihedral* (Chap. IV, § 1, no. 2) *of order* $2m$. *It consists of the rotations $\rho_{2n\theta}$ and the products $\rho_{2n\theta}s$ for $n \in \mathbf{Z}$. The transforms of* D *and* D′ *by the elements of* W *are the transforms of* D *by the rotations $\rho_{n\theta}$ for $n \in \mathbf{Z}$.*

The Corollary to Prop. 6 shows that $s's$ is of order m, which gives the first assertion. The elements of W are thus of the form $(s's)^n = \rho_{2n\theta}$ or $(s's)^n s = \rho_{2n\theta}s$; the last assertion follows from this, since $\mathrm{D}' = \rho_\theta(\mathrm{D})$.

COROLLARY. *Let* C *be the open angular sector formed by the union of the open half-lines Δ_1 starting at the origin and such that* $0 < (\widehat{\Delta, \Delta_1}) < \theta$. *Then* *no transform of* D *or* D′ *by an element of* W *meets* C *if and only if* m *is finite and*

$$\theta = \pi/m.$$

If $m = \infty$, the image of the set $n\theta$ $(n \in \mathbf{Z})$ is dense in $\mathbf{R}/2\pi\mathbf{Z}$ (*General Topology*, Chap. VII, § 1, Prop. 11); the union of the transforms of D by the elements of W is thus dense in V and meets C. If m is finite and if $\theta = k\pi/m$ with $1 < k < m$, the integers k and m being relatively prime, there exists an integer h such that $hk \equiv 1$ mod. m; then $(\widehat{\mathrm{D}, \rho_{h\theta}(\mathrm{D})}) \equiv \pi/m \pmod{\pi}$, and $\rho_{h\theta}(\mathrm{D})$ meets C. This shows that the condition is necessary. The converse is immediate.

Remark. Assume that m is finite and that $\theta = \pi/m$. If $n \in \mathbf{Z}$, let C_n be the union of the open half-lines Δ_1 starting at 0 such that

$$n\theta < (\widehat{\Delta, \Delta_1}) < (n+1)\theta.$$

The C_n for $-m \leqslant n < m$ are connected open subsets forming a partition of $\mathrm{E} - \bigcup_n \mathrm{D}_n$ (where $\mathrm{D}_n = \rho_{n\theta}(\mathrm{D})$). These are therefore the *chambers* determined in E by the system of m lines D_n $(1 \leqslant n \leqslant m)$. We have $\mathrm{C}_{2k} = \rho_{2k\theta}(\mathrm{C})$ and $\mathrm{C}_{2k-1} = \rho_{2k\theta}s(\mathrm{C})$. Moreover, $\mathrm{C}_n = \mathrm{C}$ if and only if $n \in 2m\mathbf{Z}$. Consequently, *the group* W *permutes the chambers* C_n *simply-transitively.*

We show finally that, *if* $w \in \mathrm{W}$ *is such that the chambers* C *and* $w(\mathrm{C})$ *are on opposite sides of the line* D, *then* $l(sw) = l(w) - 1$ (the lengths being taken with respect to $\mathrm{S} = \{s, s'\}$). Indeed, the assumption implies that $w(\mathrm{C}) = \mathrm{C}_n$ with $-m \leqslant n < 0$. If $n = -2k$, we have $w = (ss')^k$ and $sw = s'(ss')^{k-1}$, so $l(w) = 2k$ and $l(sw) = 2k - 1$ (Chap. IV, § 1, no. 2, *Remark*). If $n = -2k+1$, we have

$$w = (ss')^{k-1}s \quad \text{and} \quad sw = (s's)^{k-1},$$

hence $l(w) = 2k - 1$ and $l(sw) = 2k - 2$. Q.E.D.

§ 3. GROUPS OF DISPLACEMENTS GENERATED BY REFLECTIONS

In this paragraph, we denote by E a *real* affine space of finite dimension d, and by T the space of translations of E. We assume that T is provided with a scalar product (that is, a *non-degenerate*, positive, symmetric bilinear form), denoted by $(t|t')$. For $t \in \mathrm{T}$, put $\| t \| = (t|t)^{1/2}$. The function $d(x, y) = \| x - y \|$ is a distance on E, which defines the topology of E (§ 1).

We denote by $\mathfrak{H}$ a set of hyperplanes of E and by W the group of displacements of the euclidean space E generated by the orthogonal reflections

s_{H} with respect to the hyperplanes $\mathrm{H} \in \mathfrak{H}$ (§ 2, no. 4). We assume that the following conditions are satisfied:

(D1) *For any* $w \in \mathrm{W}$ *and any* $\mathrm{H} \in \mathfrak{H}$, *the hyperplane* $w(\mathrm{H})$ *belongs to* $\mathfrak{H}$;
(D2) *The group* W, *provided with the discrete topology, acts properly on* E.

Since E is locally compact, it follows from the *Remark* of § 4, no. 5 of *General Topology*, Chap. III, that condition (D2) is equivalent to the following condition:

(D′2) *For any two compact subsets* K *and* L *of* E, *the set of* $w \in \mathrm{W}$ *such that* $w(\mathrm{K})$ *meets* L *is finite.*

1. PRELIMINARY RESULTS

Lemma 1. The set of hyperplanes $\mathfrak{H}$ *is locally finite.*

Indeed, let K be a compact subset of E. If a hyperplane $\mathrm{H} \in \mathfrak{H}$ meets K, the set $s_{\mathrm{H}}(\mathrm{K})$ also meets K, since every point of $\mathrm{K} \cap \mathrm{H}$ is fixed by s_{H}. The set of $\mathrm{H} \in \mathfrak{H}$ meeting K is thus finite by (D′2).

We can thus apply to E and $\mathfrak{H}$ the definitions and results of § 1. We shall call the chambers, facets, walls, etc. defined in E by $\mathfrak{H}$ simply the chambers, facets, walls, etc. relative to W. Any displacement $w \in \mathrm{W}$ permutes the chambers, facets, walls, etc.

Lemma 2. Let C *be a chamber.*

(i) *For any* $x \in \mathrm{E}$, *there exists an element* $w \in \mathrm{W}$ *such that* $w(x) \in \overline{\mathrm{C}}$.

(ii) *For any chamber* C′, *there is an element* $w \in \mathrm{W}$ *such that* $w(\mathrm{C}') = \mathrm{C}$.

(iii) *The group* W *is generated by the set of orthogonal reflections with respect to the walls of* C.

Let $\mathfrak{M}$ be the set of walls of C and let $\mathrm{W}_{\mathfrak{M}}$ be the subgroup of W generated by the reflections with respect to the walls of C.

(i) Let $x \in \mathrm{E}$ and let J be the orbit of x under the group $\mathrm{W}_{\mathfrak{M}}$. It suffices to prove that J meets $\overline{\mathrm{C}}$.

Let a be a point of C; there is a closed ball B with centre a meeting J; since B is compact, property (D′2) of no. 1 shows that $\mathrm{B} \cap \mathrm{J}$ is finite. Hence, there exists a point y of J such that

$$d(a, y) \leqslant d(a, y') \quad \text{for all } y' \text{ in J.} \tag{1}$$

We shall prove that $y \in \overline{\mathrm{C}}$. For this, it suffices to show that if H is a wall of C then $y \in \overline{\mathrm{D}_{\mathrm{H}}(\mathrm{C})}$ (cf. § 1, no. 4, Prop. 9). Since $s_{\mathrm{H}} \in \mathrm{W}_{\mathfrak{M}}$, we have $s_{\mathrm{H}}(y) \in \mathrm{J}$ and so (fig. 1)

$$d(a, y)^2 \leqslant d(a, s_{\mathrm{H}}(y))^2 \tag{2}$$

by (1). There exist $b \in \mathrm{H}$ and two vectors t and u such that $a = b + t$ and $y = b + u$, the vector u being orthogonal to H; then $s_{\mathrm{H}}(y) = b - u$, and (2) is equivalent to $(t - u|t - u) \leqslant (t + u|t + u)$, or to $(t|u) \geqslant 0$. This inequality implies that $y \in \mathrm{D_H(C)}$.

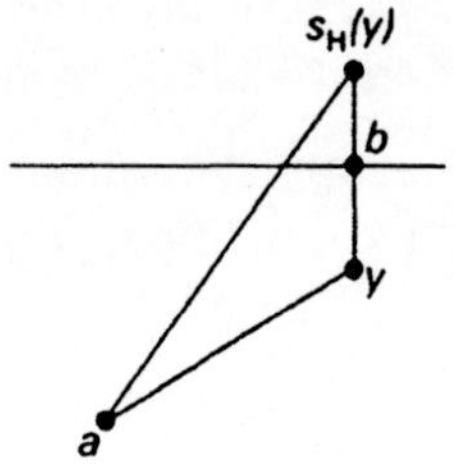

Fig. 1

(ii) Let C′ be a chamber and $a' \in \mathrm{C}'$. By what we have proved, there exists $w \in \mathrm{W}_{\mathfrak{M}}$ such that $w^{-1}(a') \in \overline{\mathrm{C}}$; hence, the chamber C′ meets $\overline{w(\mathrm{C})}$; since $\overline{w(\mathrm{C})}$ is the union of $w(\mathrm{C})$ and facets with empty interior (§ 1, no. 2, Prop. 3), we have $\mathrm{C}' = w(\mathrm{C})$.

(iii) We have to prove that $\mathrm{W} = \mathrm{W}_{\mathfrak{M}}$ and for this it suffices to prove that $s_{\mathrm{H}'} \in \mathrm{W}_{\mathfrak{M}}$ for all $\mathrm{H}' \in \mathfrak{H}$. Now H′ is a wall of at least one chamber C′ (§ 1, no. 4, Prop. 8); we have seen that there exists $w \in \mathrm{W}_{\mathfrak{M}}$ such that $\mathrm{C}' = w(\mathrm{C})$; consequently, there exists a wall H of C such that $\mathrm{H}' = w(\mathrm{H})$, hence $s_{\mathrm{H}'} = w.s_{\mathrm{H}}.w^{-1} \in \mathrm{W}_{\mathfrak{M}}$.

2. RELATION WITH COXETER SYSTEMS

THEOREM 1. *Let* C *be a chamber and let* S *be the set of reflections with respect to the walls of* C.

(i) *The pair* (W, S) *is a Coxeter system.*

(ii) *Let* $w \in \mathrm{W}$ *and let* H *be a wall of* C. *The relation* $l(s_{\mathrm{H}}w) > l(w)$ *implies that the chambers* C *and* $w(\mathrm{C})$ *are on the same side of* H.

(iii) *For any chamber* C′, *there exists a unique element* $w \in \mathrm{W}$ *such that* $w(\mathrm{C}) = \mathrm{C}'$.

(iv) *The set of hyperplanes* H *such that* $s_{\mathrm{H}} \in \mathrm{W}$ *is equal to* $\mathfrak{H}$.

Every element of S is of order 2 and Lemma 2 shows that S generates W. For any wall H of C, denote by $\mathrm{P_H}$ the set of elements $w \in \mathrm{W}$ such that the chambers C and $w(\mathrm{C})$ (which do not meet H) are on the same side of H. We shall verify conditions (A′), (B′) and (C) of Chap. IV, § 1, no. 7.

(A′) $1 \in \mathrm{P_H}$: Trivial.

(B′) $\mathrm{P_H}$ *and* $s_{\mathrm{H}}.\mathrm{P_H}$ *are disjoint*: Indeed, $w(\mathrm{C})$ and $s_{\mathrm{H}}w(\mathrm{C})$ are on opposite sides of H, so if $w(\mathrm{C})$ is on the same side of H as C, it is not on the same side as $s_{\mathrm{H}}w(\mathrm{C})$.

(C) *Let* $w \in \mathrm{P_H}$ *and let* H′ *be a wall of* C *such that* $ws_{\mathrm{H}'} \notin \mathrm{P_H}$; *then* $ws_{\mathrm{H}'} = s_{\mathrm{H}}w$: By assumption, $w(\mathrm{C})$ is on the same side of H as C and $ws_{\mathrm{H}'}(\mathrm{C})$ is on the other side. Thus, $ws_{\mathrm{H}'}(\mathrm{C})$ and $w(\mathrm{C})$ are on opposite sides of H; hence, the chambers $s_{H'}(C)$ and C are on opposite sides of the hyperplane $w^{-1}(H)$. Let a be a point of the face of C with support H′. The point $a = s_{H'}(a)$ is in the closure of the two chambers C and $s_{H'}(C)$ that are contained respectively in the two open half-spaces bounded by $w^{-1}(H)$; thus, $a \in w^{-1}(H)$, so $H' = w^{-1}(H)$. From this we deduce that $s_{H'} = w^{-1}s_H w$, hence $ws_{H'} = s_H w$.

Assertions (i) and (ii) follow from this and Prop. 6 of Chap. IV, § 1, no. 7. Moreover, we have (*loc. cit.*, condition (A))

$$\bigcap_{H \in \mathfrak{M}} P_H = \{1\}. \tag{3}$$

Lemma 2 shows that W acts transitively on the set of chambers. Moreover, if $w \in W$ is such that $w(C) = C$, then $w \in P_H$ for every wall H of C, hence $w = 1$ by (3). This proves (iii).

Finally, let H be a hyperplane such that $s_H \in W$. If H did not belong to $\mathfrak{H}$, there would be at least one chamber C′ meeting H (§1, no. 3, Prop. 7). Every point of $H \cap C'$ is invariant under s_H, and thus belongs to the chambers C′ and $s_H(C')$; thus, $C' = s_H(C')$, which contradicts (iii) since $s_H \neq 1$.

COROLLARY. *Let Σ be a set of reflections generating* W. *Then every reflection belonging to* W *is conjugate to an element of Σ.*

Let $\mathfrak{H}'$ be the set of hyperplanes of the form $w(H)$ with $w \in W$ and $H \in \mathfrak{H}$ such that $s_H \in \Sigma$. Since W is generated by the family $(s_H)_{H \in \mathfrak{H}'}$ and since $\mathfrak{H}'$ is stable under W, we can apply all the results of this no. to $\mathfrak{H}'$ instead of $\mathfrak{H}$; but Th. 1, (iv) shows that every reflection in W is of the form s_H with $H \in \mathfrak{H}'$, hence the corollary.

3. FUNDAMENTAL DOMAIN, STABILISERS

Recall (*Integration*, Chap. VII, § 2, no. 10, Def. 2) that a subset D of E is called a *fundamental domain* for the group W if every orbit of W in E meets D in exactly one point. This is equivalent to the following pair of conditions:

a) For every $x \in E$, there exists $w \in W$ such that $w(x) \in D$.

b) If $x, y \in D$ and $w \in W$ are such that $y = w(x)$, then $y = x$ (even though we may have $w \neq 1$).

We are going to prove the following three statements:

THEOREM 2. *For any chamber* C, *the closure $\overline{C}$ of* C *is a fundamental domain for the action of* W *on* E.

PROPOSITION 1. *Let* F *be a facet and* C *a chamber such that $F \subset \overline{C}$. Let $w \in W$. The following conditions are equivalent:*

(i) *$w(F)$ meets F;*

(ii) *$w(F) = F$;*

(iii) *$w(\overline{F}) = \overline{F}$;*

(iv) *w fixes at least one point of* F;
(v) *w fixes every point of* F;
(vi) *w fixes every point of* $\overline{\mathrm{F}}$;
(vii) *w belongs to the subgroup of* W *generated by the reflections with respect to the walls of* C *containing* F.

For every subset A of E, denote by W(A) the subgroup of W consisting of the elements that fix every point of A.

PROPOSITION 2. *Let* A *be a non-empty subset of* E, *let* $\mathfrak{H}_{\mathrm{A}}$ *be the set of hyperplanes* $\mathrm{H} \in \mathfrak{H}$ *containing* A, *let* A′ *be the intersection of the* $\mathrm{H} \in \mathfrak{H}_{\mathrm{A}}$, *and let* F *be a facet of* E *open in* A′ (§1, no. 3, Prop. 7). *Then* $\mathrm{W(A)} = \mathrm{W(A')} = \mathrm{W(F)}$, *and* W(A) *is generated by the reflections with respect to the hyperplanes in* $\mathfrak{H}_{\mathrm{A}}$.

We first prove the following assertion:

(I) *Let* C *be a chamber, let x and y be two points of* $\overline{\mathrm{C}}$ *and let* $w \in \mathrm{W}$ *be such that* $w(x) = y$. *Then* $x = y$ *and w belongs to the subgroup* $\mathrm{W}_{\mathfrak{N}}$, *where* $\mathfrak{N}$ *is the set of walls of* C *containing x.*

We argue by induction on the length q of w (relative to the set S of reflections with respect to the walls of C), the case $q = 0$ being obvious. If $q \geqslant 1$, there exist a wall H of C and an element $w' \in \mathrm{W}$ such that $w = s_{\mathrm{H}}w'$ and $l(w') = q - 1$. Since $l(s_{\mathrm{H}}w) < l(w)$, the chambers C and $w(\mathrm{C})$ are on opposite sides of H by Th. 1 of no. 2. Thus, $\overline{\mathrm{C}} \cap w(\overline{\mathrm{C}}) \subset \mathrm{H}$, so $y \in \mathrm{H}$. Thus $y = w'(x)$ and the induction hypothesis implies that $x = y$ and $w' \in \mathrm{W}_{\mathfrak{N}}$. Since $y \in \mathrm{H}$, it follows that $\mathrm{H} \in \mathfrak{N}$, and hence that $w = s_{\mathrm{H}}w' \in \mathrm{W}_{\mathfrak{N}}$, completing the proof of (I).

Proof of Theorem 2: this follows from (I) and Lemma 2.

Proof of Proposition 1: we know that two distinct facets are disjoint and have distinct closures (§1, no. 2, Cor. of Prop. 3). The equivalence of (i), (ii) and (iii) follows. On the other hand, it is clear that

$$\text{(vii)} \Longrightarrow \text{(vi)} \Longrightarrow \text{(v)} \Longrightarrow \text{(iv)} \Longrightarrow \text{(i)}$$

and assertion (I) shows that (i) $\Longrightarrow$ (vii).

Proof of Proposition 2: let A″ be the affine subspace of E generated by A. Clearly, $\mathrm{W(A)} = \mathrm{W(A'')}$. By Prop. 7 of §1, no. 3, there exists a point $x \in \mathrm{A''}$ that does not belong to any hyperplane $\mathrm{H} \in \mathfrak{H} - \mathfrak{H}_{\mathrm{A}}$. Let F_x be the facet containing x: it is open in A″ and Prop. 1 shows that

$$\mathrm{W}(\mathrm{F}_x) \subset \mathrm{W(A')} \subset \mathrm{W(A)} = \mathrm{W(A'')} \subset \mathrm{W}(\{x\}) = \mathrm{W}(\mathrm{F}_x),$$

hence $\mathrm{W(A)} = \mathrm{W(A')} = \mathrm{W}(\mathrm{F}_x)$. Replacing A by F, we also have

$$\mathrm{W(A)} = \mathrm{W(F)},$$

hence the proposition.

Remarks. 1) It follows from Th. 2 that, if C is a chamber and F a facet, *there exists a unique facet* F′ *contained in* $\overline{\mathrm{C}}$ *that is transformed into* F *by an element of* W.

2) It follows from Props. 1 and 2 that, for any non-empty subset A of E, there exists a point $a \in \mathrm{E}$ such that $\mathrm{W(A)} = \mathrm{W}(\{a\})$; moreover, the group W(A) is a *Coxeter group* (Th. 1).

3) Let C be a chamber of E and S the set of reflections with respect to the walls of C. Let $w \in \mathrm{W}$ and let $(s_1, \ldots, s_q)$ be a reduced decomposition of w with respect to S. If $x \in \overline{\mathrm{C}}$ is fixed by w, then $s_j(x) = x$ for all j: this follows from Prop. 1 above and Cor. 1 of Prop. 7 of Chap. IV, § 1.

4. COXETER MATRIX AND COXETER GRAPH OF W

Let C be a chamber, S = S(C) the set of orthogonal reflections with respect to the walls of C and $\mathrm{M} = (m(s, s'))$ the Coxeter matrix of the Coxeter system (W, S) (Chap. IV, § 1, no. 9): recall that $m(s, s')$ is the order (finite or infinite) of the element ss' of W (for $s, s' \in \mathrm{S}$). If C′ is another chamber, the unique element $w \in \mathrm{W}$ such that $w(\mathrm{C}) = \mathrm{C}'$ defines a bijection

$$s \mapsto f(s) = wsw^{-1}$$

from S to S′ = S(C′), and we have $m(f(s), f(s')) = m(s, s')$. It follows that, if W acts on the set X of pairs (C, s), where C is a chamber and $s \in \mathrm{S(C)}$, by $w.(\mathrm{C}, s) = (w(\mathrm{C}), wsw^{-1})$, each orbit i of W in X meets each of the sets $\{\mathrm{C}\} \times \mathrm{S(C)}$ in exactly one point, which we denote by $(\mathrm{C}, s_i(\mathrm{C}))$. Thus, if I is the set of orbits and $i, j \in \mathrm{I}$, the number $m_{ij} = m(s_i(\mathrm{C}), s_j(\mathrm{C}))$ is independent of the choice of chamber C. The matrix $\mathrm{M(W)} = (m_{ij})_{i,j \in \mathrm{I}}$ is a Coxeter matrix called the *Coxeter matrix* of W. The Coxeter graph associated to M(W) (Chap. IV, § 1, no. 9) is called the *Coxeter graph* of W.

Let C be a chamber. For any $i \in \mathrm{I}$, denote by $\mathrm{H}_i(\mathrm{C})$ the wall of C such that $s_i(\mathrm{C})$ is the reflection with respect to $\mathrm{H}_i(\mathrm{C})$ and by $e_i(\mathrm{C})$ the unit vector orthogonal to $\mathrm{H}_i(\mathrm{C})$ on the same side of $\mathrm{H}_i(\mathrm{C})$ as C. The map $i \mapsto \mathrm{H}_i(\mathrm{C})$ is called the *canonically indexed family of walls of* C.

PROPOSITION 3. *Let* C *be a chamber and let* $i, j \in \mathrm{I}$ *with* $i \neq j$. *Put* $s_i = s_i(\mathrm{C})$, $\mathrm{H}_i = \mathrm{H}_i(\mathrm{C})$, $e_i = e_i(\mathrm{C})$ *and define* s_j, H_j *and* e_j *similarly.*

(i) *If* H_i *and* H_j *are parallel, then* $m_{ij} = \infty$ *and* $e_i = -e_j$.

(ii) *If* H_i *and* H_j *are not parallel, then* m_{ij} *is finite and*

$$(e_i | e_j) = -\cos(\pi / m_{ij}). \tag{4}$$

(iii) *We have* $(e_i | e_j) \leqslant 0$.

If H_i and H_j are parallel, $s_i s_j$ is a translation (§ 2, no. 4, Prop. 5), so $m_{ij} = \infty$. Moreover, either $e_i = e_j$ or $e_i = -e_j$. Now, there exists a point a (resp. a') in the closure of C that belongs to H_i (resp. H_j) but not to H_j

(resp. H_i). Then $(a' - a|e_i) > 0$ and $(a - a'|e_j) > 0$, which excludes the case $e_i = e_j$ and proves (i).

Assume now that H_i and H_j are not parallel. Choose an origin $a \in H_i \cap H_j$ and identify T with E by the bijection $t \mapsto a+t$. Let V be the plane orthogonal to $H_i \cap H_j$ and passing through a. Put $\Gamma = V \cap D_{H_i}(C) \cap D_{H_j}(C)$ (where $D_H(C)$ denotes the open half-space bounded by H and containing C (§1, no. 1)) and let D (resp. D′) be the half-line in V contained in $H_i \cap V$ (resp. $H_j \cap V$) and in the closure of Γ. For a suitable orientation of V, the set Γ is the union of the open half-lines Δ in V such that

$$0 < (\widehat{D, \Delta}) < (\widehat{D, D'}).$$

Let W′ be the subgroup of W generated by s_i and s_j. For any $w \in W'$, the hyperplanes $w(H_i)$ and $w(H_j)$ belong to $\mathfrak{H}$, contain $H_i \cap H_j$ and do not meet C. It follows that they do not meet Γ (§ 1, no. 5, Prop. 10). The Cor. of Prop. 7 of § 2, no. 5 thus implies (ii).

Finally, assertion (iii) follows immediately from (i) and (ii), since $m_{ij} \geqslant 2$ for $i \neq j$.

Remark. Formula (4) is actually valid for all $i, j \in I$: in fact, $\pi/m_{ij} = 0$ if $m_{ij} = \infty$, and if $i = j$ then $m_{ij} = 1$ and $(e_i|e_j) = 1$.

5. SYSTEMS OF VECTORS WITH NEGATIVE SCALAR PRODUCTS

Lemma 3. Let q be a positive quadratic form on a real vector space V *and let* B *be the associated symmetric bilinear form. Let $a_1, \ldots, a_n$ be elements of* V *such that* $B(a_i, a_j) \leqslant 0$ *for* $i \neq j$.

(i) *If $c_1, \ldots, c_n$ are real numbers such that* $q\left(\sum_i c_i a_i\right) = 0$, *then*

$$q\left(\sum_i |c_i| a_i\right) = 0.$$

(ii) *If q is non-degenerate and if there exists a linear form f on* V *such that $f(a_i) > 0$ for all i, the vectors $a_1, \ldots, a_n$ are linearly independent.*

The relation $B(a_i, a_j) \leqslant 0$ for $i \neq j$ immediately implies that

$$q\left(\sum_i |c_i| a_i\right) \leqslant q\left(\sum_i c_i a_i\right),$$

hence (i). If q is non-degenerate, the relation $\sum_i c_i a_i = 0$ thus implies that

$$\sum_i |c_i| a_i = 0;$$

it follows that, for any linear form f on V, we have $\sum_i |c_i| f(a_i) = 0$, and hence $c_i = 0$ for all i if we also have $f(a_i) > 0$ for all i. This proves (ii).

Lemma 4. Let $Q = (q_{ij})$ *be a real, symmetric, square matrix of order* n *such that:*

a) $q_{ij} \leqslant 0$ *for* $i \neq j$*;*

b) there does not exist a partition of $\{1, 2, \ldots, n\}$ *into two non-empty subsets* I *and* J *such that* $(i, j) \in \mathrm{I} \times \mathrm{J}$ *implies* $q_{ij} = 0$*;*

c) the quadratic form $q(x_1, \ldots, x_n) = \sum_{i,j} q_{ij} x_i x_j$ *on* $\mathbf{R}^n$ *is positive.*

Then:

(i) *The kernel* N *of* q *is of dimension* 0 *or* 1*. If* $\dim \mathrm{N} = 1$*,* N *is generated by a vector all of whose coordinates are* > 0*.*

(ii) *The smallest eigenvalue of* Q *is of multiplicity* 1 *and a corresponding eigenvector has all its coordinates* > 0 *or all its coordinates* < 0*.*

Since q is a positive quadratic form, the kernel N of q is the set of isotropic vectors for q (*Algebra*, Chap. IX, § 7, no. 1, Cor. of Prop. 2). Let $a_1, \ldots, a_n$ be the canonical basis of $\mathbf{R}^n$. If $\sum_i c_i a_i \in \mathrm{N}$, Lemma 3 shows that we also have $\sum_i |c_i| a_i \in \mathrm{N}$, and hence $\sum_i q_{ji} |c_i| = 0$ for all j. Let I be the set of i such that $c_i \neq 0$. If $j \notin \mathrm{I}$, then $q_{ji}|c_i| \leqslant 0$ for $i \in \mathrm{I}$ and $q_{ji}|c_i| = 0$ for $i \notin \mathrm{I}$, so $q_{ji} = 0$ for $j \notin \mathrm{I}$ and $i \in \mathrm{I}$. Assumption *b*) thus implies that either $\mathrm{I} = \varnothing$ or $\mathrm{I} = \{1, \ldots, n\}$. Consequently, every non-zero vector in N has all its coordinates $\neq 0$. If $\dim \mathrm{N} \geqslant 2$, the intersection of N with the hyperplane with equation $x_i = 0$ would be of dimension $\geqslant 1$, contrary to what we have just shown. The preceding argument also shows that, if $\dim \mathrm{N} = 1$, then N contains a vector all of whose coordinates are > 0. This proves (i).

On the other hand, we know that the eigenvalues of Q are real (*Algebra*, Chap. IX, § 7, no. 3, Prop. 5) and positive since q is positive. Let λ be the smallest of them. The matrix $\mathrm{Q}' = \mathrm{Q} - \lambda \mathrm{I}_n$ is then the matrix of a degenerate positive form q' and the off-diagonal elements of Q′ are the same as those of Q. Consequently, Q′ satisfies conditions *a*), *b*) and *c*) of the statement of the lemma. Since the kernel N′ of q' is the eigenspace of Q corresponding to the eigenvalue λ, assertion (ii) follows from (i).

Lemma 5. Let $e_1, \ldots, e_n$ *be vectors generating* T *such that:*

a) $(e_i | e_j) \leqslant 0$ *for* $i \neq j$*;*

b) there does not exist a partition of $\{1, \ldots, n\}$ *into two non-empty subsets* I *and* J *such that* $(e_i | e_j) = 0$ *for* $i \in \mathrm{I}$ *and* $j \in \mathrm{J}$.

Then there are two possibilities:

1) $(e_1, \ldots, e_n)$ *is a basis of* T*;*

2) $n = \dim \mathrm{T} + 1$*; there exists a family* $(c_i)_{1 \leqslant i \leqslant n}$ *of real numbers* > 0 *such that* $\sum_i c_i e_i = 0$*, and any family* $(c'_i)_{1 \leqslant i \leqslant n}$ *of real numbers such that* $\sum_i c'_i e_i = 0$ *is proportional to* $(c_i)_{1 \leqslant i \leqslant n}$.

Put $q_{ij} = (e_i | e_j)$. The matrix $\mathrm{Q} = (q_{ij})$ then satisfies the hypotheses of Lemma 4: conditions *a*) and *b*) of Lemma 4 are the same as conditions *a*) and *b*) above, and *c*) is satisfied since $\sum_{i,j} q_{ij} x_i x_j = \| \sum_i x_i e_i \|^2$. The kernel N of the quadratic form q on $\mathbf{R}^n$, with matrix Q, is the set of $(c_1, \dots, c_n) \in \mathbf{R}^n$ such that $\sum_i c_i e_i = 0$. If $\mathrm{N} = \{0\}$, the e_i are linearly dependent and we are in case 1). If $\dim \mathrm{N} > 0$, Lemma 4 (i) shows that we are in case 2).

Lemma 6. Let $(e_1, \dots, e_n)$ *be a basis of* T *such that* $(e_i|e_j) \leqslant 0$ *for* $i \neq j$.

(i) *If* $x = \sum_i c_i e_i \in \mathrm{T}$ *is such that* $(x|e_i) \geqslant 0$ *for all* i, *then* $c_i \geqslant 0$ *for all* i.

(ii) *If* x *and* y *are two elements of* T *such that* $(x|e_i) \geqslant 0$ *and* $(y|e_i) \geqslant 0$ *for all* i, *then* $(x|y) \geqslant 0$. *If* $(x|e_i) > 0$ *and* $(y|e_i) > 0$ *for all* i, *then* $(x|y) > 0$.

Under the hypotheses of (i), assume that $c_i < 0$ for some i. Let f be the linear form on T defined by $f(e_i) = 1$ and

$$f(e_j) = -c_i / \left(\sum_{k=1}^{n} |c_k| \right) \quad \text{for} \quad j \neq i.$$

The vectors $-x, e_1, \dots, e_n$ then satisfy the hypotheses of Lemma 3 (ii) (taking for q the metric form on T). We conclude that they are linearly independent, which is absurd. Hence (i). Moreover, if $x = \sum_i c_i e_i \in \mathrm{T}$ and if $y \in \mathrm{T}$, then $(x|y) = \sum_i c_i (e_i|y)$, so (ii) follows immediately from (i).

6. FINITENESS THEOREMS

Lemma 7. Let A *be a set of unit vectors in* T. *If there exists a real number* $\lambda < 1$ *such that* $(a|a') \leqslant \lambda$ *for* $a, a' \in \mathrm{A}$ *and* $a \neq a'$, *then the set* A *is finite.*

For $a, a' \in \mathrm{A}$ such that $a \neq a'$, we have

$$\| a - a' \|^2 = 2 - 2(a|a') \geqslant 2 - 2\lambda.$$

Now, the unit sphere S of T being compact, there exists a finite covering of S by sets of diameter $< (2 - 2\lambda)^{1/2}$ and each of these sets contains at most one point of A, hence the lemma.

Denote by $\mathrm{U}(w)$ the automorphism of T associated to the affine map $w \in \mathrm{W}$ from E to itself. We have

$$w(x + t) = w(x) + \mathrm{U}(w).t \quad \text{for} \quad t \in \mathrm{T} \text{ and } x \in \mathrm{E}.$$

This defines a homomorphism U from the group W to the orthogonal group of T; the kernel of U is the set of translations belonging to W.

THEOREM 3. (i) *The set of walls of a chamber is finite.*

(ii) *The set of directions of hyperplanes belonging to* $\mathfrak{H}$ *is finite.*

(iii) *The group* U(W) *is finite.*

Assertion (i) follows immediately from Prop. 3, (iii) and Lemma 7.

We prove (ii). Let C be a chamber and $\mathfrak{M}$ the set of its walls. The facets of $\overline{\mathrm{C}}$ (relative to $\mathfrak{H}$) are the same as those relative to $\mathfrak{M}$ (§ 1, no. 4, Prop. 9).

Since $\mathfrak{M}$ is finite, they are finite in number. Since a facet meets only finitely many hyperplanes belonging to $\mathfrak{H}$, the set of hyperplanes belonging to $\mathfrak{H}$ and meeting $\overline{C}$ is finite, hence so is the set A(C) of unit vectors in T orthogonal to some hyperplane belonging to $\mathfrak{H}$ and meeting $\overline{C}$. Consequently, there exists a real number $\lambda < 1$ such that $(a|a') \leqslant \lambda$ for $a, a' \in A(C)$ and $a \neq a'$.

Let A be the set of unit vectors in T orthogonal to a hyperplane belonging to $\mathfrak{H}$. Let $a, a' \in A$ with $a \neq a'$. If a and a' are parallel, then $a = -a'$ and $(a|a') = -1$. Otherwise, let $H \in \mathfrak{H}$ (resp. $H' \in \mathfrak{H}$) be such that a (resp. a') is orthogonal to H (resp. H′). We have $H \cap H' \neq \varnothing$, and if $x \in H \cap H'$ there exists an element $w \in W$ such that $x \in w(\overline{C})$. The vectors $U(w).a$ and $U(w).a'$ then belong to A(C), we have

$$(a|a') = (U(w).a|U(w).a') \leqslant \lambda,$$

and the set A is finite by Lemma 7. Hence (ii).

Now let $w \in W$ be such that $U(w).a = a$ for all $a \in A$. Then $U(w).t = t$ for all t belonging to the subspace of T generated by A. On the other hand, if $t \in T$ is orthogonal to A, we have $U(s_H).t = t$ for all $H \in \mathfrak{H}$, hence $U(w).t = t$ and finally $U(w) = 1$. Since $U(w)(A) = A$ for all $w \in W$, we deduce that U(W) is isomorphic to a group of permutations of the finite set A, hence (iii).

PROPOSITION 4. *Let* C *be a chamber and* $\mathfrak{N}$ *a set of walls of* C. *Let* $W_{\mathfrak{N}}$ *be the subgroup of* W *generated by the orthogonal reflections with respect to the elements of* $\mathfrak{N}$. *For* $H \in \mathfrak{N}$, *denote by* e_H *the unit vector orthogonal to* H *on the same side of* H *as* C. *The following conditions are equivalent:*

(i) *The group* $W_{\mathfrak{N}}$ *is finite.*

(ii) *There exists a point of* E *invariant under every element of* $W_{\mathfrak{N}}$.

(iii) *The hyperplanes belonging to* $\mathfrak{N}$ *have non-empty intersection.*

(iv) *The family of vectors* $(e_H)_{H \in \mathfrak{N}}$ *is free in* T.

By property (D2) at the beginning of § 3, the stabiliser in W of every point of E is finite, so (ii) implies (i).

Since the group $W_{\mathfrak{N}}$ is generated by the set of reflections with respect to the hyperplanes belonging to $\mathfrak{N}$, the fixed points of $W_{\mathfrak{N}}$ are the points of E belonging to every hyperplane $H \in \mathfrak{N}$, hence the equivalence of (ii) and (iii).

Assume that there exists a point a of E such that $a \in H$ for all $H \in \mathfrak{N}$ and let $t \in T$ be such that $a + t \in C$. Since $(e_H|e_{H'}) \leqslant 0$ for $H, H' \in \mathfrak{N}$ such that $H \neq H'$ (Prop. 3), and since $(t|e_H) > 0$ for all $H \in \mathfrak{N}$, Lemma 3 (ii) implies that the e_H for $H \in \mathfrak{N}$ are linearly independent. Consequently, (iii) implies (iv).

Suppose finally that the family $(e_H)_{H \in \mathfrak{N}}$ is free. Let a be a point of E. For any hyperplane $H \in \mathfrak{N}$, there exists a real number c_H such that H consists of the points $a + t$ of E with $(t|e_H) = c_H$. Since the family (e_H) is free, there exists $t \in T$ such that $(t|e_H) = c_H$ for all $H \in \mathfrak{N}$, and the point $a + t$ of E belongs to all the hyperplanes $H \in \mathfrak{N}$. Thus, (iv) implies (iii).

Remarks. 1) Since W is generated by reflections with respect to the walls of the chamber C, the preceding proposition gives a criterion for W to be finite. We shall return to this question in no. 9.

2) Let F be a finite-dimensional real affine space and G a group of automorphisms of F. For all $g \in G$, denote by $U(g)$ the automorphism of the space of translations V of F associated to g. Assume that the image U(G) is a *finite* subgroup of **GL**(V); then V has a scalar product invariant under U(G) (*Integration*, Chap. VII, § 3, no. 1, Prop. 1). If, in addition, G acts properly on F when it is provided with the discrete topology, and if it is generated by reflections, we can apply to G the results of this paragraph.

7. DECOMPOSITION OF THE LINEAR REPRESENTATION OF W ON T

Let I be the set of vertices of the Coxeter graph of W (no. 4) and let J be a subset of I such that no vertex in J is linked to any vertex in I − J. Ley C be a chamber, s the canonical bijection from I to the set of reflections with respect to the walls of C, and let $W_{J,C}$ be the subgroup generated by the image $s(J)$. It follows from Chap. IV, § 1, no. 9, Prop. 8, that W is the *direct product* of the two subgroups $W_{J,C}$ and $W_{I-J,C}$. Let C′ be another chamber and s' the corresponding injection of I into W. We have seen (no. 4) that if $w \in W$ transforms C into C′, then $s'(i) = ws(i)w^{-1}$ for $i \in I$. Since $W_{J,C}$ is normal in W, it follows that $s'(i) \in W_{J,C}$ for all $i \in J$. We deduce that the *subgroup* $W_{J,C}$ *does not depend on* C. We denote it simply by W_J from now on.

The definition of $W_{J,C}$ clearly extends to an arbitrary subset J of I. But if there exist a vertex in J and a vertex in I − J that are *linked*, then $W_{J,C}$ is not normal and depends on the choice of C.

Let T_J^0 be the subspace of T consisting of the vectors invariant under every element of $U(W_J)$ and let T_J be the subspace orthogonal to T_J^0. Since W_J is a normal subgroup of W, it is clear that T_J^0 is invariant under U(W), and hence so is T_J.

PROPOSITION 5. *Let* $J_1, \dots, J_s$ *be the sets of vertices of the connected components of the Coxeter graph of* W. *For* $1 \leqslant p \leqslant s$, *put*

$$W_p = W_{J_p}, \quad T_p = T_{J_p}, \quad T'_p = T^0_{J_p}, \quad \text{and} \quad T_0 = \bigcap_{1 \leqslant p \leqslant s} T'_p.$$

(i) *The group* W *is the direct product of the groups* W_p $(1 \leqslant p \leqslant s)$.

(ii) *The space* T *is the orthogonal direct sum of the subspaces* $T_0, T_1, \dots$ $\dots, T_s$, *which are all stable under* U(W).

(iii) *For all* q *such that* $1 \leqslant q \leqslant s$, *the subspace* T'_q *of* T *consists of the vectors invariant under* $U(W_q)$; *it is the direct sum of the* T_p *for* $1 \leqslant p \leqslant s$ *and* $p \neq q$.

(iv) *Let* C *be a chamber. The subspace* T_p *(for* $1 \leqslant p \leqslant s$*) is generated by the vectors* $e_i(C)$ *for* $i \in J_p$ (in the notation of no. 4).

(v) *The representations of* W *in the subspaces* T_p *(*$1 \leqslant p \leqslant s$*) are absolutely irreducible, non-trivial, and pairwise inequivalent.*

Assertion (i) follows from Chap. IV, § 1, no. 9. On the other hand, we have already seen that the subspaces T_p are invariant under U(W), and so is T_0. Let C be a chamber; since W_p is generated by the reflections $s_i(C)$ for $i \in J_p$, it is clear that T'_p is the subspace orthogonal to the $e_i(C)$ for $i \in J_p$, hence (iv). Moreover, if $i \in J_p$, $j \in J_q$ with $p \neq q$, then $m_{ij} = 2$ since $\{i, j\}$ is not an edge of the Coxeter graph of W, so $(e_i|e_j) = 0$. Assertion (ii) is now immediate. And assertion (iii) follows, since T'_q is the orthogonal complement of T_q.

Finally, let V be a subspace of T_p invariant under $U(W_p)$. For all $i \in J_p$, either $e_i \in V$ or e_i is orthogonal to V (§ 2, no. 2, Prop. 3). Let A (resp. B) be the set of $i \in J_p$ such that $e_i \in V$ (resp. e_i is orthogonal to V). Clearly $(e_i|e_j) = 0$ for $i \in A$ and $j \in B$, and since J_p is connected, it follows that either $A = \varnothing$ and $V = \{0\}$, or $A = J_p$ and $V = T_p$. Consequently, the representation of W_p on T_p is irreducible, hence absolutely irreducible (§ 2, no. 1, Prop. 1). It is non-trivial by the very definition of T_p. Finally, the last assertion in (v) follows immediately from (iii).

If the subspace T_0 of vectors in T invariant under U(W) reduces to $\{0\}$, then W is said to be *essential*; if the representation U of W on T is irreducible, then W is said to be *irreducible*.

COROLLARY. *Assume that* $W \neq \{1\}$. *Then* W *is irreducible if and only if it is essential and its Coxeter graph is connected.*

Remark. Under the hypotheses of Prop. 5, the subspaces T_p for $0 \leqslant p \leqslant s$ are the isotypical components of the linear representation U of W on T (*Algebra*, Chap. VIII, § 3, no. 4). It follows (*loc. cit.*, Prop. 11) that every vector subspace V of T stable under W is the direct sum of the subspaces $V \cap T_p$ for $0 \leqslant p \leqslant s$; moreover (*loc. cit.*, Prop. 10), every endomorphism commuting with the operators $U(w)$ for $w \in W$ leaves stable each of the T_p for $0 \leqslant p \leqslant s$ and induces on them a homothety for $1 \leqslant p \leqslant s$. In particular, the bilinear forms Φ on T invariant under W are the bilinear forms given by

$$\Phi\left(\sum_k t_k, \sum_k t'_k\right) = \Phi_0(t_0, t'_0) + \sum_{1 \leqslant p \leqslant s} a_p(t_p|t'_p),$$

where Φ_0 is a bilinear form on T_0 and a_p (for $1 \leqslant p \leqslant s$) is a real number: indeed, such a form Φ can be written uniquely in the form $(t, t') \mapsto (A(t)|t')$, where A is an endomorphism of T commuting with the $U(w)$ for $w \in W$.

8. PRODUCT DECOMPOSITION OF THE AFFINE SPACE E

We retain the notation of Prop. 5. For $0 \leqslant p \leqslant s$, let E_p be the set of orbits of the group T'_p in E, and let φ_p be the canonical map from E to E_p. The action of T on E passes to the quotient; in particular, T_p acts on E_p and it is immediate (for example by taking an origin in E) that E_p is an affine space admitting T_p as its space of translations. Put $\mathrm{E}' = \mathrm{E}_0 \times \cdots \times \mathrm{E}_s$; this is an affine space having $\mathrm{T} = \mathrm{T}_0 \oplus \cdots \oplus \mathrm{T}_s$ as its space of translations. Let $\varphi : \mathrm{E} \to \mathrm{E}'$ be the product map of the φ_p; since φ commutes with the action of T, this is a bijection and even an isomorphism of affine spaces. In what follows, we identify E and E′ by means of φ; the map φ_p is then identified with the canonical projection of E′ onto E_p.

Since W leaves T'_p stable, the action of W on E passes to the quotient and defines an action of W on E_p (for $0 \leqslant p \leqslant s$), and hence by restriction an action of W_p on E_p (for $1 \leqslant p \leqslant s$). On the other hand, let C be a chamber, let $i \in \mathrm{I}$ and let p be the integer such that $i \in \mathrm{J}_p$. For any $x \in \mathrm{E}$, we have

$$s_i(\mathrm{C})(x) = x - \lambda.e_i(\mathrm{C}) \quad \text{with} \quad \lambda \in \mathbf{R}.$$

Since $e_i \in \mathrm{T}'_q$ for $q \neq p$, it follows that

$$\varphi_q(w(x)) = \varphi_q(x) \quad \text{for} \quad x \in \mathrm{E},\ w \in \mathrm{W}_p,\ 0 \leqslant q \leqslant s \text{ and } q \neq p.$$

Consequently, if $w = w_1 \dots w_s \in \mathrm{W}$ with $w_p \in \mathrm{W}_p$ for $1 \leqslant p \leqslant s$, then

$$w((x_0, \dots, x_s)) = (x_0, w_1(x_1), \dots, w_s(x_s)) \tag{5}$$

for all $x_p \in \mathrm{E}_p$ for $0 \leqslant p \leqslant s$. In other words, *the action of* W *on* $\mathrm{E} = \mathrm{E}'$ *is exactly the product of the actions of the* W_p *on* E_p (we put $\mathrm{W}_0 = \{1\}$). It follows that W_p acts faithfully on E_p and that W_p *can be identified with a group of displacements of the euclidean space* E_p (the space T_p of translations of E_p being provided, of course, with the scalar product induced by that on T).

PROPOSITION 6. (i) *The group* W_p *is a group of displacements of the euclidean affine space* E_p*; it is generated by reflections; provided with the discrete topology, it acts properly on* E_p*; it is irreducible.*

(ii) *Let* $\mathfrak{H}_p$ *be the set of hyperplanes* H *of* E_p *such that* $s_\mathrm{H} \in \mathrm{W}_p$. *The set* $\mathfrak{H}$ *consists of the hyperplanes of the form*

$$\mathrm{H} = \mathrm{E}_0 \times \mathrm{E}_1 \times \cdots \times \mathrm{E}_{p-1} \times \mathrm{H}_p \times \mathrm{E}_{p+1} \times \cdots \times \mathrm{E}_s,$$

with $p = 1, \dots, s$ *and* $\mathrm{H}_p \in \mathfrak{H}_p$.

(iii) *Every chamber* C *is of the form* $\mathrm{E}_0 \times \mathrm{C}_1 \times \cdots \times \mathrm{C}_s$, *where for each* p *the set* C_p *is a chamber defined in* E_p *by the set of hyperplanes* $\mathfrak{H}_p$*; moreover, the walls of* C_p *are the hyperplanes* $\varphi_p(\mathrm{H}_i(\mathrm{C}))$ *for* $i \in \mathrm{J}_p$.

Let C be a chamber. Put $\mathrm{H}_i = \mathrm{H}_i(\mathrm{C})$, $e_i = e_i(\mathrm{C})$ and $s_i = s_i(\mathrm{C})$ for $i \in \mathrm{I}$ (in the notation of no. 4).

(i) Let i be in J_p; since $e_i \in T_p$ and T is the direct sum of the mutually orthogonal subspaces $T_0, T_1, \ldots, T_s$, the hyperplane of T orthogonal to e_i is of the form $L_i + T'_p$, where L_i is the hyperplane of T_p orthogonal to e_i. The affine hyperplane H_i of E is of the form $L_i + T'_p + x$, with $x \in E$, and we have

$$H_i = E_0 \times E_1 \times \cdots \times E_{p-1} \times H'_i \times E_{p+1} \times \cdots \times E_s \tag{6}$$

with $H'_i = L_i + \varphi_p(x) = \varphi_p(H_i)$. It is now immediate that s_i acts in E_p by the reflection associated to the hyperplane H'_i of E_p. Thus, the group W_p is a group of displacements generated by reflections in E_p; the verification of the properness criterion (D′2) is immediate. Finally, Prop. 5, (v) shows that W_p is irreducible. This proves (i).

(ii) By the Cor. of Th. 1, the set $\mathfrak{H}_p$ consists of the hyperplanes of the form $w_p(H'_i)$ for i in J_p and w_p in W_p. Further, if $w = w_1 \ldots w_s$ with $w_p \in W_p$ for all p, formulas (5) and (6) imply that

$$w(H_i) = E_0 \times E_1 \times \cdots \times E_{p-1} \times w_p(H'_i) \times E_{p+1} \times \cdots \times E_s, \tag{7}$$

from which (ii) follows immediately.

(iii) Let i be in J_p; by formula (6), the open half-space D_i bounded by H_i and containing C is of the form

$$D_i = E_0 \times E_1 \times \cdots \times E_{p-1} \times D'_i \times E_{p+1} \times \cdots \times E_s,$$

where D'_i is an open half-space bounded by H'_i in E_p. Put $C_p = \bigcap_{i \in J_p} D'_i$; since $C = \bigcap_{i \in I} D_i$, it follows immediately that

$$C = E_0 \times C_1 \times \cdots \times C_s;$$

consequently, none of the sets C_p is empty, and since C does not meet any hyperplane belonging to $\mathfrak{H}$, the set C_p does not meet any hyperplane belonging to $\mathfrak{H}_p$. Prop. 5 of § 1, no. 3 now shows that C_p is one of the chambers defined by $\mathfrak{H}_p$ in E_p. By using Prop. 4 of § 1, no. 2, it is easy to see that the walls of C_p are the hyperplanes $H'_i = \varphi_p(H_i)$ for $i \in J_p$.

9. STRUCTURE OF CHAMBERS

Let C be a chamber, let $\mathfrak{M}$ be the set of walls of C, and for $H \in \mathfrak{M}$ let e_H be the unit vector orthogonal to H on the same side of H as C.

PROPOSITION 7. *Assume that the group* W *is essential and finite. Then:*

(i) *There exists a unique point a of* E *invariant under* W.

(ii) *The family $(e_H)_{H \in \mathfrak{M}}$ is a basis of* T.

(iii) *The chamber* C *is the open simplicial cone with vertex a defined by the basis $(e'_H)_{H \in \mathfrak{M}}$ of* T *such that $(e_H | e'_{H'}) = \delta_{HH'}$.*

(i) By Prop. 4 of no. 6, there exists a point $a \in \mathrm{E}$ invariant under W. Let $t \in \mathrm{T}$ be such that $t + a$ is invariant under W. For all $w \in \mathrm{W}$,

$$\mathrm{U}(w).t + a = w(t+a) = t + a,$$

so $\mathrm{U}(w).t = t$; since W is essential, this implies that $t = 0$, showing the uniqueness of a.

(ii) Since W is essential, $\mathrm{T} = \mathrm{T}_1$ in the notation of no. 7, and Prop. 5, (iv) shows that the family $(e_{\mathrm{H}})_{\mathrm{H}\in\mathfrak{M}}$ generates the vector space T. The existence of a point of E invariant under W shows that the family $(e_{\mathrm{H}})_{\mathrm{H}\in\mathfrak{M}}$ is free (no. 6, Prop. 4).

(iii) Let a be the unique point of E invariant under W. Since $(e_{\mathrm{H}})_{\mathrm{H}\in\mathfrak{M}}$ is a basis of T, and since the scalar product is a non-degenerate bilinear form on T, there exists a unique basis $(e'_{\mathrm{H}})_{\mathrm{H}\in\mathfrak{M}}$ of T such that $(e_{\mathrm{H}}|e'_{\mathrm{H}'}) = \delta_{\mathrm{HH}'}$ for H, H' in $\mathfrak{M}$. Every point x of E can be written uniquely in the form $x = t + a$ with $t = \sum_{\mathrm{H}\in\mathfrak{M}} \xi_{\mathrm{H}}.e'_{\mathrm{H}}$ and the ξ_{H} real. Then x belongs to C if and only if, for every hyperplane $\mathrm{H} \in \mathfrak{M}$, x is on the same side of H as e_{H}, or in other words $(t|e_{\mathrm{H}}) = \xi_{\mathrm{H}}$ is strictly positive. Hence (iii).

PROPOSITION 8. *Assume that the group* W *is essential, irreducible and infinite. Then:*

(i) *No point of* E *is invariant under* W.

(ii) *We have* $\mathrm{Card}\,\mathfrak{M} = \dim \mathrm{T} + 1$, *and there exist real numbers* $c_{\mathrm{H}} > 0$ *such that* $\sum_{\mathrm{H}\in\mathfrak{M}} c_{\mathrm{H}}.e_{\mathrm{H}} = 0$. *If the real numbers* c'_{H} *are such that* $\sum_{\mathrm{H}\in\mathfrak{M}} c'_{\mathrm{H}}.e_{\mathrm{H}} = 0$, *there exists a real number* ξ *such that* $c'_{\mathrm{H}} = \xi c_{\mathrm{H}}$ *for all* H *in* $\mathfrak{M}$.

(iii) *The chamber* C *is an open simplex.*

Assertion (i) follows from Prop. 4. On the other hand, since W is essential, the vectors $(e_{\mathrm{H}})_{\mathrm{H}\in\mathfrak{M}}$ generate T. We have $(e_{\mathrm{H}}|e_{\mathrm{H}'}) \leqslant 0$ for $\mathrm{H}, \mathrm{H}' \in \mathfrak{M}$ and $\mathrm{H} \neq \mathrm{H}'$ (Prop. 3) and, since W is irreducible, there does not exist a partition of $\mathfrak{M}$ into two disjoint subsets $\mathfrak{M}'$ and $\mathfrak{M}''$ such that $\mathrm{H}' \in \mathfrak{M}'$ and $\mathrm{H}'' \in \mathfrak{M}''$ imply that $(e_{\mathrm{H}'}|e_{\mathrm{H}''}) = 0$. We can thus apply Lemma 5 of no. 5, and case 1) of that lemma is excluded; indeed, the e_{H} are not linearly independent, since W has no fixed point. Assertion (ii) follows.

We now prove (iii). Number the walls of C as $\mathrm{H}_0, \mathrm{H}_1, \dots, \mathrm{H}_d$ and put $t_m = e_{\mathrm{H}_m}$. By (ii), the vectors $t_1, \dots, t_d$ form a basis of T, so the hyperplanes $\mathrm{H}_1, \dots, \mathrm{H}_d$ have a point a_0 in common, and there exists a basis $(t'_1, \dots, t'_d)$ of T such that $(t_m|t'_n) = \delta_{mn}$; moreover, again by (ii) there exist real numbers $c_1 > 0, \dots, c_d > 0$ such that

$$t_0 = -(c_1.t_1 + \dots + c_d.t_d).$$

Since the vector t_0 is orthogonal to the hyperplane H_0, there exists a real number c such that H_0 is the set of points $x = t + a_0$ of E with $(t|t_0) = -c$.

Every point of E can be written uniquely in the form $x = t + a_0$ with $t = \xi_1.t'_1 + \dots + \xi_d.t'_d$ and $\xi_1, \dots, \xi_d$ real. The point x belongs to C if and only if it is on the same side of H_m as t_m for $0 \leqslant m \leqslant d$; this translates into the inequalities $(t|t_1) > 0, \ldots, (t|t_d) > 0$, and $(t|t_0) > -c$, or equivalently by $\xi_1 > 0, \ldots, \xi_d > 0$, $c_1\xi_1 + \cdots + c_d\xi_d < c$. Since C is non-empty, $c > 0$. Put $a_m = a_0 + \frac{c}{c_m}.t'_m$ for $1 \leqslant m \leqslant d$; then the chamber C consists of the points of E of the form $a_0 + \sum_{m=1}^{d} \lambda_m.(a_m - a_0)$ with $\lambda_1 > 0, \ldots, \lambda_d > 0$ and $\lambda_1 + \cdots + \lambda_d < 1$, so C is the open simplex with vertices $a_0, \ldots, a_d$. Q.E.D.

Remarks. 1) Identify E with $E_0 \times E_1 \times \cdots \times E_s$ and W with $W_1 \times \cdots \times W_s$ as in no. 8. By Prop. 6, the chamber C is then identified with

$$E_0 \times C_1 \times \cdots \times C_s,$$

where C_p is a chamber in E_p with respect to the set of hyperplanes $\mathfrak{H}_p$. By Props. 7 and 8, each of the chambers $C_1, \ldots, C_s$ is an open simplicial cone or an open simplex.

2) Assume that W is irreducible and essential. If H and H′ are two walls of C, then $m_{HH'} = +\infty$ if and only if $e_H = -e_{H'}$ (Prop. 3). By Props. 7 and 8, this can happen only if H and H′ are the only walls of C and E is of dimension 1. Thus, the only case in which one of the $m_{HH'}$ is infinite is that in which E is of dimension 1 and the group W is generated by the reflections associated to two distinct points (cf. § 2, no. 4).

In the general case, the entries of the Coxeter matrix associated to W are finite unless at least one of $E_1, \ldots, E_s$ is of the preceding type.

10. SPECIAL POINTS

Let L be the set of translations belonging to W and let Λ be the set of $t \in T$ such that the translation $x \mapsto t + x$ belongs to L. It is immediate that Λ is stable under U(W) and that L is a normal subgroup of W. Since W acts properly on E, the same holds for L, and it follows easily that Λ is a discrete subgroup of T. For any point x of E, denote by W_x the stabiliser of x in W.

PROPOSITION 9. *Let $a \in E$. The following conditions are equivalent:*

(i) *We have* $W = W_a.L$*;*

(ii) *The restriction of the homomorphism* U *to* W_a *is an isomorphism from* W_a *to* U(W)*;*

(iii) *For every hyperplane* $H \in \mathfrak{H}$*, there exists a hyperplane* $H' \in \mathfrak{H}$ *parallel to* H *and such that* $a \in H'$.

It is clear that (i) ⇔ (ii), since L is the kernel of U and $L \cap W_a = \{1\}$.

Assume (i) and let $H \in \mathfrak{H}$; then $s_H \in W_a.L$ so there exists a vector $t \in \Lambda$ such that $a = s_H(a) + t$; the vector t is orthogonal to H, and if $H' = H + \frac{1}{2}t$ then $s_{H'}(x) = s_H(x) + t$ for all $x \in E$ (cf. § 2, no. 4, Prop. 5). Since $t \in \Lambda$ and $s_H \in W$, we have $s_{H'} \in W$, and so $H' \in \mathfrak{H}$; we also have $a = s_{H'}(a)$, and so $a \in H'$. Thus, (i) implies (iii).

Assume (iii). Let $H \in \mathfrak{H}$; take H' as in (iii). Then $s_{H'}(a) = a$, so $s_{H'} \in W_a$; since H is parallel to H', the element $w = s_{H'}s_H$ of W is a translation (§ 2, no. 4, Prop. 5), so $w \in L$; then $s_H = s_{H'}w \in W_a.L$. Since W is generated by the family $(s_H)_{H\in\mathfrak{H}}$, it follows that $W = W_a.L$ and hence (iii) implies (i).

DEFINITION 1. *A point a of* E *is special for* W *if it satisfies the equivalent conditions in Prop. 9.*

It is clear that the set of special points of E is stable under W.

PROPOSITION 10. *There exists a special point for* W.

By Prop. 6 of no. 8, we need only consider the case when W is essential.

The group U(W) of automorphisms of T is finite (cf. no. 6, Th. 3) and $U(s_H)$ is an orthogonal reflection for every hyperplane H; moreover, U(W) is generated by the family $(U(s_H))_{H\in\mathfrak{H}}$. By Prop. 7 of no. 9, there exists a basis $(e_i)_{i\in I}$ of T such that the group U(W) is generated by the set of reflections $(s_i)_{i\in I}$ defined by

$$s_i(t) = t - 2(t|e_i).e_i.$$

The Cor. of Th. 1 of no. 2 shows that every reflection $s \in U(W)$ is of the form $s = U(s_H)$ with $H \in \mathfrak{H}$. We can thus find in $\mathfrak{H}$ a family of hyperplanes $(H_i)_{i\in I}$ such that $s_i = U(s_{H_i})$ for all i. Since the vectors e_i are linearly independent, there exists $a \in E$ such that $a \in H_i$ for all $i \in I$. We have $s_{H_i} \in W_a$, so $U(W) = U(W_a)$, which means that $W = W_a.L$ since L is the kernel of U. Thus, a is special.

When W is finite and essential, there is only one special point for W, namely the unique point invariant under W. Thus, the consideration of special points is interesting mainly when W is infinite.

PROPOSITION 11. *Assume that* W *is essential. Let a be a special point for* W. *The chambers relative to* W_a *are the open simplicial cones with vertex a. For every chamber* C′ *relative to* W_a, *there exists a unique chamber* C *relative to* W *contained in* C′ *and such that* $a \in \overline{C}$. *The union of the* $w'(\overline{C})$ *for* $w' \in W_a$ *is a closed neighbourhood of a in* E. *Every wall of* C′ *is a wall of* C. *If* W *is infinite and irreducible, the walls of* C *are the walls of* C′ *together with an affine hyperplane not parallel to the walls of* C′.

Let $\mathfrak{H}'$ be the set of $H \in \mathfrak{H}$ containing a. The group W_a is generated by the s_H for $H \in \mathfrak{H}'$ (no. 3, Prop. 2). The chambers relative to W_a are the open simplicial cones with vertex a (no. 9, Prop. 7). Let C′ be such a chamber and let U be a non-empty open ball with centre a not meeting any element of $\mathfrak{H} - \mathfrak{H}'$. Since $a \in \overline{C'}$, there exists a point b in $U \cap C'$. Then $b \notin H$ for all $H \in \mathfrak{H}$, so b belongs to a chamber C relative to $\mathfrak{H}$. Since $\mathfrak{H}' \subset \mathfrak{H}$, we have $C \subset C'$. The set $U \cap C'$ does not meet any $H \in \mathfrak{H}$ and is convex, so $U \cap C' \subset C$; thus $a \in \overline{C}$. Conversely, let C_1 be a chamber relative to W contained in C′ and such that

$a \in \overline{C}_1$; then C_1 meets U and $U \cap C_1 \subset U \cap C' = U \cap C$; the chambers C and C_1, having a point in common, must coincide. For any $w' \in W_a$, we have $w'(U) = U$, so

$$U \cap w'(C) = w'(U \cap C) = w'(U \cap C') = U \cap w'(C');$$

since the union of the $w'(C)$ for $w' \in W_a$ is dense in E, the union of the $U \cap w'(C) = U \cap w'(C')$ is dense in U, and the union of the $w'(\overline{C})$ for $w' \in W_a$ thus contains U. Finally, if H is a wall of C′, there exist a point $c \in U \cap H$ and an open neighbourhood $V \subset U$ of c such that $V \cap C'$ is the intersection of V and the open half-space bounded by H containing C′; since $V \cap C' = V \cap U \cap C' = V \cap U \cap C = V \cap C$, it follows that H is a wall of C. If W is infinite and irreducible, C is an open simplex (no. 9, Prop. 8) and so has one more wall than the open simplicial cone C′.

COROLLARY. *Assume that* W *is essential.*

(i) *If $a \in E$ is special, there exists a chamber* C *such that a is an extremal point of* $\overline{C}$.

(ii) *If* C *is a chamber, there exists an extremal point of* $\overline{C}$ *that is special.*

The first assertion follows from Prop. 11. The second follows from the first and the fact that W acts transitively on the set of chambers.

However, an extremal point of $\overline{C}$ is not necessarily a special point for W (cf. Chap. VI, Plate X, Systems B_2 and G_2).

Remark. 1) Assume that W is essential, irreducible and infinite and retain the notation of Prop. 11. Since U is an isomorphism from W_a to U(W), it follows that the Coxeter graph of the group of displacements U(W) (which is generated by the reflections $U(s_H)$ for $H \in \mathfrak{H}$) can be obtained from the Coxeter graph of W by omitting the vertex i corresponding to the unique wall of C that is not a wall of C′.

PROPOSITION 12. *Assume that* W *is essential. Let a be a special point, let* $L(a)$ *be the set of its transforms under the group of translations* L, *and let* C *be a chamber. Then* $\overline{C}$ *meets* $L(a)$ *in a unique point; this point is an extremal point of* $\overline{C}$.

There exists a chamber C_1 such that a is an extremal point of $\overline{C}_1$ (Cor. of Prop. 11). Every chamber is of the form $C = tw'(C_1)$ with $w' \in W_a$ and $t \in L$ since $W = W_a.L$; thus $tw'(a) = t(a) \in L(a)$ is an extremal point of $\overline{C}$. On the other hand, $\overline{C}$ cannot contain two distinct points of $L(a)$ since $\overline{C}$ is a fundamental domain for W (no. 3, Th. 2).

Remark. 2) The set $L(a)$ is contained in the set of special points, but in general is distinct from it (cf. Chap. VI, § 2, no. 2 and Plates I to VI).

§ 4. GEOMETRIC REPRESENTATION OF A COXETER GROUP

In this paragraph, all the vector spaces considered are *real* vector spaces.

1. FORM ASSOCIATED TO A COXETER GROUP

Let S be a set and let $M = (m(s,s'))_{s,s' \in S}$ be a *Coxeter matrix* (Chap. IV, § 1, no. 9) of type S. Recall that this means:

(1) The elements of M are integers or $+\infty$.
(2) M is symmetric.
(3) $m(s,s) = 1$ for all s.
(4) $m(s,s') \geqslant 2$ for $s \neq s'$.

Let $E = \mathbf{R}^{(S)}$, let $(e_s)_{s \in S}$ be the canonical basis of E, and let B_M be the bilinear form on E such that

$$B_M(e_s, e_{s'}) = -\cos\frac{\pi}{m(s,s')}.$$

The form B_M is *symmetric*. It is called the *associated form* of the matrix M. We have

$$B_M(e_s, e_s) = 1 \quad \text{and} \quad B_M(e_s, e_{s'}) \leqslant 0 \quad \text{if} \quad s \neq s'.$$

Let $s \in S$ and let f_s be the linear form $x \mapsto 2B_M(e_s, x)$. We denote by σ_s the *pseudo-reflection* defined by the pair (e_s, f_s) (cf. § 2, no. 1); since $\langle e_s, f_s \rangle = 2$, it is a *reflection* (§ 2, no. 2). We have

$$\sigma_s(x) = x - 2B_M(e_s, x).e_s$$

and in particular

$$\sigma_s(e_{s'}) = e_{s'} + 2\cos\frac{\pi}{m(s,s')}.e_s.$$

Since e_s is not isotropic for B_M, the space E is the direct sum of the line $\mathbf{R}e_s$ and the hyperplane H_s orthogonal to e_s. Since σ_s is equal to -1 on $\mathbf{R}e_s$ and to 1 on H_s, it follows that σ_s *preserves* the form B_M. When S is finite and B_M is non-degenerate (a case to which we shall return in no. 8), it follows that σ_s is an *orthogonal reflection* (§ 2, no. 3).

2. THE PLANE $E_{s,s'}$ AND THE GROUP GENERATED BY σ_s AND $\sigma_{s'}$

In this number, we denote by s and s' two elements of S with $s \neq s'$. Put $m = m(s, s')$ and denote by $E_{s,s'}$ the plane $\mathbf{R}e_s \oplus \mathbf{R}e_{s'}$.

PROPOSITION 1. *The restriction of* B_M *to* $E_{s,s'}$ *is positive, and it is non-degenerate if and only if* m *is finite.*

Let $z = xe_s + ye_{s'}$, with $x, y \in \mathbf{R}$, be an element of $E_{s,s'}$. We have

$$B_M(z,z) = x^2 - 2xy\cos\frac{\pi}{m} + y^2$$
$$= \left(x - y.\cos\frac{\pi}{m}\right)^2 + y^2\sin^2\frac{\pi}{m},$$

which shows that B_M is positive on $E_{s,s'}$, and that it is non-degenerate there if and only if $\sin\frac{\pi}{m} \neq 0$. The proposition follows.

The reflections σ_s and $\sigma_{s'}$ leave $E_{s,s'}$ stable. We are going to determine the order of the restriction of $\sigma_s\sigma_{s'}$ to $E_{s,s'}$. We distinguish two cases:

a) $m = +\infty$.

Let $u = e_s + e_{s'}$. We have $B_M(u, e_s) = B_M(u, e_{s'}) = 0$, so u is invariant under σ_s and $\sigma_{s'}$. Moreover,

$$\sigma_s(\sigma_{s'}(e_s)) = \sigma_s(e_s + 2e_{s'}) = 3e_s + 2e_{s'} = 2u + e_s,$$

hence

$$(\sigma_s\sigma_{s'})^n(e_s) = 2nu + e_s \quad \text{for all} \quad n \in \mathbf{Z}.$$

It follows that the restriction of $\sigma_s\sigma_{s'}$ to $E_{s,s'}$ is of *infinite order.*

b) m *is finite.*

The form B_H provides $E_{s,s'}$ with the structure of a *euclidean plane.* Since the scalar product of e_s and $e_{s'}$ is equal to $-\cos\frac{\pi}{m} = \cos\left(\pi - \frac{\pi}{m}\right)$, we can orient $E_{s,s'}$ so that the angle between the half-lines $\mathbf{R}_+e_s$ and $\mathbf{R}_+e_{s'}$ is equal to $\pi - \frac{\pi}{m}$. If D and D′ denote the lines orthogonal to e_s and $e_{s'}$,

$$(\widehat{D', D}) = \pi - (\widehat{D, D'}) = \frac{\pi}{m}.$$

Now, the restrictions $\overline{\sigma}_s$ and $\overline{\sigma}_{s'}$ of σ_s and $\sigma_{s'}$ to $E_{s,s'}$ are the *orthogonal symmetries* with respect to D and D′. By the Cor. to Prop. 6 of § 2, no. 5, it follows that $\overline{\sigma}_s\overline{\sigma}_{s'}$ *is the rotation with angle* $\frac{2\pi}{m}$. In particular, its order is m.

We now return to E:

PROPOSITION 2. *The subgroup of* **GL**(E) *generated by* σ_s *and* $\sigma_{s'}$ *is a dihedral group of order* $2m(s, s')$.

Since σ_s and $\sigma_{s'}$ are of order 2, and are distinct, it is enough to show that their product $\sigma_s\sigma_{s'}$ is of order $m(s, s')$. When $m(s, s')$ is infinite, this follows from *a*) above. When $m(s, s')$ is finite, it follows from Prop. 1 that E is the direct sum of $E_{s,s'}$ and its orthogonal complement $V_{s,s'}$; since σ_s and $\sigma_{s'}$ are the identity on $V_{s,s'}$, and since the restriction of $\sigma_s\sigma_{s'}$ to $E_{s,s'}$ is of order $m(s, s')$ by *b*), the order of $\sigma_s\sigma_{s'}$ is indeed equal to $m(s, s')$.

3. GROUP AND REPRESENTATION ASSOCIATED TO A COXETER MATRIX

We retain the notation of the preceding numbers. Let $W = W(M)$ be the group defined by the *family of generators* $(g_s)_{s\in S}$ and the *relations*[1]

$$(g_s g_{s'})^{m(s,s')} = 1, \qquad \text{for } s, s' \in S,\ m(s, s') \neq +\infty.$$

PROPOSITION 3. *There exists a unique homomorphism*

$$\sigma : W \to \mathbf{GL}(E)$$

such that $\sigma(g_s) = \sigma_s$ *for all* $s \in S$. *The elements of* $\sigma(W)$ *preserve the bilinear form* B_M.

To prove the existence and uniqueness of σ, it is enough to show that $(\sigma_s\sigma_{s'})^{m(s,s')} = 1$ if $m(s, s') \neq +\infty$. Now, if $s = s'$, this follows from the fact that σ_s is of order 2; if $s \neq s'$, it follows from what we proved in no. 2. Finally, since the reflections σ_s preserve B_M, so do the elements of $\sigma(W)$.

Remark. 1) We shall see in no. 4 that σ is *injective*; the group W can thus be identified with the subgroup of $\mathbf{GL}(E)$ generated by the σ_s.

PROPOSITION 4. *a*) *The map* $s \mapsto g_s$ *from* S *to* W *is injective.*

b) *Each of the* g_s *is of order 2.*

c) *If* $s, s' \in S$, $g_s g_{s'}$ *is of order* $m(s, s')$.

Assertion *a*) follows from the fact that the composite map

$$s \mapsto g_s \mapsto \sigma_s$$

from S to $\mathbf{GL}(E)$ is injective.

For *b*) (resp. *c*)), we remark that the order of g_s (resp. the order of $g_s g_{s'}$) is *at most* 2 (resp. *at most* $m(s, s')$). Since we have seen in no. 2 that the order of σ_s (resp. of $\sigma_s\sigma_{s'}$) is 2 (resp. $m(s, s')$), we must have equality.

In view of *a*), S can be *identified* with a subset of W by means of the map $s \mapsto g_s$.

---

[1] This means that, if L_S denotes the free group on S, W is the quotient of L_S by the smallest normal subgroup of L_S containing the elements $(ss')^{m(s,s')}$, for $m(s, s') \neq +\infty$.

COROLLARY. *The pair* (W, S) *is a Coxeter system with matrix* M.

This is simply the content of properties *b*) and *c*), together with the definition of W.

Remark. 2) We have thus shown that *every Coxeter matrix corresponds to a Coxeter group.*

4. CONTRAGREDIENT REPRESENTATION

Let E^* be the dual of E. Since W acts on E via σ, it also acts, by transport of structure, on E^*. The corresponding representation

$$\sigma^* : W \to \mathbf{GL}(E^*)$$

is called the *contragredient representation* of σ. We have

$$\sigma^*(w) = {}^t\sigma(w^{-1}) \text{ for all } w \in W.$$

If $x^* \in E^*$ and $w \in W$, we denote by $w(x^*)$ the transform of x^* by $\sigma^*(w)$.

If $s \in S$, denote by A_s the set of $x^* \in E^*$ such that $x^*(e_s) > 0$. Let C be the intersection of the A_s, $s \in S$. When S is *finite*, C is an *open simplicial cone* in E^* (§ 1, no. 6).

THEOREM 1 (Tits). *If* $w \in W$ *and* $C \cap w(C) \neq \varnothing$, *then* $w = 1$.

We indicate immediately several consequences of this theorem:

COROLLARY 1. *The group* W *acts simply-transitively on the set of* $w(C)$ *for* $w \in W$.

This is clear.

COROLLARY 2. *The representations* σ *and* σ^* *are injective.*

Indeed, if $\sigma^*(w) = 1$, then $w(C) = C$, so $w = 1$ by the theorem. The injectivity of σ follows from that of σ^*.

COROLLARY 3. *If* S *is finite,* $\sigma(W)$ *is a discrete subgroup of* $\mathbf{GL}(E)$ *(provided with its canonical* Lie *group structure); similarly,* $\sigma^*(W)$ *is a discrete subgroup of* $\mathbf{GL}(E^*)$.

Let $x^* \in C$. The set U of $g \in \mathbf{GL}(E^*)$ such that $g(x^*) \in C$ is a neighbourhood of the identity element in $\mathbf{GL}(E^*)$; by the theorem,

$$\sigma^*(W) \cap U = \{1\};$$

thus, $\sigma^*(W)$ is a discrete subgroup of $\mathbf{GL}(E^*)$. By transport of structure, it follows that $\sigma(W)$ is discrete in $\mathbf{GL}(E)$.

Proof of Theorem 1.

If $w \in \mathrm{W}$, denote by $l(w)$ the *length of* w with respect to S (Chap. IV, § 1, no. 1).

We are going to prove the following assertions, where n denotes an integer $\geqslant 0$:

(P_n) *Let* $w \in \mathrm{W}$, *with* $l(w) = n$, *and* $s \in \mathrm{S}$. *Then:*
either $w(\mathrm{C}) \subset \mathrm{A}_s$;
or $w(\mathrm{C}) \subset s(\mathrm{A}_s)$ *and* $l(sw) = l(w) - 1$.

(Q_n) *Let* $w \in \mathrm{W}$, *with* $l(w) = n$, *and* $s, s' \in \mathrm{S}$, $s \neq s'$. *Let* $\mathrm{W}_{s,s'}$ *be the subgroup of* W *generated by* s *and* s'. *There exists* $u \in \mathrm{W}_{s,s'}$ *such that*

$$w(\mathrm{C}) \subset u(\mathrm{A}_s \cap \mathrm{A}_{s'}) \quad \text{and} \quad l(w) = l(u) + l(u^{-1}w).$$

These assertions are trivial for $n = 0$. We prove them by induction on n, according to the scheme

$$((\mathrm{P}_n) \text{ and } (\mathrm{Q}_n)) \Longrightarrow (\mathrm{P}_{n+1}) \quad \text{and} \quad ((\mathrm{P}_{n+1}) \text{ and } (\mathrm{Q}_n)) \Longrightarrow (\mathrm{Q}_{n+1}).$$

Proof that $((\mathrm{P}_n) \text{ and } (\mathrm{Q}_n)) \Longrightarrow (\mathrm{P}_{n+1})$.

Let $w \in \mathrm{W}$, with $l(w) = n + 1$, and $s \in \mathrm{S}$. We can write w in the form $w = s'w'$ with $s' \in \mathrm{S}$ and $l(w') = n$. If $s' = s$, (P_n) applied to w' shows that $w'(\mathrm{C}) \subset \mathrm{A}_s$, hence $w(\mathrm{C}) \subset s(\mathrm{A}_s)$ and $l(sw) = l(w') = l(w) - 1$. If $s' \neq s$, (Q_n) applied to w' shows that there exists $u \in \mathrm{W}_{s,s'}$ such that

$$w'(\mathrm{C}) \subset u(\mathrm{A}_s \cap \mathrm{A}_{s'}) \quad \text{and} \quad l(w') = l(u) + l(u^{-1}w').$$

We have $w(\mathrm{C}) = s'w'(\mathrm{C}) \subset s'u(\mathrm{A}_s \cap \mathrm{A}_{s'})$.

Lemma 1. Let $s, s' \in \mathrm{S}$, *with* $s \neq s'$, *and let* $v \in \mathrm{W}_{s,s'}$. *Then* $v(\mathrm{A}_s \cap \mathrm{A}_{s'})$ *is contained in either* A_s *or in* $s(\mathrm{A}_s)$, *and in the second case* $l(sv) = l(v) - 1$.

The proof will be given in no. 5.

We apply the lemma to the element $v = s'u$. There are two possibilities: either

$$s'u(\mathrm{A}_s \cap \mathrm{A}_{s'}) \subset \mathrm{A}_s \quad \text{and } \textit{a fortiori} \quad w(\mathrm{C}) \subset \mathrm{A}_s,$$

or

$$s'u(\mathrm{A}_s \cap \mathrm{A}_{s'}) \subset s(\mathrm{A}_s) \quad \text{and } \textit{a fortiori} \quad w(\mathrm{C}) \subset s(\mathrm{A}_s).$$

Moreover, in the second case, $l(ss'u) = l(s'u) - 1$. Hence

$$\begin{aligned} l(sw) = l(ss'w') = l(ss'u.u^{-1}w') &\leqslant l(ss'u) + l(u^{-1}w') \\ = l(s'u) + l(u^{-1}w') - 1 &\leqslant l(w) - 1, \end{aligned}$$

and we know that this implies that $l(sw) = l(w) - 1$.

Proof that $((\mathrm{P}_{n+1})$ and $(\mathrm{Q}_n)) \Longrightarrow (\mathrm{Q}_{n+1})$.

Let $w \in \mathrm{W}$, with $l(w) = n+1$, and $s, s' \in \mathrm{S}$, $s \neq s'$. If $w(\mathrm{C})$ is contained in $\mathrm{A}_s \cap \mathrm{A}_{s'}$, condition (Q_{n+1}) is satisfied with $u = 1$. For if not, suppose for example that $w(\mathrm{C})$ is not contained in A_s. By (P_{n+1}), $w(\mathrm{C}) \subset s(\mathrm{A}_s)$ and $l(sw) = n$. By (Q_n), applied to sw, there exists $v \in \mathrm{W}_{s,s'}$ such that

$$sw(\mathrm{C}) \subset v(\mathrm{A}_s \cap \mathrm{A}_{s'}) \quad \text{and} \quad l(sw) = l(v) + l(v^{-1}sw).$$

Then

$$w(\mathrm{C}) \subset sv(\mathrm{A}_s \cap \mathrm{A}_{s'})$$

and

$$\begin{aligned} l(w) &= 1 + l(sw) = 1 + l(v) + l(v^{-1}sw) \\ &\geqslant l(sv) + l((sv)^{-1}w) \geqslant l(w), \end{aligned}$$

so the inequalities above must be equalities. It follows that (Q_{n+1}) is satisfied with $u = sv$.

Proof of the theorem.

Let $w \in \mathrm{W}$, with $w \neq 1$. We can write w in the form sw' with $s \in \mathrm{S}$ and $l(w') = l(w) - 1$. By (P_n), applied to w' and $n = l(w')$, we have $w'(\mathrm{C}) \subset \mathrm{A}_s$, since the case $w'(\mathrm{C}) \subset s(\mathrm{A}_s)$ is excluded because $l(sw') = l(w) = l(w') + 1$. So $w(\mathrm{C}) = sw'(\mathrm{C}) \subset s(\mathrm{A}_s)$, and since A_s and $s(\mathrm{A}_s)$ are disjoint, we have $\mathrm{C} \cap w(\mathrm{C}) = \varnothing$. Q.E.D.

5. PROOF OF LEMMA 1

Let $\mathrm{E}^*_{s,s'}$ be the dual of the plane $\mathrm{E}_{s,s'} = \mathbf{R}e_s \oplus \mathbf{R}e_{s'}$ (no. 2). The transpose of the injection $\mathrm{E}_{s,s'} \to \mathrm{E}$ is a surjection

$$p : \mathrm{E}^* \to \mathrm{E}^*_{s,s'}$$

that commutes with the action of the group $\mathrm{W}_{s,s'}$. It is clear that A_s, $\mathrm{A}_{s'}$ and $\mathrm{A}_s \cap \mathrm{A}_{s'}$ are the *inverse images under* p of corresponding subsets of $\mathrm{E}^*_{s,s'}$ (considered as the space of the contragredient representation of the Coxeter group $\mathrm{W}_{s,s'}$). Moreover, since the length of an element of $\mathrm{W}_{s,s'}$ is the same with respect to $\{s, s'\}$ and with respect to S (Chap. IV, § 1, no. 8), *we are reduced finally to the case where* $\mathrm{S} = \{s, s'\}$; if $m = m(s, s')$, the group W is then a *dihedral* group of order $2m$.

We now distinguish two cases:

a) $m = +\infty$.

Let $(\varepsilon, \varepsilon')$ be the dual basis of $(e_s, e_{s'})$. Then

$$\begin{aligned} s.\varepsilon = -\varepsilon + 2\varepsilon', \quad s'.\varepsilon = \varepsilon, \\ s.\varepsilon' = \varepsilon', \quad s'.\varepsilon' = 2\varepsilon - \varepsilon'. \end{aligned}$$

Let D be the affine line of E^* containing ε and ε'; the formulas above show that D is stable under s and s' and that the restriction of s (resp. s') to D is the reflection with respect to the point ε' (resp. ε). Let

$$\theta : \mathbf{R} \to \mathrm{D}$$

be the affine bijection $t \mapsto \theta(t) = t\varepsilon + (1-t)\varepsilon'$. Let I_n be the image under θ of the open interval $]n, n+1[$, and let C_n be the union of the $\lambda \mathrm{I}_n$ for $\lambda > 0$. Then $\mathrm{C}_0 = \mathrm{C}$; moreover, by the *Remark* of § 2, no. 4, applied to the affine space D, the I_n are permuted simply-transitively by W; hence so are the C_n. If $v \in \mathrm{W}$, $v(\mathrm{C})$ is equal to one of the C_n, hence is contained in A_s if $n \geqslant 0$ and in $s(\mathrm{A}_s)$ if $n < 0$. In the second case, I_0 and I_n are on opposite sides of the point ε'; hence $l(sv) = l(v) - 1$ (*loc. cit.*).

b) m is finite.

The form $\mathrm{B_M}$ is then non-degenerate (no. 2) so we can identify E^* with E. We have seen that E can be oriented so that the angle between the half-lines $\mathbf{R}_+ e_s$ and $\mathbf{R}_+ e_{s'}$ is equal to $\pi - \frac{\pi}{m}$. Let D (resp. D′) be the half-line obtained from $\mathbf{R}_+ e_s$ (resp. $\mathbf{R}_+ e_{s'}$) by a rotation of $\pi/2$ (resp. $-\pi/2$), cf. Fig. 2. The chamber C is the set of $x \in \mathrm{E}$ whose scalar product with e_s and $e_{s'}$ is > 0; this is the open angular sector with origin D′ and extremity D. By the *Remark* of § 2, no 5, every element v of W transforms C into an angular sector that is on the same side of D as C (i.e. is contained in A_s) or on the opposite side (i.e. contained in $s(\mathrm{A}_s)$), and in the latter case

$$l(sv) = l(v) - 1,$$

which completes the proof of the lemma.

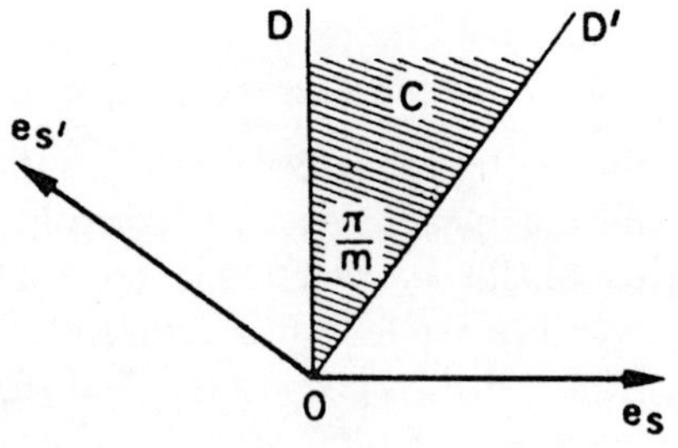

Fig. 2

6. FUNDAMENTAL DOMAIN OF W IN THE UNION OF THE CHAMBERS

We retain the notation of no. 4. For $s \in S$, denote by H_s the hyperplane of E^* orthogonal to e_s, by $\overline{A_s}$ the set of $x^* \in E^*$ such that $\langle x^*, e_s \rangle \geqslant 0$ and by $\overline{C}$ the intersection of the $\overline{A_s}$ for $s \in S$. For the weak topology $\sigma(E^*, E)$ defined by the duality between E^* and E (*Topological Vector Spaces*, Chap. II, §6, no. 2), the $\overline{A_s}$ are closed half-spaces and $\overline{C}$ is a closed convex cone. Moreover, $\overline{C}$ is the *closure* of C; indeed, if $x^* \in \overline{C}$ and $y^* \in C$, then $x^* + ty^* \in C$ for every real number $t > 0$ and $x^* = \lim_{t \to 0}(x^* + ty^*)$.

For $X \subset S$, put

$$C_X = \left(\bigcap_{s \in X} H_s \right) \cap \left(\bigcap_{s \in S - X} A_s \right).$$

We have $C_X \subset \overline{C}$, $C_\varnothing = C$ and $C_S = \{0\}$. The sets C_X, for $X \in \mathfrak{B}(S)$, form a *partition* of $\overline{C}$.

On the other hand, recall (Chap. IV, § 1, no. 8) that W_X denotes the subgroup of W generated by X. Clearly $w(x^*) = x^*$ for $w \in W_X$ and $x^* \in C_X$.

PROPOSITION 5. *Let* $X, X' \subset S$ *and* $w, w' \in W$. *If* $w(C_X) \cap w'(C_{X'}) \neq \varnothing$, *then* $X = X'$, $wW_X = w'W_{X'}$ *and* $w(C_X) = w'(C_{X'})$.

We are reduced immediately to the case $w' = 1$. The proof is by induction on the length n of w. If $n = 0$, the assertion is clear. If $l(w) > 0$, there exists $s \in S$ such that $l(sw) = l(w) - 1$ and then (cf. the end of no. 4) $w(C) \subset s(A_s)$, hence $w(\overline{C}) \subset s(\overline{A_s})$. Since $\overline{C} \subset \overline{A_s}$, it follows that

$$\overline{C} \cap w(\overline{C}) \subset H_s.$$

Then $s(x^*) = x^*$ for all $x^* \in \overline{C} \cap w(\overline{C})$, and *a fortiori* for all

$$x^* \in C_{X'} \cap w(C_X).$$

Consequently, the relation $C_{X'} \cap w(C_X) \neq \varnothing$ implies on the one hand that $C_{X'} \cap H_s \neq \varnothing$, and hence that $s \in X'$, and on the other hand that $C_{X'} \cap sw(C_X) \neq \varnothing$. The induction hypothesis then implies that $X = X'$ and $swW_X = W_{X'} = W_X$, so $sw \in W_X$ and $w \in W_X$ since $s \in W_X$. It follows that $wW_X = W_{X'}$ and that $w(C_X) = C_X = C_{X'}$.

COROLLARY. *Let* X *be a subset of* S *and* x^* *an element of* C_X. *The stabiliser of* x^* *in* W *is* W_X.

Now let U be the union of the $w(\overline{C})$ for $w \in W$, and let $\mathfrak{F}$ be the set of subsets of U of the form $w(C_X)$, with $X \subset S$ and $w \in W$. By the above, $\mathfrak{F}$ is a *partition* of U.

PROPOSITION 6. (i) *The cone* U *is convex.*

(ii) *Every closed segment contained in* U *meets only finitely many elements of* $\mathfrak{F}$.

(iii) *The cone* $\overline{\mathrm{C}}$ *is a fundamental domain for the action of* W *on* U.

To prove (iii), it is enough to show that, if $x^*, y^* \in \overline{\mathrm{C}}$ and $w \in \mathrm{W}$ are such that $w(x^*) = y^*$, then $x^* = y^*$. Now there exist two subsets X and Y of S such that $x^* \in \mathrm{C_X}$ and $y^* \in \mathrm{C_Y}$; we have $w(\mathrm{C_X}) \cap \mathrm{C_Y} \neq \varnothing$, and Prop. 5 shows that $\mathrm{X} = \mathrm{Y}$ and $w \in \mathrm{W_X}$, which implies that $x^* = y^*$.

Now let $x^*, y^* \in \mathrm{U}$; we shall show that *the segment* $[x^*y^*]$ *is covered by finitely many elements of* $\mathfrak{F}$, which will establish both (i) and (ii). By transforming x^* and y^* by the same element of W, we can assume that $x^* \in \overline{\mathrm{C}}$. Let $w \in \mathrm{W}$ be such that $y^* \in w(\overline{\mathrm{C}})$. We argue by induction on the length of w. For $s \in \mathrm{S}$, the relation $w(\overline{\mathrm{C}}) \not\subset \overline{\mathrm{A}_s}$ is equivalent to $w(\mathrm{C}) \not\subset \mathrm{A}_s$ and hence to $l(sw) < l(w)$ (cf. no. 4). Prop. 7 of no. 8 of Chap. IV, § 1 now implies that there exist only finitely many $s \in \mathrm{S}$ such that $w(\overline{\mathrm{C}}) \not\subset \overline{\mathrm{A}_s}$. The set T of $s \in \mathrm{S}$ such that $\langle y^*, e_s \rangle < 0$ is thus finite. On the other hand, the intersection $\overline{\mathrm{C}} \cap [x^*y^*]$ is a closed segment $[x^*z^*]$. If $z^* = y^*$, that is if $y^* \in \overline{\mathrm{C}}$, there exist subsets X and Y of S such that $x^* \in \mathrm{C_X}$ and $y^* \in \mathrm{C_Y}$. The open segment $]x^*y^*[$ is then contained in $\mathrm{C_{X\cap Y}}$, so $[x^*y^*] \subset \mathrm{C_X} \cup \mathrm{C_Y} \cup \mathrm{C_{X\cap Y}}$. If $z^* \neq y^*$, there exists an $s \in \mathrm{T}$ such that $z^* \in \mathrm{H}_s$. Then $w(\mathrm{C}) \not\subset \mathrm{A}_s$ and $l(sw) < l(w)$. The induction hypothesis thus implies that the segment $[z^*y^*] = s([z^*(s(y^*))])$ is covered by a finite number of elements of $\mathfrak{F}$, and hence so is

$$[x^*y^*] = [x^*z^*] \cup [z^*y^*]$$

since $[x^*z^*] \subset \overline{\mathrm{C}}$.

7. IRREDUCIBILITY OF THE GEOMETRIC REPRESENTATION OF A COXETER GROUP

We retain the notation of the preceding nos., and assume that S is *finite*.

PROPOSITION 7. *Assume that* (W, S) *is irreducible* (Chap. IV, § 1, no. 9). *Let* E^0 *be the subspace of* E *orthogonal to* E *with respect to* $\mathrm{B_M}$. *The group* W *acts trivially on* E^0, *and every subspace of* E *distinct from* E *and stable under* W *is contained in* E^0.

If $x \in \mathrm{E}^0$, then $\sigma_s(x) = x - 2\mathrm{B_M}(e_s, x)e_s = x$ for all $s \in \mathrm{S}$. Since W is generated by S, it follows that W acts trivially on E^0.

Let E' be a subspace of E stable under W. Let $s, s' \in \mathrm{S}$ be two elements that are *linked* in the graph Γ of (W, S) (Chap. IV, § 1, no. 9); recall that this means that $m(s, s') \geqslant 3$. Suppose that $e_s \in \mathrm{E}'$. Then $\sigma_{s'}(e_s) \in \mathrm{E}'$ and since the coefficient of $e_{s'}$ in $\sigma_{s'}(e_s)$ is non-zero, we have $e_{s'} \in \mathrm{E}'$. Since Γ is connected, it follows that, if E' contains one of the e_s it contains them all and coincides with E. Except in this case, it follows from Prop. 3 of § 2, no. 2

that, for all $s \in S$, E' is contained in the hyperplane H_s orthogonal to e_s. Since the intersection of the H_s is equal to E^0, this proves the proposition.

COROLLARY. *Assume that* (W, S) *is irreducible. Then:*

a) If B_M *is non-degenerate, the* W*-module* E *is absolutely simple.*

b) If B_M *is degenerate, the* W*-module* E *is not semi-simple.*

In case *a*), Prop. 7 shows that E is simple, hence also absolutely simple (§ 2, no. 1, Prop. 1).

In case *b*), $E^0 \neq 0$, $E \neq E^0$ (since $B_M \neq 0$), and Prop. 7 shows that E^0 has no complement stable under W; thus, the W-module E is not semi-simple.

8. FINITENESS CRITERION

We retain the notation of the preceding nos., and assume that S is finite.

THEOREM 2. *The following properties are equivalent:*

(1) W *is finite.*

(2) *The form* B_M *is positive and non-degenerate.*

(1) $\Longrightarrow$ (2). Let $S = \bigcup_i S_i$ be the decomposition of S into connected components (Chap. IV, § 1, no. 9), and let $W = \prod_i W_i$ be the corresponding decomposition of W. The space E can be identified with the direct sum of the spaces $E_i = \mathbf{R}^{S_i}$, and B_M can be identified with the direct sum of the corresponding forms B_{M_i}. We are thus reduced to the case when (W, S) is *irreducible*. Since W is assumed to be finite, E is a semi-simple W-module (Appendix, Prop. 2). By the Cor. to Prop. 5, it follows that E is absolutely simple. Let B' be a positive non-degenerate form on E, and let B'' be the sum of its transforms under W. Since B'' is invariant under W, it is proportional to B_M (§ 2, no. 1, Prop. 1); since $B_M(e_s, e_s) = 1$ for all $s \in S$, the coefficient of proportionality is > 0, and since B'' is positive so is B_M, which proves (2).

(2) $\Longrightarrow$ (1). If B_M is positive non-degenerate, the orthogonal group $\mathbf{O}(B_M)$ is *compact* (*Integration*, Chap. VII, § 3, no. 1). Since $\sigma(W)$ is a *discrete* subgroup of $\mathbf{O}(B_M)$ (Cor. 3 of Th. 1), it follows that $\sigma(W)$ is finite, hence so is W. Q.E.D.

The following result has been established in the course of the proof:

COROLLARY. *If* (W, S) *is irreducible and finite,* E *is an absolutely simple* W*-module.*

The finiteness criterion provided by Th. 2 permits the classification of all *finite* Coxeter groups (cf. Chap. VI, § 4). We restrict ourselves here to the following preliminary result:

PROPOSITION 8. *If* W *is finite, the graph of* (W, S) *is a forest* (Chap. IV, Appendix).

If not, this graph would contain a circuit $(s_1, \dots, s_n)$, $n \geqslant 3$. Putting $m_i = m(s_1, s_{i+1})$, $1 \leqslant i < n$, and $m_n = m(s_n, s_1)$, this means that $m_i \geqslant 3$ for all i. Let

$$x = e_{s_1} + \cdots + e_{s_n}.$$

Then $B_M(x, x) = n + 2 \sum_{i<j} B_M(e_{s_i}, e_{s_j})$. Now[2]

$$B_M(e_{s_i}, e_{s_{i+1}}) = -\cos\frac{\pi}{m_i} \leqslant -\cos\frac{\pi}{3} \leqslant -\frac{1}{2},$$

and similarly for $B_M(e_{s_n}, e_{s_1})$. Since the other terms in the sum are $\leqslant 0$, we obtain

$$B_M(x, x) \leqslant n - n = 0,$$

contrary to the fact that B_M is positive non-degenerate.

COROLLARY. *If* (W, S) *is irreducible and finite, its graph is a tree.*

Indeed, a connected forest is a tree.

Comparison with the results of § 3.

First of all let (W, S) be a finite Coxeter group. Denote by $(x|y)$ the form $B_M(x, y)$; by Th. 2, this is a scalar product on E. For all $s \in S$, let H_s be the hyperplane associated to the orthogonal reflection σ_s, and let $\mathfrak{H}$ be the family of hyperplanes $w(H_s)$, for $s \in S$, $w \in W$. Let C_0 be the set of $x \in E$ such that $(x|e_s) > 0$ for all $s \in S$. Finally, identify W (by means of σ) with a subgroup of the orthogonal group $\mathbf{O}(E)$ of the space E.

PROPOSITION 9. *With the preceding notations,* W *is the subgroup of* $\mathbf{O}(E)$ *generated by the reflections with respect to the hyperplanes of* $\mathfrak{H}$. *It is an essential group* (§ 3, no. 7) *and* C_0 *is a chamber of* E *relative to* $\mathfrak{H}$.

The first assertion is trivial. On the other hand, if $x \in E$ is invariant under W, it is orthogonal to all the e_s, and hence is zero; this shows that W is essential. Finally, the isomorphism $E \to E^*$ defined by B_M transforms C_0 to the set C of no. 4; the property (P_n) proved there shows that, for all

---

[2] The roots of the equation $z^3 - 1 = 0$ are 1 and $\frac{-1 \pm i\sqrt{3}}{2}$. Thus $\cos\frac{2\pi}{3} = -\frac{1}{2}$ and consequently $\cos\frac{\pi}{3} = \frac{1}{2}$. Note also that $\sin\frac{2\pi}{3} = \frac{\sqrt{3}}{2}$, hence

$$\sin\frac{\pi}{3} = \frac{\sqrt{3}}{2}, \quad \cos\frac{\pi}{6} = -\cos\frac{5\pi}{6} = \frac{\sqrt{3}}{2}, \quad \sin\frac{\pi}{6} = \sin\frac{5\pi}{6} = \frac{1}{2}.$$

Similarly, the roots of the equation $z^2 - i = 0$ are $\pm\frac{1+i}{\sqrt{2}}$, so

$$\cos\frac{\pi}{4} = \sin\frac{\pi}{4} = \frac{\sqrt{2}}{2} \text{ and consequently } \sin\frac{3\pi}{4} = -\cos\frac{3\pi}{4} = \frac{\sqrt{2}}{2}.$$

$w \in \mathrm{W}$ and all $s \in \mathrm{S}$, $w(\mathrm{C}_0)$ does not meet H_s. It follows that C_0 is contained in the complement U of the union of the hyperplanes of $\mathfrak{H}$, and since C_0 is connected, open and closed in U, it is a *chamber* of E relative to $\mathfrak{H}$. Q.E.D.

We can apply to W and C_0 all the properties proved in § 3. In particular, $\overline{\mathrm{C}_0}$ is a *fundamental domain* for the action of W on E (in other words, the cone U defined in no. 6 is equal to the whole of E).

Conversely, let E be a finite dimensional real vector space, provided with a scalar product $(x|y)$ and let W be an essential finite group of displacements of E leaving 0 fixed; assume that W is *generated by reflections.* Let C_0 be a chamber of E with respect to W (cf. § 3), and let S be the set of orthogonal reflections relative to the walls of C_0. Then (W, S) is a *finite Coxeter system* (§ 3, no. 2, Th. 1). Moreover, if $s \in \mathrm{S}$, denote by H_s the wall of C_0 corresponding to s, and denote by e_s the unit vector orthogonal to H_s and on the same side of H_s as C_0. If $(m(s,s'))$ denotes the Coxeter matrix of (W, S), Props. 3 and 7 of § 3 show that

$$(e_s|e_{s'}) = -\cos(\pi/m(s,s'))$$

and that the e_s form a basis of E. *The natural representation of* W *on* E *can thus be identified with the representation* σ *of no. 3.*

9. CASE IN WHICH $\mathrm{B_M}$ IS POSITIVE AND DEGENERATE

In this number, we assume that S is finite, that (W, S) is *irreducible*, and that the form $\mathrm{B_M}$ is *positive* and *degenerate.*

Lemma 2. The orthogonal complement E^0 *of* E *for* $\mathrm{B_M}$ *is of dimension 1; it is generated by an element* $v = \sum_{s \in \mathrm{S}} v_s e_s$ *with* $v_s > 0$ *for all* s.

This follows from Lemma 4 of § 3, no. 5, applied to the matrix with entries $\mathrm{B_M}(e_s, e_{s'})$.

Let $v = \sum_s v_s e_s$ be the vector satisfying the conditions of Lemma 2 and such that $\sum_s v_s = 1$, and let A be the affine hyperplane of E^* consisting of the $y^* \in \mathrm{E}^*$ such that $\langle v, y^*\rangle = 1$. If T denotes the orthogonal complement of v in E^*, A has a natural structure of an affine space with space of translations T. Moreover, the form $\mathrm{B_M}$ defines by passage to the quotient a non-degenerate scalar product on E/E^0, hence also on its dual T; this gives a *euclidean structure* on the affine space A (*Algebra*, Chap. IX, § 6, no. 6).

Let G be the subgroup of $\mathbf{GL}(\mathrm{E})$ consisting of the automorphisms leaving v and $\mathrm{B_M}$ invariant; if $g \in \mathrm{G}$, the contragredient map ${}^t g^{-1}$ leaves A and T stable, and defines by restriction to A a *displacement* $i(g)$ of A (cf. § 3). It is immediate that this gives an *isomorphism* from G to the group of displacements of A. Moreover, the stabiliser G_a of a point a of A can be identified with the orthogonal group of the Hilbert space T and is thus *compact.* On the other hand, G is a locally compact group countable at infinity and A is a Baire space: it follows (*Integration*, Chap. VII, Appendix, Lemma 2) that the map $\psi : g \mapsto g(a)$ defines a homeomorphism from G/G_a to A. Thus G *acts properly on* A (*General Topology,* Chap. III, § 4, no. 2, Prop. 5). Since W is a subgroup of G, it can be identified with a group of displacements of A. We are going to show that this group satisfies the assumptions of § 3. More precisely:

PROPOSITION 10. *The group* W *provided with the discrete topology acts properly on* A; *it is generated by orthogonal reflections; it is infinite, irreducible and essential* (§ 3, no. 7). *The intersection* $C \cap A$ *is a chamber of* A *for* W. *If* L_s *denotes the hyperplane of* A *formed by the intersection of* A *with the hyperplane of* E^* *orthogonal to* e_s, *the* L_s *for* $s \in S$ *are the walls of* $C \cap A$. *If* ε_s *is the unit vector of* T *orthogonal to* L_s *on the same side of* L_s *as* $C \cap A$, *then* $(\varepsilon_s|\varepsilon_t) = -\cos(\pi/m(s,t))$ *(for* $s, t \in S$*) and the Coxeter matrix of* W (§ 3, no. 4) *is identified with* M.

By Cor. 3 of Th. 1, W is discrete in $\mathbf{GL}(E)$, and hence in G, and acts properly on A. Let $s \in S$. Since $\operatorname{Card} S \geqslant 2$, the hyperplane of E^* orthogonal to e_s is not orthogonal to v and its intersection L_s with A is indeed a hyperplane. The displacement corresponding to s is thus a displacement of order 2 leaving fixed all the points of L_s: it is necessarily the orthogonal reflection associated to L_s. It follows that W is generated by orthogonal reflections. Th. 2 now shows that it is infinite and Prop. 7 that it is essential and irreducible.

Since C is an open simplicial cone, whose walls are the hyperplanes with equations $\langle x^*, e_s\rangle = 0$ (for $s \in S$), the intersection $C \cap A$ is a convex, hence connected, open and closed subset of the complement of the union of the L_s in A. Moreover, $C \cap A$ is non-empty, for if $x^* \in C$ we have $\langle x^*, v\rangle = \sum_s v_s \langle x^*, e_s\rangle > 0$ and $\langle x^*, v\rangle^{-1} x^* \in C \cap A$. It follows that $C \cap A$ is a chamber of A relative to the system of the L_s. Moreover, $w(C \cap A) \cap L_s = \varnothing$ for all $w \in W$ (cf. no. 4, property (P_n)) and it follows that $C \cap A$ is a chamber of A relative to the system consisting of the transforms of the L_s by the elements of W; by the Cor. of Th. 1 of § 3, no. 2, it follows that $C \cap A$ is a chamber of A relative to W.

Let a_s^* be the vertex of the simplex $C \cap A$ not in L_s. We have

$$\langle a_s^*, e_t\rangle = 0$$

for $s, t \in S$ and $s \neq t$, and

$$\langle a_s^*, e_s\rangle = v_s^{-1}\langle a_s^*, v\rangle = v_s^{-1}.$$

Let ε_s be the vector in T defined by the relations:

$$(\varepsilon_s | a_s^* - a_t^*) = v_s^{-1} \text{ for } t \in S,\ t \neq s.$$

The vector ε_s is orthogonal to L_s and is on the same side of the hyperplane L_s as $C \cap A$. Moreover

$$(\varepsilon_s|a_s^* - a_t^*) = \langle e_s, a_s^* - a_t^* \rangle \quad \text{for all} \quad s,t \in S$$

which shows that ε_s is the image of the class of e_s under the isomorphism from E/E^0 to T given by the quadratic form B_M. It follows that

$$(\varepsilon_s|\varepsilon_t) = B_M(e_s, e_t).$$

Consequently ε_s is a unit vector and the last assertion of Prop. 10 is proved.

The euclidean affine space A provided with the group W is called *the space associated to the Coxeter matrix* M and we denote it by A_M.

Proposition 10 admits a converse:

PROPOSITION 11. *Let* W *be a group of displacements of a euclidean affine space* A, *satisfying the assumptions of* § 3. *Assume that* W *is infinite, essential and irreducible. Then the form* B_M *attached to the Coxeter matrix* M *of* W *is positive degenerate and there exists a unique isomorphism from the affine space* A_M *associated to* M *to* A, *commuting with the action of* W. *This isomorphism transforms the scalar product of* A_M *into a multiple of the scalar product of* A.

Let C_0 be a chamber of A and let S be the set of orthogonal reflections with respect to the walls of C_0. If η_s denotes the unit vector orthogonal to the hyperplane N_s associated to the reflection s and on the same side of N_s as C_0 (§3, Prop. 3), the form B_M is such that $B_M(e_s, e_t) = (\eta_s|\eta_t)$ for $s, t \in S$. It is thus *positive*. Since the η_s are linearly dependent (§ 3, no. 9, Prop. 8), it is *degenerate*.

We can thus apply the preceding constructions to M. With the same notation as above, $(\varepsilon_s|\varepsilon_t) = (\eta_s|\eta_t)$ and there exists a unique isomorphism φ of Hilbert spaces from T to the space of translations of A such that $\varphi(\varepsilon_s) = \eta_s$. Let a and b be two distinct vertices of C_0 and s_0 the reflection in S such that $a \notin N_{s_0}$. Put $\lambda = (\eta_s|a - b)$ and let ψ be the affine bijection from A_M to A defined by

$$\psi(a_{s_0} + x) = a + v_{s_0}\lambda\varphi(x) \quad \text{for} \quad x \in T.$$

It is then immediate that $\psi(L_s) = N_s$ for all $s \in S$ and that ψ transforms the scalar product of A_M into a multiple of that on A. It follows at once that ψ commutes with the action of W. Finally, the uniqueness of ψ is evident, for a_s for example is the unique point of A_M invariant under the reflections $t \in S$, $t \neq s$.

§ 5. INVARIANTS IN THE SYMMETRIC ALGEBRA

1. POINCARÉ SERIES OF GRADED ALGEBRAS

Let K be a commutative ring with unit element, not reduced to 0. Let M be a graded K-module of type $\mathbf{Z}$, and M_n the set of homogeneous elements of M of degree n. Assume that each M_n is *free and of finite type.* Then the rank $\mathrm{rk}_K(M_n)$ is defined for all n (*Commutative Algebra*, Chap. II, § 5, no. 3).

DEFINITION 1. *If there exists* $n_0 \in \mathbf{Z}$ *such that* $M_n = 0$ *for* $n \leqslant n_0$*, the formal series* $\sum_{n \geqslant n_0} \mathrm{rk}_K(M_n)T^n$*, which is an element of* $\mathbf{Q}((T))$*, is called the Poincaré series of* M *and denoted by* $P_M(T)$.

Let M′ be another graded K-module of type $\mathbf{Z}$, and $(M'_n)_{n\in\mathbf{Z}}$ its grading. Assume that M'_n is zero for n less than a certain number. Then

$$P_{M\oplus M'}(T) = P_M(T) + P_{M'}(T) \tag{1}$$

and, if $M \otimes_K M'$ is provided with the total grading (*Algebra*, Chap. II, § 11, no. 5),

$$P_{M\otimes M'}(T) = P_M(T)P_{M'}(T). \tag{2}$$

PROPOSITION 1. *Let* $S = \bigoplus_{n\geqslant 0} S_n$ *be a commutative graded* K*-algebra with a system of generators* $(x_1, x_2, \ldots, x_m)$ *consisting of homogeneous and algebraically independent elements. Let* d_i *be the degree of* x_i*, and assume that* $d_i > 0$ *for all* i*. Then the* S_n *are free and of finite rank over* K*, and*

$$P_S(T) = \prod_{i=1}^{m} (1 - T^{d_i})^{-1}. \tag{3}$$

Indeed, S can be identified with the tensor product $K[x_1] \otimes \cdots \otimes K[x_m]$, provided with the total grading. The Poincaré series of $K[x_i]$ is

$$\sum_{n\geqslant 0} T^{nd_i} = (1 - T^{d_i})^{-1},$$

and it suffices to apply (2).

Under the assumptions of Prop. 1, we shall say that S is a *graded polynomial algebra over* K.

COROLLARY. *The degrees* d_i *are determined up to order by* S.

Indeed, the inverse of $P_S(T)$ is the polynomial $N(T) = \prod_{i=1}^{m}(1 - T^{d_i})$, which is thus uniquely determined. If q is an integer $\geqslant 1$ and if $\zeta \in \mathbf{C}$ is a primitive qth root of unity, the multiplicity of the root ζ of N(T) is equal to the number of d_i that are multiples of q. This number is zero for q sufficiently large. The number of d_i equal to q is thus determined uniquely by descending induction.

The integers d_i are called the *characteristic degrees* of S. The number of them is equal to the transcendence degree of S over K when K is a field; we shall also call it the transcendence degree of S over K in the general case. It is the multiplicity of the root 1 of the polynomial N(T).

Let $\mathrm{S} = \bigoplus_{n\geqslant 0} \mathrm{S}_n$ be a commutative graded K-algebra, and $\mathrm{R} = \bigoplus_{n\geqslant 0} \mathrm{R}_n$ a graded subalgebra of S. *Assume that each* R_n *is free and of finite type, and that the* R*-module* S *admits a finite basis consisting of homogeneous elements* $z_1, z_2, \dots, z_\mathrm{N}$ *of degrees* $f_1, f_2, \dots, f_\mathrm{N}$. Then, if M denotes the graded K-module $\sum_{j=1}^{\mathrm{N}} \mathrm{K}z_j$, the graded K-module S is isomorphic to $\mathrm{R}\otimes_\mathrm{K} \mathrm{M}$, so each S_n is free and of finite type and

$$\mathrm{P_S(T)} = \mathrm{P_M(T)P_R(T)} = \left(\sum_{j=1}^{\mathrm{N}} \mathrm{T}^{f_j}\right) \mathrm{P_R(T)}. \tag{4}$$

PROPOSITION 2. *Retain the preceding notation and assume that* S *and* R *are graded polynomial algebras.*

(i) R *and* S *have the same transcendence degree* r *over* K.

(ii) *Let* $p_1, \dots, p_r$ *(resp.* $q_1, \dots, q_r$*) be the characteristic degrees of* S *(resp.* R*). Then*

$$\prod_{i=1}^{r} (1 - \mathrm{T}^{q_i}) = \left(\sum_{j=1}^{\mathrm{N}} \mathrm{T}^{f_j}\right) \prod_{i=1}^{r} (1 - \mathrm{T}^{p_i}).$$

(iii) $\mathrm{N}p_1p_2\dots p_r = q_1q_2\dots q_r$.

Formula (4) shows first of all that the multiplicity of the root 1 is the same in the polynomials $\mathrm{P_S(T)}^{-1}$ and $\mathrm{P_R(T)}^{-1}$ and, taking (3) into account, proves both (i) and (ii).

It follows from (ii) that

$$\prod_{i=1}^{r} (1 + \mathrm{T} + \mathrm{T}^2 + \dots + \mathrm{T}^{q_i - 1}) = \left(\sum_{j=1}^{\mathrm{N}} \mathrm{T}^{f_j}\right) \prod_{i=1}^{r} (1 + \mathrm{T} + \mathrm{T}^2 + \dots + \mathrm{T}^{p_\mathrm{I} - 1}).$$

Putting $\mathrm{T} = 1$ in this relation gives (iii).

Remark. Let $\mathrm{S} = \mathrm{K}[\mathrm{X}_1, \dots, \mathrm{X}_n]$ be a graded polynomial algebra over K, d_i the degree of X_i and $\mathrm{F}(\mathrm{X}_1, \dots, \mathrm{X}_n)$ a homogeneous element of degree m of S. Then

$$\sum_{i=1}^{n} d_i \mathrm{X}_i \frac{\partial \mathrm{F}}{\partial \mathrm{X}_i} = m\mathrm{F}. \tag{5}$$

Indeed, it is immediate that the K-linear map D from S to S that transforms every homogeneous element z of degree p into pz is a derivation of S. Thus

$$mF(X_1,\ldots,X_n) = D(F(X_1,\ldots,X_n)) = \sum_{i=1}^{n} D(X_i)\frac{\partial F}{\partial X_i} = \sum_{i=1}^{n} d_i X_i \frac{\partial F}{\partial X_i}.$$

2. INVARIANTS OF A FINITE LINEAR GROUP: MODULAR PROPERTIES

Let K be a commutative ring, V a K-module, and G a group acting on V. We know that every automorphism of V extends uniquely to an automorphism of the symmetric algebra $S = \mathbf{S}(V)$, and thus G acts on this algebra. If $x \in S$ and $g \in G$, we denote by $g_S.x$ the transform of x by g. Let R be the subalgebra S^G of S formed by the elements invariant under G.

Assume that G is finite, V is of finite type, and K is noetherian. Then S is an R-*module of finite type*, and R is a K-algebra of finite type (*Commutative Algebra*, Chap. V, § 1, no. 9, Th. 2). Assume that S is integral and let N be its field of fractions. The field of fractions L of R is the set of elements of N invariant under G (*loc. cit.*, Cor. of Prop. 23), so N is a G*alois* extension of L. Every element of N can be written z/t with $z \in S$ and $t \in R$ (*loc. cit.*, Prop. 23). By *Algebra*, Chap. II, §7, no. 10, Cor. 3 of Prop. 26, the rank of the R-module S is $[N : L]$. Assume that G acts faithfully on V. The Galois group of N over L can then be identified with G, so $[N : L] = \mathrm{Card}\, G$; thus

$$\mathrm{rk}_R(S) = [N : L] = \mathrm{Card}(G). \tag{6}$$

For any graded algebra $A = A_0 \oplus A_1 \oplus \cdots \oplus A_n \oplus \cdots$, denote by A_+ the ideal $\bigoplus_{n>0} A_n$.

THEOREM 1. *Let* K *be a commutative field,* V *a finite dimensional vector space over* K, $S = \mathbf{S}(V)$ *the symmetric algebra of* V, G *a finite group of automorphisms of* V, *and* R *the graded subalgebra of* S *consisting of the elements invariant under* G. *Assume that* G *is generated by pseudo-reflections* (§ 2, no. 1) *and that* $q = \mathrm{Card}(G)$ *is coprime to the characteristic of* K. *Then the* R-*module* S *has a basis consisting of* q *homogeneous elements.*

a) Since every submodule of $S/(R_+S)$ is free over $R_0 = K$, it is enough to show (in view of *Algebra*, Chap. II, § 11, no. 4, Prop. 7) that the canonical homomorphism from $R_+ \otimes_R S$ to S is injective. For any R-module E, denote by T(E) the R-module $\mathrm{Ker}(R_+ \otimes_R E \to E)$ (*in other words, $T(E) = \mathrm{Tor}_1^R(R/R_+, E)_*$). If E, E' are two R-modules and u is a homomorphism from E to E', the homomorphism $1 \otimes u$ from $R_+ \otimes E$ to $R_+ \otimes E'$ defines by restriction to T(E) a homomorphism from T(E) to $T(E')$ that we denote by $T(u)$. If u' is a homomorphism from E' to an R-module E'', we have $T(u' \circ u) = T(u') \circ T(u)$. Thus, if G acts R-linearly on E, then G acts on T(E).

b) The group G acts R-linearly on S, and hence also on T(S). Moreover, T(S) has a natural structure of graded S-module. We show first that, if $g \in \mathrm{G}$, then g transforms every element x of T(S) into an element congruent to x modulo $\mathrm{S}_1\mathrm{T(S)}$. It is enough to do this when g is a pseudo-reflection. Then there exists a non-zero vector v in V such that $g(x) - x \in \mathrm{K}v$ for all $x \in \mathrm{V}$. Since V generates S, it follows that g_S acts trivially on $\mathrm{S}/\mathrm{S}v$. Thus, for any $y \in \mathrm{S}$, there exists an element $h(y)$ in S such that

$$g_\mathrm{S}(y) - y = h(y)v.$$

Since S is integral and v is non-zero, this element is determined uniquely by y; it is immediate that h is an endomorphism of degree -1 of the R-module S. Thus, $g_\mathrm{S} - 1_\mathrm{S} = m_v \circ h$, where m_v denotes the homothety with ratio v in S. Hence,

$$\mathrm{T}(g_\mathrm{S}) - 1_{\mathrm{T(S)}} = \mathrm{T}(g_\mathrm{S} - 1_\mathrm{S}) = \mathrm{T}(m_v) \circ \mathrm{T}(h),$$

the image of which is contained in $v\mathrm{T(S)}$, proving our assertion.

c) We show that any element of T(S) invariant under G is zero. Indeed, let Q be the endomorphism of the R-module S defined by

$$\mathrm{Q}(y) = q^{-1} \sum_{g \in \mathrm{G}} g_\mathrm{S}(y)$$

for all $y \in \mathrm{S}$. Then $\mathrm{Q(S)} = \mathrm{R}$. We can thus write $\mathrm{Q} = i \circ \mathrm{Q}'$, where Q' is a homomorphism from the R-module S to the R-module R and i denotes the canonical injection of R into S. Thus $\mathrm{T(Q)} = \mathrm{T(i)} \circ \mathrm{T(Q')}$ and $\mathrm{T(Q')} = 0$ since $\mathrm{T(R)} = \mathrm{Ker}(\mathrm{R}_+ \otimes \mathrm{R} \to \mathrm{R}) = 0$. Thus

$$0 = \mathrm{T(Q)} = q^{-1} \sum_{g \in \mathrm{G}} \mathrm{T}(g_\mathrm{S}).$$

But $q^{-1} \sum_{g \in \mathrm{G}} \mathrm{T}(g_\mathrm{S})$ leaves fixed the elements of T(S) invariant under G. These elements are therefore zero.

d) Assume that $\mathrm{T(S)} \neq 0$. There exists in T(S) a homogeneous element $u \neq 0$ of minimum degree. By *b*), u is invariant under G. By *c*), $u = 0$. This is a contradiction, so $\mathrm{T(S)} = 0$. Q.E.D.

Remarks. 1) It follows from *Algebra*, Chap. II, §11, no. 4, Prop. 7 that, if $(z_1, \dots, z_q)$ is a family of homogeneous elements of S whose canonical images in $\mathrm{S}/(\mathrm{R}_+\mathrm{S})$ form a basis of $\mathrm{S}/(\mathrm{R}_+\mathrm{S})$ over K, then $(z_1, \dots, z_q)$ is a basis of S over R.

2) Let g be a pseudo-reflection of V, whose order $n \geqslant 2$ is finite and coprime to the characteristic of K. By Maschke's theorem (Appendix, Prop. 2), V can be decomposed as $\mathrm{D} \oplus \mathrm{H}$, where H is the hyperplane consisting of the elements of V invariant under g and D is a line on which g acts by multiplication by a primitive nth root of unity. When $\mathrm{K} = \mathbf{R}$, this is possible only when $n = 2$, and g is then a *reflection*; in this case, the groups to which Th. 1

applies are the *finite Coxeter groups.* (For $K = \mathbf{C}$, on the other hand, Th. 1 applies to certain groups that are not Coxeter groups.)[3]

THEOREM 2. *Retain the assumptions and notation of Theorem* 1.

(i) *There exists a graded vector subspace of* S *forming a complement to* R_+S *in* S *and stable under* G.

(ii) *Let* U *be such a complement. The canonical homomorphism from* $U \otimes_K R$ *to* S *is an isomorphism of* G*-modules, and the representation of* G *in* U *(resp.* S*) is isomorphic to the regular representation of* G *on* K *(resp.* R*).*

Indeed, for any integer $n \geqslant 0$, the K-vector spaces S_n and $(R_+S) \cap S_n$ are stable under G, and it follows from Maschke's theorem (Appendix, Prop. 2) that there exists a G-stable complement U_n of $(R_+S) \cap S_n$ in S_n. Then $\sum_{n \geqslant 0} U_n$ is a G-stable complement of R_+S in S, hence (i).

Let U be a graded vector subspace of S forming a complement of R_+S in S and stable under G. By Remark 1, every basis of the K-vector space U is also a basis of the R-module S, and consequently is a basis of the field of fractions N of S over the field of fractions L of R. Thus, the L-vector space N can be identified with $U \otimes_K L$. Since U is stable under G, this identification is compatible with the action of G. The group algebra L[G] of G over L can be identified with the algebra $K[G] \otimes_K L$. The Galois extension N of L admits a normal basis (*Algebra*, Chap. V, § 10, no. 9, Th. 6), which can be interpreted as saying that N, considered as an L[G]-module, is isomorphic to the module of the regular representation of G over L. Since U is finite dimensional over K, it follows from the Appendix, Prop. 1, that the K[G]-module U is isomorphic to the regular representation of G over K. Our assertions follow immediately from this.

3. INVARIANTS OF A FINITE LINEAR GROUP: RING-THEORETIC PROPERTIES

THEOREM 3. *We retain the assumptions and notation of Th.* 1. *In the set of systems of generators of the ideal* R_+ *of* R *consisting of homogeneous elements, choose a minimal element* $(\alpha_1, \ldots, \alpha_l)$. *Let* k_i *be the degree of* α_i. *Assume that the* k_i *are coprime to the characteristic exponent of* K. *Then* $l = \dim V$, *the* α_i *generate the* K*-algebra* R, *and are algebraically independent over* K. *In particular,* R *is a graded* K*-algebra of polynomials of transcendence degree* l *over* K.

The assumption made about the k_i is superfluous, but is irrelevant for the applications to finite Coxeter groups, since then $K = \mathbf{R}$. Cf. no. 5, where we shall give another proof of Th. 3.

[3] A classification of such groups can be found in G. C. SHEPHARD and J. A. TODD, Finite unitary reflection groups, *Canadian J. of Maths.*, Vol. VI (1954), p. 274-304.

Th. 3 follows from Prop. 2 (i), Th. 1 and the following lemma:

Lemma 1. Let K *be a commutative field,* S *a graded* K*-algebra of polynomials, and* R *a graded subalgebra of* S *of finite type such that the* R*-module* S *admits a basis* $(z_\lambda)_{\lambda \in \Lambda}$ *consisting of homogeneous elements. In the set of systems of generators of the ideal* R_+ *of* R *consisting of homogeneous elements, choose a minimal element* $(\alpha_1, \ldots, \alpha_s)$*. Assume that, for all* i*, the degree* k_i *of* α_i *is coprime to the characteristic exponent* p *of* K*. Then the* α_i *generate the* K*-algebra* R *and are algebraically independent over* K*.*

By *Algebra*, Chap. II, § 11, no. 4, Prop. 7, the assumption made about the α_i is equivalent to saying that they are homogeneous and that their images in the K-vector space $R_+/(R_+)^2$ form a basis of this space. This condition is invariant under extension of the base field; we can thus reduce to the case where the latter is *perfect.*

The family $(\alpha_1, \ldots, \alpha_s)$ generates the algebra R by *Commutative Algebra*, Chap. III, § 1, no. 2, Prop. 1. We argue by contradiction and assume that this family is not algebraically independent over K.

1) We show first of all that there exist families

$$(\beta_i)_{1 \leqslant i \leqslant s}, \quad (y_k)_{1 \leqslant k \leqslant r}, \quad (d_{ik})_{1 \leqslant i \leqslant s,\, 1 \leqslant k \leqslant r}$$

of homogeneous elements of S with the following properties:

$$\beta_i \in R \text{ for all } i, \text{ and the } \beta_i \text{ are not all zero;} \tag{7}$$

$$\deg y_k > 0 \text{ for all } k; \tag{8}$$

$$\alpha_i = \sum_{k=1}^{r} d_{ik} y_k \quad \text{for all } i; \tag{9}$$

$$\sum_{i=1}^{s} \beta_i d_{ik} = 0 \quad \text{for all } k. \tag{10}$$

Let $X_1, \ldots, X_s$ be indeterminates and give $K[X_1, \ldots, X_s]$ with the graded algebra structure for which X_i has degree k_i. There exist non-zero homogeneous elements $H(X_1, \ldots, X_s)$ of $K[X_1, \ldots, X_s]$ such that $H(\alpha_1, \ldots, \alpha_s) = 0$; choose H to be of minimum degree. If $\partial H/\partial X_i \neq 0$, the polynomial $\frac{\partial H}{\partial X_i}(\alpha_1, \ldots, \alpha_s)$ is a non-zero homogeneous element of R; if $p \neq 1$, H is not of the form H_1^p with $H_1 \in K[X_1, \ldots, X_s]$. Take

$$\beta_i = k_i \frac{\partial H}{\partial X_i}(\alpha_1, \ldots, \alpha_s).$$

Since K is perfect, the polynomials $\partial H/\partial X_i \in K[X_1, \ldots, X_s]$ are not all zero (*Algebra*, Chap. V, § 1, no. 3, Prop. 4); in view of the assumption made about the k_i, neither are the β_i.

On the other hand, S can be identified with a graded algebra of polynomials $K[x_1, \ldots, x_r]$ for appropriate indeterminates $x_1, \ldots, x_r$ with suitable degrees $m_i > 0$. Let D_k be the partial derivative with respect to x_k on S. Take

$d_{ik} = k_i^{-1}\mathrm{D}_k(\alpha_i)$. Then the equality (10) holds because its left-hand side is $\mathrm{D}_k(\mathrm{H}(\alpha_1,\ldots,\alpha_s))$. On the other hand, if we put $y_1 = m_1x_1,\ldots,y_r = m_rx_r$, the equality (9) follows from the equality (5) of no. 1.

2) Let $\mathfrak{b}$ be the ideal of R generated by the β_i; there exists a subset J of

$$\mathrm{I} = \{1, 2, \ldots, s\}$$

such that $(\beta_i)_{i\in\mathrm{J}}$ is a minimal system of generators of $\mathfrak{b}$. Then $\mathrm{J} \neq \varnothing$ since $\mathfrak{b} \neq 0$. We shall deduce from (9) and (10) that, if $i \in \mathrm{J}$, α_i is an R-linear combination of the α_j for $j \neq i$, which will contradict the minimality of $(\alpha_1,\ldots,\alpha_s)$ and will complete the proof.

There exist homogeneous elements γ_{ji} of R ($i \in \mathrm{J}$, $j \in \mathrm{I}-\mathrm{J}$) such that

$$\beta_j = \sum_{i\in\mathrm{J}} \gamma_{ji}\beta_i \quad (j \in \mathrm{I}-\mathrm{J}). \tag{11}$$

Taking (11) into account, formula (10) gives

$$\sum_{i\in\mathrm{J}} \beta_i \left(d_{ik} + \sum_{j\in\mathrm{IJ}} \gamma_{ji}d_{jk}\right) = 0. \tag{12}$$

Put

$$u_{ik} = d_{ik} + \sum_{j\in\mathrm{I}-\mathrm{J}} \gamma_{ji}d_{jk}. \tag{13}$$

Thus

$$\sum_{i\in\mathrm{J}} \beta_i u_{ik} = 0. \tag{14}$$

Write $u_{ik} = \sum_{\lambda\in\Lambda} \delta_{ik\lambda}z_\lambda$, where the $\delta_{ik\lambda}$ belong to R. Relation (14) implies that $\sum_{i\in\mathrm{J}} \beta_i\delta_{ik\lambda} = 0$ for all k and λ. If one of the $\delta_{ik\lambda}$ had a non-zero homogeneous component of degree 0, the preceding equality would imply that one of the β_i ($i \in \mathrm{J}$) is an R-linear combination of the others, contradicting the minimality of $(\beta_i)_{i\in\mathrm{J}}$. Thus $\delta_{ik\lambda} \in \mathrm{R}_+$ and consequently $u_{ik} \in \mathrm{R}_+\mathrm{S}$ for all i and k. Thus, there exist $u_{ikh} \in \mathrm{S}$ such that $u_{ik} = \sum_{h=1}^{s} u_{ikh}\alpha_h$, in other words, by (13),

$$d_{ik} + \sum_{j\in\mathrm{I}-\mathrm{J}} \gamma_{ji}d_{jk} = \sum_{h=1}^{s} u_{ikh}\alpha_h. \tag{15}_{ik}$$

Multiply both sides of $(15)_{ik}$ by y_k and add for i in J fixed and $k = 1, 2, \ldots, r$; in view of (9), we find that

$$\alpha_i + \sum_{j\in\mathrm{I}-\mathrm{J}} \gamma_{ji}\alpha_j = \sum_{h=1}^{s}\sum_{k=1}^{r} u_{ikh}y_k\alpha_h.$$

Take the homogeneous components of degree k_i of both sides. Since $\deg y_k > 0$, α_i is an S-linear combination of the α_j for $j \neq i$. Since S is free over R and $\alpha_1,\ldots,\alpha_s \in \mathrm{R}$, it follows that α_i is an R-linear combination of the α_j with $j \neq i$ (*Commutative Algebra*, Chap. I, § 3, no. 5, Prop. 9 *d*)).

COROLLARY. *With the assumptions and notation of Th. 3, the product of the characteristic degrees of* R *is* Card(G).

Indeed, $\mathrm{rk}_{\mathrm{R}}(\mathrm{S}) = \mathrm{Card}(\mathrm{G})$ (formula (6), no. 2). The characteristic degrees of S are equal to 1. Then the corollary follows from no. 1, Prop. 2 (iii).

Lemma 2. Let K *be a commutative field,* V *a finite dimensional vector space over* K, $\mathrm{S} = \bigoplus_{n \geqslant 0} \mathrm{S}_n$ *the symmetric algebra of* V, s *an endomorphism of* V, *and* $s^{(n)}$ *the canonical extension of* s *to* S_n. *Then, with* T *denoting an indeterminate, we have in* K[[T]]

$$\sum_{n=0}^{\infty} \mathrm{Tr}(s^{(n)})\mathrm{T}^n = (\det(1 - s\mathrm{T}))^{-1}.$$

Extending the base field if necessary, we can assume that K is algebraically closed. Let $(e_1, \dots, e_r)$ be a basis of V with respect to which the matrix of s is lower triangular, and let $\lambda_1, \dots, \lambda_r$ be the diagonal elements of this matrix. With respect to the basis $(e_1^{i(1)} \dots e_r^{i(r)})_{i(1)+\cdots+i(r)=n}$ of S_n, ordered lexicographically, the matrix of $s^{(n)}$ is lower triangular and its diagonal elements are the products $\lambda_1^{i(1)} \dots \lambda_r^{i(r)}$. Thus

$$\mathrm{Tr}(s^{(n)}) = \sum_{i(1)+\cdots+i(r)=n} \lambda_1^{i(1)} \dots \lambda_r^{i(r)},$$

and consequently

$$\begin{aligned}\sum_{n=0}^{\infty} \mathrm{Tr}(s^{(n)})\mathrm{T}^n &= \left(\sum_{n=0}^{\infty} \lambda_1^n \mathrm{T}^n\right)\left(\sum_{n=0}^{\infty} \lambda_2^n \mathrm{T}^n\right) \dots \left(\sum_{n=0}^{\infty} \lambda_r^n \mathrm{T}^n\right)\\ &= (1-\lambda_1\mathrm{T})^{-1}(1-\lambda_2\mathrm{T})^{-1}\dots(1-\lambda_r\mathrm{T})^{-1}\\ &= (\det(1 - s\mathrm{T}))^{-1}.\end{aligned}$$

Lemma 3. Let K, V *and* S *be as in* Lemma 2, G *a finite group of automorphisms of* V, q *the order of* G, *and* R *the graded subalgebra of* S *consisting of the elements invariant under* G. *Assume that* K *is of characteristic* 0. *Then the Poincaré series of* R *is*

$$q^{-1} \sum_{g \in \mathrm{G}} (\det(1 - g\mathrm{T}))^{-1}.$$

Indeed, the endomorphism $f = q^{-1} \sum_{g \in \mathrm{G}} g^{(n)}$ is a projection of S_n onto R_n, so $\mathrm{Tr}(f) = \dim_{\mathrm{K}} \mathrm{S}_n^{\mathrm{G}}$. Thus, the Poincaré series of R is

$$q^{-1} \sum_{g \in \mathrm{G}} \left(\sum_{n=0}^{\infty} (\mathrm{Tr} g^{(n)}) \mathrm{T}^n\right),$$

and it suffices to apply Lemma 2.

PROPOSITION 3. *With the assumptions and notation of Th. 3, let* H *be the set of pseudo-reflections belonging to* G *and distinct from 1. Assume that* K *is of characteristic 0. Then* $\mathrm{Card}(\mathrm{H}) = \sum_{i=1}^{l}(k_i - 1)$.

By Prop. 3 of the Appendix, we can assume that K is algebraically closed. For any $g \in \mathrm{G}$, let $\lambda_1(g), \ldots, \lambda_l(g)$ be its eigenvalues. Since every $g \in \mathrm{G}$ is diagonalizable (Appendix, Prop. 2), $g = 1$ if and only if all of the $\lambda_i(g)$ are equal to 1, and $g \in \mathrm{H}$ if and only if the number of $\lambda_i(g)$ equal to 1 is $l - 1$ (we then denote by $\lambda(g)$ the eigenvalue distinct from 1). Prop. 1 of no. 1 and Lemma 3 prove that

$$q \prod_{i=1}^{l} (1 - \mathrm{T}^{k_i})^{-1} = \sum_{g \in \mathrm{G}} (\det(1 - g\mathrm{T}))^{-1} \tag{16}$$

in K[[T]], and hence in K(T). Consequently, we have in K(T)

$$q \frac{(1-\mathrm{T})^{l-1}}{\prod_{i=1}^{l}(1 - \mathrm{T}^{k_i})} = \frac{1}{1-\mathrm{T}} + \sum_{g \in \mathrm{H}} \frac{1}{1 - \lambda(g)\mathrm{T}} + \sum_{g \neq 1,\, g \notin \mathrm{H}} \frac{(1-\mathrm{T})^{l-1}}{\det(1 - g\mathrm{T})},$$

which can be written

$$\frac{q - \prod_{i=1}^{l}(1 + \mathrm{T} + \cdots + \mathrm{T}^{k_i - 1})}{(1-\mathrm{T})\prod_{i=1}^{l}(1 + \mathrm{T} + \cdots + \mathrm{T}^{k_i - 1})} \tag{17}$$

$$= \sum_{g \in \mathrm{H}} \frac{1}{1 - \lambda(g)\mathrm{T}} + \sum_{g \neq 1,\, g \notin \mathrm{H}} \frac{(1-\mathrm{T})^{l-1}}{\det(1 - g\mathrm{T})}.$$

It follows that $q - \prod_{i=1}^{l}(1 + \mathrm{T} + \cdots + \mathrm{T}^{k_i - 1})$ vanishes for $\mathrm{T} = 1$, so $q = k_1 k_2 \ldots k_l$, which we knew already by the Cor. of Th. 3. This granted, let Q(T) be the polynomial $(1-\mathrm{T})^{-1}(q - \prod_{i=1}^{l}(1+\mathrm{T}+\cdots+\mathrm{T}^{k_i-1}))$. Differentiating the equality $(1-\mathrm{T})\mathrm{Q}(\mathrm{T}) = q - \prod_{i=1}^{l}(1 + \mathrm{T} + \cdots + \mathrm{T}^{k_i-1})$ and putting $\mathrm{T} = 1$, we see that $-\mathrm{Q}(1)$ is the value for $\mathrm{T} = 1$ of

$$-\frac{d}{dt}\left(\prod_{i=1}^{l}(1 + \mathrm{T} + \cdots + \mathrm{T}^{k_i-1})\right)$$

$$= -\sum_{i=1}^{l}\left((1 + 2\mathrm{T} + \cdots + (k_i - 1)\mathrm{T}^{k_i-2})\prod_{j \neq i}(1 + \mathrm{T} + \cdots + \mathrm{T}^{k_j-1})\right)$$

so

$$\mathrm{Q}(1) = \sum_{i=1}^{l} \frac{(k_i - 1)k_i}{2} \prod_{j \neq i} k_j = \left(\prod_{j=1}^{l} k_j\right) \left(\sum_{i=1}^{l} \frac{k_i - 1}{2}\right).$$

Returning to (17), we have on the other hand

$$\mathrm{Q}(1) = \left(\prod_{j=1}^{l} k_j\right) \left(\sum_{g \in \mathrm{H}} \frac{1}{1 - \lambda(g)}\right).$$

Thus,

$$\sum_{i=1}^{l} \frac{k_i - 1}{2} = \sum_{g \in \mathrm{H}} \frac{1}{1 - \lambda(g)}. \tag{18}$$

Now the elements of G that leave fixed the points of a given hyperplane leave stable a complementary line of the hyperplane (Appendix, Prop. 2), and so form a cyclic subgroup G′ of G by *Algebra*, Chap. V, § 11, no. 1, Th. 1. Let t be the order of G′; the values of $\lambda(g)$ for $g \in \mathrm{G}'$ are $\theta, \theta^2, \ldots, \theta^{t-1}$ with θ a primitive tth root of unity. We have $\frac{1}{1-\theta^i} + \frac{1}{1-\theta^{t-i}} = 1$, so $\sum_{g \in \mathrm{G}',\, g \neq 1} \frac{1}{1-\lambda(g)} = \frac{1}{2}(t-1) = \frac{1}{2}\mathrm{Card}(\mathrm{H} \cap \mathrm{G}')$. The equality (18) thus proves the proposition.

Remark. When K = **R**, G is a Coxeter group and H is the set of reflections belonging to G, we know (§ 3) that the elements of H are in one-to-one correspondence with the *walls* of V.

PROPOSITION 4. *With the assumptions and notation of Th.* 3, *assume that* K *is of characteristic* $\neq 2$. *Then* $-1 \in \mathrm{G}$ *if and only if the characteristic degrees* $k_1, \ldots, k_l$ *of* R *are all even.*

Let f be the automorphism of the algebra S that extends the automorphism -1 of V. Then $f(z) = (-1)^{\deg z} z$ for all homogeneous z in S. Thus, if $-1 \in \mathrm{G}$, every homogeneous element of odd degree of R is zero, and the k_i are all even. Conversely, if the k_i are all even, every element of R is invariant under f, and Galois theory shows that $-1 \in \mathrm{G}$.

4. ANTI-INVARIANT ELEMENTS

We retain the assumptions and notation of Th. 3, and assume that K is of characteristic 0. An element z of S is said to be *anti-invariant* under G if

$$g(z) = (\det g)^{-1} z$$

for all $g \in \mathrm{G}$.

Let H be the set of pseudo-reflections belonging to G and distinct from 1. For all $g \in \mathrm{H}$, there exist $e_g \in \mathrm{V}$ and $f_g \in \mathrm{V}^*$ such that

$$g(x) = x + f_g(x) e_g \qquad \text{for all } x \in \mathrm{V}.$$

PROPOSITION 5. (i) *Let* D *be the element* $\prod_{g\in H} e_g$ *of* S. *The elements of* S *which are anti-invariant under* G *are the elements of* RD.

(ii) *Identify* S *with the polynomial algebra* $K[X_1,\ldots,X_l]$ *by choosing a basis* $(X_1,\ldots,X_l)$ *of* V, *and let* $(P_1,\ldots,P_l)$ *be algebraically independent homogeneous elements of* S *generating the algebra* R *(Th. 3). Then the jacobian* $J = \det\left(\frac{\partial P_i}{\partial X_j}\right)$ *is of the form* λD, *where* $\lambda \in K^*$.

a) With the notation in (ii), we have

$$dP_1 \wedge dP_2 \wedge \ldots \wedge dP_l = J\, dX_1 \wedge dX_2 \wedge \ldots \wedge dX_l,$$

so, for all $g \in G$,

$$\begin{aligned} g(J)(\det g)\, dX_1 \wedge \ldots \wedge dX_l &= g(J)\, d(gX_1) \wedge \ldots \wedge d(gX_l) \\ &= g(dP_1 \wedge \ldots \wedge dP_l) = dP_1 \wedge \ldots \wedge dP_l = J\, dX_1 \wedge \ldots \wedge dX_l, \end{aligned}$$

hence J is anti-invariant under G. On the other hand, the field of fractions N of S is a Galois extension of the field of fractions E of R (no. 2); if Δ is a derivation of E with values in an extension field Ω of N, Δ extends to a derivation of N with values in Ω (*Algebra*, Chap. V, § 16, no. 4, Th. 3); since the P_i are algebraically independent, it follows that $dP_1 \wedge \ldots \wedge dP_l \neq 0$, hence $J \neq 0$.

b) Let z be an element of S anti-invariant under G. We show that z is divisible by D in S. Let a be a non-zero vector in V. The elements of G that leave Ka stable leave stable a complementary hyperplane L (Appendix, Prop. 2); an element of G leaving Ka stable is 1 or a pseudo-reflection with vector a if and only if it induces 1 on L; the pseudo-reflections with vector a belonging to G thus constitute, together with 1, a cyclic subgroup G′ of G; let t be its order. There exists a basis $(X_1,\ldots,X_l)$ of V such that $a = X_1$, $X_2 \in L,\ldots,X_l \in L$, and z can be identified with a polynomial $P(X_1,\ldots,X_l)$ with coefficients in K. From $g(z) = (\det g)^{-1}z$ for $g \in G'$, we see that X_1 only appears in $P(X_1,\ldots,X_l)$ with exponents congruent to -1 modulo t. Thus, $P(X_1,\ldots,X_l)$ is divisible by $X_1^{t-1} = a^{t-1}$. Now D is, up to a scalar factor, the product of the a^{t-1} for those $a \in V$ such that $t > 1$, and these elements of S are mutually coprime. Since S is factorial, z is divisible by D.

c) By *a*) and *b*), J is divisible by D in S. Now

$$\deg J = \sum_{i=1}^{l} (k_i - 1) = \mathrm{Card}(H)$$

(Prop. 3), so $\deg J = \deg D$, hence $J = \lambda D$ with $\lambda \in K$. Since $J \neq 0$, $\lambda \in K^*$. This proves (ii).

d) Parts *a*) and *c*) of the proof show that D is anti-invariant under G. Next, if $y \in R$, it is clear that yD is anti-invariant under G. Finally, if $z \in S$ is anti-invariant under G, we have seen in *b*) that there exists $y \in S$ such that $z = y$D. Since S is integral, $y \in R$. This proves (i).

*5. COMPLEMENTS[4]

Lemma 4. Let K *be a commutative field,* V *a finite dimensional vector space over* K, G *a finite group of automorphisms of* V *whose order* q *is invertible in* K, S *the symmetric algebra of* V, *and* R *the subalgebra of* S *consisting of the elements invariant under* G. *A prime ideal* B *of height 1 of* S *is ramified over* $\mathfrak{p} = \mathrm{B} \cap \mathrm{R}$ *(Commutative Algebra) if and only if there exist a non-zero element* a *of* V *and a non-zero element* f *of* V^* *such that* $\mathrm{B} = \mathrm{S}a$ *and the pseudo-reflection* $s_{a,f}$ *belongs to* G. *The decomposition group* $\mathcal{G}^{\mathrm{Z}}(\mathrm{B})$ *is then the subgroup of elements of* G *leaving* Ka *stable, and the inertia group* $\mathcal{G}^{\mathrm{T}}(\mathrm{B})$ *is the cyclic subgroup* H_a *of* G *consisting of the pseudo-reflections of* G *with vector* a. *The residue field* S(B) *of* S *at* B *is separable over the residue field* $\mathrm{R}(\mathfrak{p})$ *of* R *at* $\mathfrak{p}$, *and the ramification index* $e(\mathrm{B}/\mathfrak{p})$, *equal to the coefficient of* B, *augmented by* 1, *in the divisor* $\mathrm{div}(\mathrm{D}_{\mathrm{S}/\mathrm{R}})$ *of the different, is equal to* $\mathrm{Card}(\mathrm{H}_a)$.

To say that B is ramified over R means that its inertia group $\mathcal{G}^{\mathrm{T}}(\mathrm{B})$ does not reduce to the identity, in other words that there exists $g \neq 1$ in G such that $g(z) \equiv z$ (mod. B) for all $z \in \mathrm{S}$. Since S is a factorial ring, B is a principal ideal Sa, and a must divide all the elements $g(z) - z$ ($z \in \mathrm{S}$); now, for $z \in \mathrm{V}$, these elements are homogeneous of degree 1 and are all non-zero (since $g \neq 1$); thus, a must be homogeneous of degree 1, in other words $a \in \mathrm{V}$. Then there exists a linear form f on V such that $g = s_{a,f}$. Conversely, if g is a pseudo-reflection $s_{a,f}$ different from 1, then $g(z) \equiv z$ (mod. Sa) for all $z \in \mathrm{S}$, so g belongs to the inertia group of the prime ideal $\mathrm{B} = \mathrm{S}a$. This proves the first assertion of the lemma and the characterizations of $\mathcal{G}^{\mathrm{Z}}(\mathrm{B})$ and $\mathcal{G}^{\mathrm{T}}(\mathrm{B})$. Since q is coprime to the characteristic p of K (which is also that of S(B)), the extension S(B) of $\mathrm{R}(\mathfrak{p})$ is separable (*Commutative Algebra*, Chap. V, § 2, no. 2, Cor. of Prop. 5). The equality $e(\mathrm{B}/\mathfrak{p}) = \mathrm{Card}(\mathrm{H}_a)$ follows from this (*Commutative Algebra*). Since $e(\mathrm{B}/\mathfrak{p})$ is coprime to p, the coefficient of B in $\mathrm{div}(\mathrm{D}_{\mathrm{S}/\mathrm{R}})$ is $e(\mathrm{B}/\mathfrak{p}) - 1$ (*Commutative Algebra*). This proves the lemma.

Lemma 5. Let K *be a commutative field,* S *a graded polynomial algebra over* K, *and* R *a graded subalgebra of* S. *Then* S *is a free graded* R*-module* (*Algebra*, Chap. II, § 11, no. 2) *if and only if the following two conditions are satisfied:*

a) R *is a graded polynomial algebra over* K;

b) *if* $(\alpha_1, \ldots, \alpha_s)$ *is a system of generators of the* K*-algebra* R *consisting of algebraically independent homogeneous elements, this system is an* S*-regular sequence*[5].

[4] In this number, we use results from chapters in preparation in the book on Commutative Algebra. We indicate them by the symbol *"Commutative Algebra"*.

[5] This means that, for all $i \in \{1, 2, \ldots, s\}$, the canonical image of α_i in the ring

$$\mathrm{S}/(\mathrm{S}\alpha_1 + \cdots + \mathrm{S}\alpha_{i-1})$$

is not a zero divisor in this ring.

When S *is an* R*-module of finite type, b) is a consequence of a).*

See *Commutative Algebra* for the proof.

THEOREM 4. *Let* K *be a commutative field,* V *a finite dimensional vector space over* K*,* S *the symmetric algebra of* V*,* G *a finite group of automorphisms of* V*, and* R *the subalgebra of* S *consisting of the elements invariant under* G*. Assume that* $q = \operatorname{Card} G$ *is invertible in* K*. The following conditions are equivalent:*

(i) G *is generated by pseudo-reflections;*

(ii) S *is a free graded* R*-module;*

(iii) R *is a graded polynomial algebra over* K.

The equivalence of (ii) and (iii) follows from no. 2 and Lemma 5. The implication (i) $\Longrightarrow$ (ii) follows from Th. 1.

We show that (iii) $\Longrightarrow$ (i). Let G′ be the subgroup of G generated by the pseudo-reflections belonging to G, and let R′ be the subalgebra of S consisting of the elements invariant under G′. We have $R \subset R' \subset S$. By Lemma 4, $\operatorname{div}(D_{S/R}) = \operatorname{div}(D_{S/R'})$, so $\operatorname{div}(D_{R'/R}) = 0$. Assume then that R is a graded polynomial algebra. Since this is also the case for R′ (since G′ is generated by pseudo-reflections), Lemma 5 shows that the R-module R′ admits a homogeneous basis $(Q_1, \dots, Q_m)$; let $q_i = \deg(Q_i)$. Put

$$d = \det(\operatorname{Tr}_{R'/R}(Q_iQ_j)), \quad \text{cf. } \textit{Algebra}, \text{ Chap. IX, } \S 2.$$

The fact that $\operatorname{div}(D_{R'/R})$ is zero shows that $\operatorname{div}(d) = 0$ (*Commutative Algebra*), which means that d belongs to K^*. On the other hand $\operatorname{Tr}_{R'/R}(Q_iQ_j)$ is a homogeneous element of degree $q_i + q_j$, and d is homogeneous of degree $2\sum_i q_i$. Thus, $\sum_i q_i = 0$, i.e. $q_i = 0$ for all i, which means that $R' = R$, and so $G' = G$ by Galois theory. This proves that G is generated by pseudo-reflections. Q.E.D.

Remarks. 1) Under the assumptions of Th. 4, the product of the characteristic degrees of R is q (formula (6) and Prop. 2 (iii)), so they are coprime to the characteristic of K. This was asserted in no. 3.

2) If we do not assume that Card(G) is invertible in K, we still have the implications (ii) $\Longleftrightarrow$ (iii) (cf. Lemma 5) and (ii) $\Longrightarrow$ (i) (cf. Exerc. 8); but the implication (i) $\Longrightarrow$ (ii) is no longer true (Exerc. 9).

PROPOSITION 6. *The assumptions and notation are those of Th. 4. Let* H *be the set of pseudo-reflections belonging to* G *and distinct from* 1*. Assume that* H *generates* G*. For all* $g \in G$*, put* $g(x) = x + f_g(x)e_g$ *with* $e_g \in V$*,* $f_g \in V^*$*. Put*

$$D = \prod_{g \in H} e_g \in S.$$

(i) *The different of* S *over* R *is the principal ideal* SD.

(ii) *Identify* S *with the algebra* $K[X_1, \ldots, X_l]$ *by choosing a basis* $(X_1, \ldots, X_l)$ *of* V, *and let* $P_1, \ldots, P_l$ *be algebraically independent homogeneous elements generating the algebra* R. *Then the jacobian* $J = \det\left(\frac{\partial P_i}{\partial X_j}\right)$ *is of the form* λD *where* $\lambda \in K^*$.

(iii) $\sum_{i=1}^{l}(\deg(P_i) - 1) = \mathrm{Card}(H)$.

(iv) *The set of anti-invariant elements of* S *is* RD.

Assertion (i) follows from Lemma 4. Assertion (ii) follows from the fact that SJ is the different of S over R (*Commutative Algebra*). Assertion (iii) is obtained by writing down the fact that the homogeneous polynomials D and J are of the same degree. The proof of (iv) is then the same as that given in no. 4 (proof of Prop. 5, parts *b*) and *d*)).$_*$

§ 6. COXETER TRANSFORMATION

In this paragraph, V denotes a real vector space of finite dimension l and W denotes a finite subgroup of **GL**(V), generated by reflections and essential (§ 3, no. 7). Provide V with a scalar product $(x|y)$ invariant under W. Denote by $\mathfrak{H}$ the set of hyperplanes H of V such that the corresponding orthogonal reflection s_H belongs to W.

1. DEFINITION OF COXETER TRANSFORMATIONS

An *ordered chamber* relative to W is a pair consisting of a chamber C determined by $\mathfrak{H}$ and a bijection $i \mapsto H_i$ from $\{1, 2, \ldots, l\}$ onto the set of walls of C (cf. § 3, no. 9, Prop. 7).

DEFINITION 1. *The Coxeter transformation determined by an ordered chamber* $(C, (H_i)_{1 \leqslant i \leqslant l})$ *is the element* $c = s_{H_1} s_{H_2} \ldots s_{H_l}$ *of* W.

PROPOSITION 1. *All Coxeter transformations are conjugate in* W.

Since W permutes the chambers determined by $\mathfrak{H}$ transitively (§ 3, no. 2, Th. 1), we are reduced to proving the following: let $(C, (H_i)_{1 \leqslant i \leqslant l})$ be an ordered chamber and $\pi \in S_l$; then $s_{H_1} s_{H_2} \ldots s_{H_l}$ and $s_{H_{\pi(1)}} s_{H_{\pi(2)}} \ldots s_{H_{\pi(l)}}$ are conjugate in W. Taking into account § 4, no. 8, Prop. 8, this will follow immediately from the following lemma:

Lemma 1. Let X *be a finite forest, and* $x \mapsto g_x$ *a map from* X *to a group* Γ *such that* g_x *and* g_y *are conjugate whenever* x *and* y *are not linked in* X. *Let* $\mathcal{T}$ *be the set of total orderings on* X. *For all* $\xi \in \mathcal{T}$, *let* p_ξ *be the product in* Γ *of the sequence* $(g_x)_{x \in X}$ *defined by* ξ. *Then the elements* p_ξ *are conjugate in* Γ.

1) We proceed by induction on $n = \mathrm{Card}\,X$. The case $n = 1$ is immediate, so assume that $n \geqslant 2$. There exists in X a terminal vertex a (Chap. IV, Appendix, no. 3, Prop. 2). Let $b \in X - \{a\}$ be a vertex linked to a if one exists; if a is not linked to any vertex in $X - \{a\}$, let b in $X - \{a\}$ be arbitrary. In all cases, g_a commutes with g_x for $x \neq b$. Let $\eta \in \mathcal{T}$ be such that a is the largest element of X and b the largest element of $X - \{a\}$; we let $\xi \in \mathcal{T}$ and prove that p_ξ, p_η are conjugate.

2) Assume first that, for ξ, a is the largest element of X and b the largest element of $X - \{a\}$. Let X′ be the full subgraph $X - \{a\}$, which is a forest. Define a map $x \mapsto g'_x$ from X′ to Γ by putting $g'_x = g_x$ if $x \neq b$, $g'_b = g_b g_a$. Let ξ', η' be the restrictions of ξ, η to X′. The induction hypothesis applies, so $p_{\xi'}$ and $p_{\eta'}$ are conjugate. But it is clear that $p_{\xi'} = p_\xi$, $p_{\eta'} = p_\eta$, proving the lemma in this case.

3) Assume that a is the largest element of X for ξ. Let X_1 (resp. X_2) be the set of elements of $X - \{a\}$ strictly larger (resp. smaller) than b; let ξ_i be the restriction of ξ to X_i. Then

$$p_\xi = p_{\xi_1} g_b p_{\xi_2} g_a = p_{\xi_1} g_b g_a p_{\xi_2},$$

and this element is conjugate to $p_{\xi_2} p_{\xi_1} g_b g_a$. We are thus reduced to case 2).

4) In the general case, let X_3 (resp. X_4) be the set of elements of X strictly larger (resp. smaller) than a; let ξ_i be the restriction of ξ to X_i. Then $p_\xi = p_{\xi_3} g_a p_{\xi_4}$, and this element is conjugate to $p_{\xi_4} p_{\xi_3} g_a$. We are thus reduced to case 3).

It follows from Prop. 1 that all the Coxeter transformations are of the same order $h = h(W)$. This number is called the *Coxeter number* of W.

Remark. Let $W_1, \dots, W_m$ be essential finite groups acting in the spaces $V_1, \dots, V_m$ and generated by reflections. Let C_j be a chamber relative to W_j. Let W be the group $W_1 \times \cdots \times W_m$ acting in the space $V_1 \times \cdots \times V_m$. Then $C_1 \times \cdots \times C_m$ is a chamber relative to W. The Coxeter transformations of W defined by C are the products $c_1 c_2 \dots c_m$, where c_j is a Coxeter transformation of W_j defined by C_j.

2. EIGENVALUES OF A COXETER TRANSFORMATION

Since all Coxeter transformations are conjugate (no. 1, Prop. 1), they all have the same characteristic polynomial P(T). Let h be the Coxeter number of W. Then

$$P(T) = \prod_{j=1}^{l} \left(T - \exp\frac{2i\pi m_j}{h} \right),$$

where $m_1, m_2, \dots, m_l$ are integers such that

$$0 \leqslant m_1 \leqslant m_2 \leqslant \cdots \leqslant m_l < h.$$

DEFINITION 2. *The integers* $m_1, m_2, \dots, m_l$ *are called the exponents of* W.

Let C be a chamber determined by $\mathfrak{H}$, $H_1, \dots, H_l$ its walls, and put $s_i = s_{H_i}$. Denote by e_i the unit vector orthogonal to H_i and on the same side of H_i as C. By Prop. 2 of the Appendix of Chap. IV, we can assume that the H_i are numbered so that $e_1, e_2, \dots, e_r$ are pairwise orthogonal and $e_{r+1}, e_{r+2}, \dots, e_l$ are pairwise orthogonal. Then $s' = s_1 s_2 \dots s_r$ is the orthogonal symmetry with respect to the subspace

$$V' = H_1 \cap H_2 \cap \dots \cap H_r,$$

$s'' = s_{r+1} s_{r+2} \dots s_l$ is the orthogonal symmetry with respect to the subspace

$$V'' = H_{r+1} \cap H_{r+2} \cap \dots \cap H_l,$$

and $c = s's''$ is a Coxeter transformation. Since $(e_1, \dots, e_l)$ is a basis of V, V is the direct sum of V′ and V″.

We deduce first that 1 *is not an eigenvalue of* c. For if $x \in V$ is such that $c(x) = x$, then $s'(x) = s''(x)$, so $x - s'(x) = x - s''(x)$ is orthogonal to V′ and V″, and hence is zero. Thus, $x = s'(x) = s''(x) \in V' \cap V'' = \{0\}$.

Consequently,

$$0 < m_1 \leqslant m_2 \leqslant \dots \leqslant m_l < h. \tag{1}$$

The characteristic polynomial of c has real coefficients. Thus, for all j, the power of $T - \exp\frac{2i\pi m_j}{h}$ in P(T) is equal to that of $T - \exp\frac{2i\pi(h-m_j)}{h}$. Hence

$$m_j + m_{l+1-j} = h \quad (1 \leqslant j \leqslant l). \tag{2}$$

Adding the equalities (2) we obtain

$$m_1 + m_2 + \dots + m_l = \frac{1}{2} lh. \tag{3}$$

Lemma 2. Assume that W *is irreducible and that* $\dim V \geqslant 2$. *With the preceding notation, there exist two linearly independent vectors* z', z'' *such that*

(i) *the plane* P *generated by* z', z'' *is stable under* s' *and* s'';

(ii) $s'|P$ *and* $s''|P$ *are orthogonal reflections with respect to* $\mathbf{R}z'$ *and* $\mathbf{R}z''$;

(iii) $z', z'' \in \overline{C}$, *and* $P \cap C$ *is the set of linear combinations of* z', z'' *with coefficients* > 0.

Let $(e^1, \dots, e^l)$ be the basis of V such that $(e^i|e_j) = \delta_{ij}$. Then C is the open simplicial cone determined by the e^i (§ 3, no. 9, Prop. 7). It is clear that V′ is generated by $e^{r+1}, \dots, e^l$ and V″ by $e^1, \dots, e^r$. Let q be the endomorphism of V such that $q(e^1) = e_1, \dots, q(e^l) = e_l$. Its matrix with respect to $(e^1, \dots, e^l)$ is $Q = ((e_i|e_j))$. We have $(e_i|e_j) \leqslant 0$ for $i \neq j$ (§ 3, no. 4, Prop. 3). Since W is irreducible, there does not exist any partition $\{1, 2, \dots, l\} = I_1 \cup I_2$ such that $(e_i|e_j) = 0$ for $i \in I_1$ and $j \in I_2$. Thus (§ 3, no. 5, Lemma 4) Q has an eigenvector $(a_1, \dots, a_l)$ all of whose coordinates are > 0; let a be the corresponding eigenvalue. Put

$$z = a_1 e^1 + \cdots + a_l e^l,$$
$$z'' = a_1 e^1 + \cdots + a_r e^r \in \mathrm{V}'' \cap \overline{\mathrm{C}},$$
$$z' = a_{r+1} e^{r+1} + \cdots + a_l e^l \in \mathrm{V}' \cap \overline{\mathrm{C}},$$

and let P be the plane generated by z' and z''. Then $\mathrm{P} \cap \mathrm{C}$ is the set of linear combinations of z' and z'' with coefficients > 0. The relation $q(z) = az$ gives $\sum_{j=1}^{l} a_j e_j = \sum_{j=1}^{l} a a_j e^j$; scalar multiplying by e_k (where $k \leqslant r$) gives $a_k + \sum_{j=r+1}^{l} a_j (e_j|e_k) = a a_k$; thus

$$\begin{aligned}
(a-1)z'' &= \sum_{k=1}^{r} \left(\sum_{j=r+1}^{l} a_j (e_j|e_k) \right) e^k \\
&= \sum_{j=r+1}^{l} a_j \left(\sum_{k=1}^{r} (e_j|e_k) e^k \right) \\
&= \sum_{j=r+1}^{l} a_j \left(-e^j + \sum_{k=1}^{l} (e_j|e_k) e^k \right) \\
&= - \sum_{j=r+1}^{l} a_j e^j + \sum_{j=r+1}^{l} a_j e_j \\
&= -z' + \sum_{j=r+1}^{l} a_j e_j .
\end{aligned}$$

Thus, $(a-1)z'' + z'$ is orthogonal to $e^1, \ldots, e^r$, that is, to V''. Hence, s'' leaves stable the plane generated by z'' and $(a-1)z'' + z'$, that is, P. Similarly, s' leaves P stable. Since $z' \in \mathrm{P} \cap \mathrm{V}'$ and $z'' \in \mathrm{P} \cap \mathrm{V}''$, $s'|\mathrm{P}$ and $s''|\mathrm{P}$ are the reflections with respect to $\mathbf{R}z'$ and $\mathbf{R}z''$.

THEOREM 1. *Assume that* W *is irreducible. Then:*

(i) $m_1 = 1$, $m_l = h - 1$.

(ii) $\mathrm{Card}(\mathfrak{H}) = \frac{1}{2} l h$.

We retain the preceding notation. The restriction of $c = s's''$ to P is the rotation with angle $2(\widehat{z'', z'})$ (§2, no. 5, Cor. of Prop. 6). Since c is of order h, the h elements $1, c, \ldots, c^{h-1}$ of W are pairwise distinct; the elements $s', s'c, \ldots, s'c^{h-1}$ are thus pairwise distinct, and are distinct from the preceding elements since $c^i|\mathrm{P}$ is a rotation and $s'c^j|\mathrm{P}$ is a reflection. The set

$$\{1, c, \ldots, c^{h-1}, s', s'c, \ldots, s'c^{h-1}\}$$

is the subgroup W′ of W generated by s' and s'', and induces on P the group W″ generated by the orthogonal reflections with respect to $\mathbf{R}z', \mathbf{R}z''$. The transform of C by an element of W′ is either disjoint from $-\mathrm{C}$ or equal to $-\mathrm{C}$. Thus, the transform of $\mathrm{P} \cap \mathrm{C}$ by an element of W″ is either disjoint from $-(\mathrm{P} \cap \mathrm{C})$ or equal to $-(\mathrm{P} \cap \mathrm{C})$. Hence, for a suitable orientation of P, there exists an integer $m > 0$ such that $\widehat{(z'', z')} = \frac{\pi}{m}$ (§ 2, no. 5, Cor. of Prop. 7). Moreover, the sets $g'(\mathrm{C})$, for $g' \in \mathrm{W}'$, are pairwise disjoint; the sets $g''(\mathrm{P} \cap \mathrm{C})$, for $g'' \in \mathrm{W}''$, are thus pairwise disjoint; so W'' is of order $2h$. Hence $m = h$. By definition, $c|\mathrm{P}$ is a rotation with angle $\frac{2\pi}{m}$, and so has eigenvalues $\exp\frac{2i\pi}{h}, \exp\frac{2i\pi(h-1)}{h}$. This proves that $m_1 = 1, m_l = h-1$.

The transforms of $\mathbf{R}z'$ and $\mathbf{R}z''$ by W′ are h lines $\mathrm{D}_1, \dots, \mathrm{D}_h$ of P, and the points of $\mathrm{P} - (\mathrm{D}_1 \cup \dots \cup \mathrm{D}_h)$ are transforms by the elements of W′ of points of $\mathrm{P} \cap \mathrm{C}$. Thus, a hyperplane of $\mathfrak{H}$ necessarily cuts P along one of the lines D_i, and consequently is a transform by an operation of W′ of a hyperplane of $\mathfrak{H}$ containing $\mathbf{R}z'$ or $\mathbf{R}z''$.

Now, any $\mathrm{H} \in \mathfrak{H}$ that contains $\mathbf{R}z'$ is one of the hyperplanes $\mathrm{H}_1, \dots, \mathrm{H}_r$. Indeed, let e_H be the unit vector orthogonal to H and on the same side of H as C. Then $e_\mathrm{H} = \lambda_1 e_1 + \dots + \lambda_l e_l$ with the λ_i all $\geqslant 0$ (§ 3, no. 5, Lemma 6, (i)). Now $0 = (e_\mathrm{H}|z') = \lambda_{r+1}a_{r+1} + \dots + \lambda_l a_l$, so

$$\lambda_{r+1} = \dots = \lambda_l = 0, \quad \text{and} \quad e_\mathrm{H} = \lambda_1 e_1 + \dots + \lambda_r e_r.$$

Suppose that two of the λ_i were non-zero, for example λ_1 and λ_2; since $e_1, \dots, e_r$ are pairwise orthogonal, we would have

$$s_1(e_\mathrm{H}) = -\lambda_1 e_1 + \lambda_2 e_2 + \dots + \lambda_r e_r$$

and the coordinates of $s_1(e_\mathrm{H})$ would not be of the same sign, which is absurd (*loc. cit.*). Thus, e_H is proportional to one of the vectors $e_1, \dots, e_r$, which proves our assertion. Similarly, any $\mathrm{H} \in \mathfrak{H}$ that contains $\mathbf{R}z''$ is one of the hyperplanes $\mathrm{H}_{r+1}, \dots, \mathrm{H}_l$.

The number of elements of $\mathfrak{H}$ containing $\mathbf{R}z'$ or $\mathbf{R}z''$ is therefore l. If h is even, $\mathrm{Card}(\mathfrak{H})$ is thus equal to $\frac{h}{2}l$. If h is odd, $\mathrm{Card}(\mathfrak{H})$ is equal to $\frac{h-1}{2}l+r$, and also to $\frac{h-1}{2}l+(l-r)$; hence $r = l-r$, so $r = \frac{l}{2}$, and $\mathrm{Card}(\mathfrak{H}) = \frac{h-1}{2}l+\frac{l}{2} = \frac{h}{2}l$.

Remark. Retain the notation of the preceding proof. Let c' be the $\mathbf{C}$-linear extension of c to $\mathrm{V} \otimes_\mathbf{R} \mathbf{C}$, and c'' the restriction of c' to $\mathrm{P} \otimes_\mathbf{R} \mathbf{C}$. From our study of $c|\mathrm{P}$, c'' has an eigenvector x corresponding to the eigenvalue $\exp\frac{2i\pi}{h}$, and this eigenvector does not belong to any of the sets $\mathrm{D} \otimes_\mathbf{R} \mathbf{C}$, where D denotes a line of P (since D is not stable under c). Now, for any $\mathrm{H} \in \mathfrak{H}$, we have seen that $\mathrm{H} \cap \mathrm{P}$ is a line; thus, $x \notin \mathrm{H} \otimes_\mathbf{R} \mathbf{C}$.

COROLLARY. *Let* R_0 *be the set of unit vectors of* V *orthogonal to an element of* $\mathfrak{H}$. *If* W *is irreducible,*

$$\sum_{u \in \mathrm{R}_0} (x|u)^2 = h(x|x) \tag{4}$$

for all $x \in \mathrm{V}$.

Put $f(x) = \sum_{u \in \mathrm{R}_0} (x|u)^2$. It is clear that f is a positive quadratic form invariant under W, and non-degenerate since the e_i form a basis of V. Since

W is irreducible, there exists a constant β such that $f(x) = \beta(x|x)$ (§ 2, no. 1, Prop. 1). If $(x_i)_{1 \leqslant i \leqslant l}$ is an orthonormal basis of V for the scalar product $(x|y)$, then

$$\beta l = \sum_{i=1}^{l} \beta(x_i|x_i) = \sum_{i=1}^{l} f(x_i) = \sum_{i=1}^{l} \sum_{u \in \mathrm{R}_0} (x_i|u)^2$$
$$= \sum_{u \in \mathrm{R}_0} 1 = \mathrm{Card}(\mathrm{R}_0) = 2\mathrm{Card}(\mathfrak{H}) = hl.$$

Thus $\beta = h$, which proves (4).

PROPOSITION 2. *If* W *is irreducible and* h *is even, the unique element of* W *that transforms* C *to* $-$C *is* $c^{h/2}$.

We use the notation in the proof of Th. 1. Since $c|\mathrm{P}$ is a rotation through an angle $\frac{2\pi}{h}$, $c^{h/2}$ transforms z' to $-z'$, z'' to $-z''$, and hence $z' + z'' = z$ to $-z$. Now $z \in \mathrm{C}$, so the chamber $c^{h/2}(\mathrm{C})$ is necessarily $-$C.

PROPOSITION 3. *Assume that* W *is irreducible. Let* $u_1, \dots, u_l$ *be homogeneous elements of the symmetric algebra* $\mathrm{S} = \mathbf{S}(\mathrm{V})$, *algebraically independent over* **R** *and generating the algebra of elements of* S *invariant under* W (§ 5, no. 3, Th. 3). *If* p_j *is the degree of* u_j, *the exponents of* W *are* $p_1 - 1, \dots, p_l - 1$.

Put $\mathrm{V}' = \mathrm{V} \otimes_{\mathbf{R}} \mathbf{C}$, $\mathrm{S}' = \mathbf{S}(\mathrm{V}') = \mathrm{S} \otimes_{\mathbf{R}} \mathbf{C}$, and extend the scalar product on V to a hermitian form on V′. If c is a Coxeter transformation of W, there exists an orthonormal basis $(\mathrm{X}_i)_{1 \leqslant i \leqslant l}$ of V′ consisting of eigenvectors of $c \otimes 1$ (*Algebra*, Chap. IX, § 7, no. 3, Prop. 4); moreover, we can assume that, for $1 \leqslant j \leqslant l$, X_j corresponds to the eigenvalue $\exp \frac{2i\pi m_j}{h}$ of $c \otimes 1$. It is clear that S′ can be identified with the algebra $\mathbf{C}[\mathrm{X}_1, \dots, \mathrm{X}_l]$, and that we can write $u_j \otimes 1 = f_j(\mathrm{X}_1, \dots, \mathrm{X}_l)$, where f_j is a homogeneous polynomial of degree p_j in $\mathbf{C}[\mathrm{X}_1, \dots, \mathrm{X}_l]$. Put $\mathrm{D}_j = \frac{\partial}{\partial \mathrm{X}_j}$ and $\mathrm{J} = \det(\mathrm{D}_k f_j)$. Recall (§ 5, no. 4, Prop. 5) that $\mathrm{J}(\mathrm{X}_1, \dots, \mathrm{X}_l)$ is proportional to the product in S′ of $\mathrm{Card}(\mathfrak{H})$ vectors y_k of V each of which is orthogonal to a hyperplane of $\mathfrak{H}$. Since we can assume that $\mathrm{X}_1 \notin \mathrm{H} \otimes \mathbf{C}$ for all $\mathrm{H} \in \mathfrak{H}$ (*Remark*), the X_1 component of each of the vectors y_k is non-zero, so $\mathrm{J}(1, 0, \dots, 0) \neq 0$. The rule for expanding determinants now proves the existence of a permutation σ of $\{1, 2, \dots, l\}$ such that $(\mathrm{D}_{\sigma(j)} f_j)(1, 0, \dots, 0) \neq 0$ for all j. Since $\mathrm{D}_{\sigma(j)} f_j$ is homogeneous of degree $p_j - 1$, the coefficient of $\mathrm{X}_1^{p_j - 1} \mathrm{X}_{\sigma(j)}$ in $f_j(\mathrm{X}_1, \dots, \mathrm{X}_l)$ is non-zero. Now $f_j(\mathrm{X}_1, \dots, \mathrm{X}_l)$ is invariant under $c \otimes 1$, and

$$(c \otimes 1)(\mathrm{X}_1^{p_j - 1} \mathrm{X}_{\sigma(j)}) = \left(\exp \frac{2i\pi}{h} (p_j - 1 + m_{\sigma(j)}) \right) (\mathrm{X}_1^{p_j - 1} \mathrm{X}_{\sigma(j)}).$$

This proves that $p_j - 1 + m_{\sigma(j)} \equiv 0 \pmod{h}$. Now $h - m_{\sigma(j)}$ is an exponent (formula (2)). Permuting the u_j if necessary, we can assume that $p_j - 1 \equiv m_j \pmod{h}$ for all j. Since $p_j - 1 \geqslant 0$ and $m_j < h$, we have $p_j - 1 = m_j + \mu_j h$ with μ_j an integer $\geqslant 0$. By § 5, Prop. 3, we see that

$$\mathrm{Card}(\mathfrak{H}) = \sum_{j=1}^{l} (p_j - 1) = \sum_{j=1}^{l} m_j + h \sum_{j=1}^{l} \mu_j.$$

Taking into account formula (3) and Th. 1 (ii), we obtain $h \sum_{j=1}^{l} \mu_j = 0$, so $\mu_j = 0$ for all j, and finally $p_j - 1 = m_j$ for all j.

COROLLARY 1. *If* $(m_i)_{1 \leqslant i \leqslant l}$ *is the increasing sequence of exponents of* W, *the order of* W *is equal to* $(m_1 + 1)(m_2 + 1) \ldots (m_l + 1)$.

This follows from the relations $m_j + 1 = p_j$ and § 5, Cor. of Th. 3.

COROLLARY 2. *If* c *is a Coxeter transformation of* W,

$$\exp\left(\frac{2i\pi}{h}\right) \quad \text{and} \quad \exp\left(\frac{-2i\pi}{h}\right)$$

are eigenvalues of c *of multiplicity* 1.

Otherwise, there would exist two non-proportional homogeneous invariants of degree 2 in S, and hence two non-proportional quadratic forms on V^* invariant under W, contrary to § 2, no. 1, Prop. 1.

COROLLARY 3. *The homothety with ratio* -1 *of* V *belongs to* W *if and only if all the exponents of* W *are odd. In that case,* h *is even and* $c^{h/2} = -1$ *for any Coxeter transformation* c *of* W.

The first assertion follows from § 5, no. 3, Prop. 4. Assume that the exponents of W are odd. Then h is even by formula (2), and

$$\left(\exp\frac{2i\pi m_j}{h}\right)^{h/2} = \exp(i\pi m_j) = -1;$$

thus $c^{h/2} = -1$ since c is a semi-simple automorphism of V (*Algebra*, Chap. IX, § 7, no. 3, Prop. 4).

APPENDIX
COMPLEMENTS ON LINEAR REPRESENTATIONS

The following proposition generalizes Prop. 13 of Chap. 1, § 3, no. 8.

PROPOSITION 1. *Let* K *be a commutative field,* A *a* K*-algebra, and* V *and* W *two left* A*-modules that are finite dimensional vector spaces over* K*. If there exists an extension* L *of* K *such that the* $(\mathrm{A}\otimes_{\mathrm{K}}\mathrm{L})$*-modules* $\mathrm{V}\otimes_{\mathrm{K}}\mathrm{L}$ *and* $\mathrm{W}\otimes_{\mathrm{K}}\mathrm{L}$ *are isomorphic, then the* A*-modules* V *and* W *are isomorphic.*

a) Assume first that L is an extension of K of *finite degree* n. Since $\mathrm{V}\otimes_{\mathrm{K}}\mathrm{L}$ and $\mathrm{W}\otimes_{\mathrm{K}}\mathrm{L}$ are isomorphic as $(\mathrm{A}\otimes_{\mathrm{K}}\mathrm{L})$-modules, they are isomorphic as A-modules; but, as A-modules, they are isomorphic to V^n and W^n, respectively. Now V and W are A-modules of finite length; thus V (resp. W) is the direct sum of a family $(\mathrm{M}_i^{r_i})_{1\leqslant i\leqslant p}$ (resp. $(\mathrm{N}_j^{s_j})_{1\leqslant j\leqslant l}$) of submodules such that the M_i (resp. N_j) are indecomposable, and that two of the M_i (resp. N_j) with distinct indices are not isomorphic (*Algebra*, Chap. VIII, § 2, no. 2, Th. 1). Then V^n (resp. W^n) is the direct sum of the $\mathrm{M}_i^{nr_i}$ (resp. $\mathrm{N}_j^{ns_j}$); it follows (*loc. cit.*) that $p = q$ and, after a suitable permutation of the N_j, that M_i is isomorphic to N_i and nr_i is equal to ns_i for $1\leqslant i\leqslant p$. Thus, V is isomorphic to W.

b) Assume that K is an infinite field. The assumption implies that V and W have the same dimension over K. Let $(e_i)_{1\leqslant i\leqslant m}$ and $(e'_i)_{1\leqslant i\leqslant m}$ be bases of V and W over K, and (a_λ) a basis of A over K. An isomorphism $u : \mathrm{V}\otimes_{\mathrm{K}}\mathrm{L}\to\mathrm{W}\otimes_{\mathrm{K}}\mathrm{L}$ is a bijective L-linear map and at the same time an $(\mathrm{A}\otimes_{\mathrm{K}}\mathrm{L})$-homomorphism, in other words it satisfies the conditions

$$a_\lambda u(e_i) = u(a_\lambda e_i) \quad \text{for all } \lambda \text{ and all } i. \tag{1}$$

Put $a_\lambda e_i = \sum_j \gamma_{\lambda ij} e_j$, $a_\lambda e'_i = \sum_j \gamma'_{\lambda ij} e'_j$, where the $\gamma_{\lambda ij}$ and $\gamma'_{\lambda ij}$ belong to K, and $u(e_i) = \sum_j \xi_{ij} e'_j$, where the ξ_{ij} belong to L. The conditions (1) can be written

$$\sum_j \xi_{ij}\gamma'_{\lambda jk} = \sum_j \gamma_{\lambda ij}\xi_{jk} \tag{2}$$

for all λ, i, k. By assumption, the homogeneous linear equations (2) have a solution $(\xi_{ij}) \in \mathrm{L}^{m^2}$ such that $\det(\xi_{ij}) \neq 0$. Since the coefficients of the system (2) belong to K, we know (*Algebra*, Chap. II, § 8, no. 5, Prop. 6) that this system also admits non-trivial solutions in K^{m^2}; let E be the vector subspace of $\mathbf{M}_m(\mathrm{K}) = \mathrm{K}^{m^2}$, not reduced to zero, formed by these solutions. Let $(c_l)_{1 \leqslant l \leqslant p}$ be a basis of E, and put $(\xi_{ij}) = \sum_l \eta_l c_l$ for any matrix $(\xi_{ij}) \in \mathrm{E}$; then $\det(\xi_{ij})$ is a polynomial $\mathrm{P}(\eta_1, \dots, \eta_p)$ with coefficients in K. On the other hand, we know (*loc. cit.*) that the solutions of (2) in L^{m^2} are of the form $\sum_l \zeta_l c_l$, this time with $\zeta_l \in \mathrm{L}$; for such a solution, $\det(\xi_{ij})$ is equal to $\mathrm{P}(\zeta_1, \dots, \zeta_p)$. Granting this, if we had $\mathrm{P}(\eta_1, \dots, \eta_p) = 0$ for all $\eta_1, \dots \eta_p \in \mathrm{K}$, the coefficients of P would be zero since K is infinite; we would then have $\mathrm{P}(\zeta_1, \dots, \zeta_p) = 0$ for all $\zeta_1, \dots, \zeta_p \in \mathrm{L}$, which is contrary to our assumption. We can therefore find a matrix $(\xi_{ij}) \in \mathrm{E}$ such that $\det(\xi_{ij}) \neq 0$, and the corresponding linear map $\mathrm{V} \to \mathrm{W}$ is an isomorphism.

c) General Case. Let Ω be an algebraically closed extension of L, and K_0 the algebraic closure of K in Ω. The assumption implies that $\mathrm{V} \otimes_{\mathrm{K}} \Omega$ and $\mathrm{W} \otimes_{\mathrm{K}} \Omega$ are isomorphic $(\mathrm{A} \otimes_{\mathrm{K}} \Omega)$-modules. Since K_0 is infinite, part *b*) shows that $\mathrm{V} \otimes_{\mathrm{K}} \mathrm{K}_0$ and $\mathrm{W} \otimes_{\mathrm{K}} \mathrm{K}_0$ are isomorphic $(\mathrm{A} \otimes_{\mathrm{K}} \mathrm{K}_0)$-modules. Retaining the notation in *b*), the system (2) admits a solution $(\xi_{ij}) \in \mathrm{K}_0^{m^2}$ such that $\det(\xi_{ij}) \neq 0$. But the ξ_{ij} all belong to some algebraic extension K_1 of finite degree over K. The $(\mathrm{A} \otimes_{\mathrm{K}} \mathrm{K}_1)$-modules $\mathrm{V} \otimes_{\mathrm{K}} \mathrm{K}_1$ and $\mathrm{W} \otimes_{\mathrm{K}} \mathrm{K}_1$ are isomorphic, and the proof is completed by using *a*).

PROPOSITION 2 (Maschke). *Let* A *be a ring with unit element,* E *a left* A-*module,* F *a direct summand of* E, G *a group of finite order* q, *and* ρ *a linear representation of* G *on* E. *Assume that* $q.1$ *is invertible in* A *and that* F *is stable under* G. *Then there exists a complement of* F *in* E *that is stable under* G.

Let p be a projection of E onto F. For all $x \in \mathrm{E}$, put

$$f(x) = q^{-1} \sum_{s \in \mathrm{G}} \rho(s)^{-1} p(\rho(s)x).$$

We have $f(x) \in \mathrm{F}$ and $f(y) = y$ for all $y \in \mathrm{F}$, so f is a projection of E onto F. On the other hand, if $t \in \mathrm{G}$,

$$\begin{aligned} \rho(t)f(x) &= q^{-1} \sum_{s \in \mathrm{G}} \rho(st^{-1})^{-1} p(\rho(s)x) \\ &= q^{-1} \sum_{s \in \mathrm{G}} \rho(s)^{-1} p(\rho(st)x) \\ &= f(\rho(t)x). \end{aligned}$$

Thus f commutes with $\rho(\mathrm{G})$, so $\mathrm{Ker}(f)$ is a complement of F stable under G.

COROLLARY. *Let* G *be a finite group of order* q, *and* K *a commutative field whose characteristic does not divide* q. *Then the group algebra of* G *over* K *is semi-simple.*

Indeed, by Prop. 2, every module over this algebra is semi-simple.

PROPOSITION 3. *Let* A *be a commutative ring,* M *an* A*-module,* G *a finite group acting on* M*, and* A′ *an* A*-module. Assume that the order* q *of* G *is invertible in* A*. Let* M^{G} *be the set of elements of* M *invariant under* G*. Then the canonical homomorphism from* $\mathrm{M}^{\mathrm{G}} \otimes_{\mathrm{A}} \mathrm{A}'$ *to* $\mathrm{M} \otimes_{\mathrm{A}} \mathrm{A}'$ *defines an isomorphism from* $\mathrm{M}^{\mathrm{G}} \otimes_{\mathrm{A}} \mathrm{A}'$ *onto the module* $(\mathrm{M} \otimes_{\mathrm{A}} \mathrm{A}')^{\mathrm{G}}$ *of elements of* $\mathrm{M} \otimes_{\mathrm{A}} \mathrm{A}'$ *invariant under* G.

Indeed, let Q be the projection of M onto M^{G} defined by $\mathrm{Q}(x) = q^{-1} \sum_{g \in \mathrm{G}} g(x)$ for all $x \in \mathrm{M}$. If i denotes the canonical injection of M^{G} into M, $\mathrm{Q} \circ i$ is the identity map of M^{G}, so $(\mathrm{Q} \otimes 1_{\mathrm{A}'}) \circ (i \otimes 1_{\mathrm{A}'})$ is the identity map of $\mathrm{M}^{\mathrm{G}} \otimes_{\mathrm{A}} \mathrm{A}'$. Since $\mathrm{Q} \otimes 1_{\mathrm{A}'} = q^{-1} \sum_{g \in \mathrm{G}} (g \otimes 1_{\mathrm{A}'})$, the image of $i \otimes 1_{\mathrm{A}'}$ is $(\mathrm{M} \otimes \mathrm{A}')^{\mathrm{G}}$. On the other hand, $i \otimes 1_{\mathrm{A}'}$ is injective by what has been said before.

Remark. The preceding proposition applies in particular when A′ is an A-*algebra.* In that case, $\mathrm{M}^{\mathrm{G}} \otimes_{\mathrm{A}} \mathrm{A}'$ is an A′-submodule of $\mathrm{M} \otimes_{\mathrm{A}} \mathrm{A}'$.

EXERCISES

§ **2.**

1) Let K be a commutative ring with unit element, let E be an A-module, and let E^* be its dual. Denote by φ the canonical homomorphism from $E \otimes E^*$ to End(E).

a) Any element distinct from 1 in End(E) of the form

$$s_{x,y^*} = 1 - \varphi(x \otimes y^*),$$

with $x \in E$ and $y^* \in E^*$, is called a *pseudo-reflection* in E. Such an element s is called a reflection if x and y^* can be chosen so that $\langle x, y^* \rangle = 2$; show that we then have $s^2 = 1$ and $s(x) = -x$.

b) Let $x \in E$, $y^* \in E^*$ be such that $\langle x, y^* \rangle = 1$. Show that E is the direct sum of the submodule Kx generated by x and the orthogonal complement H of y^*. Show that Kx is free with basis x, and that $s = s_{2x,y^*}$ is equal to 1 on H and to -1 on Kx.

2) With the notation of Exerc. 1, show that $\det(s_{x,y^*}) = 1 - \langle x, y^* \rangle$ if E is a free K-module of finite type.

¶ 3) Let V be a complex Hilbert space with basis $e_1, \ldots, e_l$. For $1 \leqslant i \leqslant l$, let s_i be a unitary pseudo-reflection, with vector e_i, such that $s_i(e_i) = c_i e_i$, with $c_i \neq 1$; an element of V is invariant under s_i if and only if it is orthogonal to e_i. Let W be the subgroup of $\mathbf{GL}(V)$ generated by the s_i.

a) Let i be an integer $\geqslant 1$. Show that every element of $\bigwedge^i V$ invariant under W is zero. (Argue by induction on l; if V' is the subspace of V generated by $e_1, \ldots, e_{l-1}$, and if e is a non-zero vector orthogonal to V', any element of $\bigwedge^i V$ can be written in the form $a + (b \wedge e)$, with $a \in \bigwedge^i V'$ and $b \in \bigwedge^{i-1} V'$; if $a + (b \wedge e)$ is invariant under W, a and b are invariant under the subgroup W' generated by $s_1, \ldots, s_{l-1}$, and the induction hypothesis applies.)

b) Assume that W is *finite*. Show, by using *a*), that, for any endomorphism A of V,

$$\sum_{w \in W} \det(A - w) = \mathrm{Card}(W).\det(A)$$

$$\sum_{w \in W} \det(1 - Aw) = \mathrm{Card}(W).$$

Deduce that, for any $A \in \mathrm{End}(V)$, there exists $w \in W$ such that Aw has no non-zero fixed point.

c) Let Γ be the graph whose set of vertices is $[1, l]$, the arrows being the sets $\{i, j\}$ such that e_i and e_j are not orthogonal. Show that V is a simple W-module if and only if Γ is connected and non-empty.

d) Assume that V is a simple W-module. Show that the W-modules $\bigwedge^i V$ $(0 \leqslant i \leqslant l)$ are simple. (Show that there exists an integer j such that the graph $\Gamma - \{j\}$ is connected. Argue by induction on l, and apply the induction hypothesis to the subspace V' generated by the e_i, $i \neq j$.) Show that these modules are pairwise non-isomorphic[6].

§ **3.**

1) The notation and assumptions being those of no. 1, show that the chambers relative to W are open simplices if and only if W is infinite and irreducible. Show that E/W is compact if and only if W is a product of infinite irreducible groups.

2) Let V be a finite dimensional real vector space equipped with a scalar product, F a finite subgroup of the orthogonal group of V generated by reflections, Λ a discrete subgroup of V stable under F, and W the group of displacements of V generated by F and the translations by a vector belonging to Λ. Let $\mathfrak{H}$ be the set of hyperplanes H of V such that $s_H \in F$. Let R be the set of elements of Λ orthogonal to an element of $\mathfrak{H}$.

a) W is generated by reflections if and only if R generates Λ.

b) In $\mathbf{R}^2$ equipped with the scalar product $((x, y), (x', y')) \mapsto xx' + yy'$, let

$$e_1 = (1, 0), \quad e_2 = \left(-\frac{1}{2}, \frac{\sqrt{3}}{2}\right), \quad e_3 = \left(-\frac{1}{2}, -\frac{\sqrt{3}}{2}\right), \quad \Delta_i = \mathbf{R}e_i,$$

F the dihedral group generated by the s_{Δ_i}, and Λ the discrete subgroup of $\mathbf{R}^2$ generated by the e_i, a subgroup that is stable under F. Show that W is not generated by reflections.

3) Let V be a finite dimensional real vector space and W a finite subgroup of $\mathbf{GL}(V)$ generated by reflections. Show that every element of order 2 of W is a product of pairwise commuting reflections belonging to W. (Argue by induction on dim(V), and use Prop. 2.)

[6] This exercise, hitherto unpublished, was communicated to us by R. Steinberg.

4) Let V be a finite dimensional real vector space, W a finite subgroup of $\mathbf{GL}(V)$ generated by reflections, w an element of W, V′ a vector subspace of V stable under w, and k the order of the restriction $w|V'$ of w to V′. Show that there exists $x \in W$ of order k, leaving V′ stable, and such that $x|V' = w|V'$. (Let W′ be the set of elements of W leaving fixed the points of V′. This group is generated by reflections, and w permutes the chambers relative to W′; deduce that there exists $h \in W'$ such that wh leaves stable a chamber of W′; show that we can take $x = wh$.)

¶ 5) Let V be a finite dimensional real vector space, W a finite subgroup of $\mathbf{GL}(V)$ generated by reflections, C a chamber of W and S the set of walls of C. If $J \subset S$, let W_J be the subgroup of W generated by the s_H for $H \in J$, and let $\varepsilon(J) = (-1)^{\mathrm{Card}(J)}$. Show that

$$\frac{1}{\mathrm{Card}(W)} = \sum_{J \subset S} \frac{\varepsilon(J)}{\mathrm{Card}(W_J)}. \qquad (*)$$

(Let $(x|y)$ be a scalar product on V invariant under W, Σ the unit sphere of V, and μ a positive measure on Σ invariant under W and of total mass 1. If $H \in S$, let D_H be the open half-space determined by H and containing C. Let $E_H = D_H \cap \Sigma$. Then

$$(-\overline{C}) \cap \Sigma = \bigcap_{H \in S} (\Sigma - E_H),$$

so

$$\begin{aligned}\frac{1}{\mathrm{Card}(W)} &= \mu(\overline{C} \cap \Sigma) = \int_\Sigma \prod_{H \in S} (1 - \varphi_{E_H}) d\mu \\ &= \sum_{J \subset S} \varepsilon(J) \mu \left(\bigcap_{H \in J} E_H \right).\end{aligned}$$

Conclude by remarking that $\bigcap_{H \in J} E_H$ is the intersection with Σ of a chamber of W_J, and hence has measure equal to $1/\mathrm{Card}(W_J)$.)

Recover formula (*) by means of Exerc. 26 *e*) of Chap. IV, § 1 (put $t = 1$ in the identity proved in the exercise in question).

6) *a*) Let K be a commutative field, V a vector space of finite dimension n over K, φ a symmetric bilinear form on V, and N the kernel of φ. Assume that $\dim N = 1$. Show that the kernel of the extension of φ to $\bigwedge^{n-1} V$ is of dimension $n - 1$.

b) Assume in addition that $K = \mathbf{R}$ and that φ is positive. Let $(e_1, \ldots, e_n)$ be a basis of V, and $a_{ij} = \varphi(e_i, e_j)$. Assume that $a_{ij} \leqslant 0$ for $i \neq j$. Assume that there is no partition $I \cup J$ of $\{1, 2, \ldots, n\}$ such that $a_{ij} = 0$ for $i \in I, j \in J$. Let A_{ij} be the cofactor of a_{ij} in the matrix (a_{ij}). Show that $A_{ij} > 0$ for all i and j. (Let $\zeta_1 e_1 + \cdots + \zeta_n e_n$ be a vector generating N, all of whose coordinates are > 0. Show that every row and column of (A_{ij}) is proportional to $(\zeta_1, \ldots, \zeta_n)$.

Deduce that $A_{ij} = \mu\zeta_i\zeta_j$ for some constant μ. By considering the A_{ii}, show that $\mu > 0$.)

c) Show that $\zeta_1, \dots, \zeta_n$ are proportional to $\sqrt{A_{11}}, \dots, \sqrt{A_{nn}}$.

7) Let $q(\xi_1, \dots, \xi_n) = \sum_{i,j} a_{ij}\xi_i\xi_j$ $(a_{ij} = a_{ji})$ be a degenerate positive quadratic form on $\mathbf{R}^n$, such that $a_{ij} \leqslant 0$ for $i \neq j$. Assume that there is no partition $I \cup J$ of $\{1, 2, \dots, n\}$ such that $a_{ij} = 0$ for $i \in I, j \in J$.

a) Show that, if we put $\xi_i = 0$, we obtain a non-degenerate positive quadratic form with respect to $\xi_1, \dots, \xi_{i-1}, \xi_{i+1}, \dots, \xi_n$.

b) Show that $a_{ii} > 0$ for all i. (Let $(\zeta_1, \dots, \zeta_n)$ be an element of the kernel of q, with $\zeta_1 > 0, \dots, \zeta_n > 0$. Use the equality $a_{1i}\zeta_1 + \dots + a_{ni}\zeta_n = 0$.)

c) Show that if we replace one of the a_{ij} by some $a'_{ij} < a_{ij}$, the new form is non-positive. (Use the equality $\sum_{i,j} a_{ij}\zeta_i\zeta_j = 0$.)

8) Let (a_{ij}) be a real symmetric matrix with n rows and n columns.

a) Put $s_k = \sum_{i=1}^{n} a_{ik}$. Then, for all $\xi_1, \dots, \xi_n \in \mathbf{R}$,

$$\sum_{i,k} a_{ik}\xi_i\xi_k = \sum_k s_k\xi_k^2 - \frac{1}{2}\sum_{i,k} a_{ik}(\xi_i - \xi_k)^2.$$

b) Let $\zeta_1, \dots, \zeta_n \in \mathbf{R}^*$. Put $\sum_i \zeta_i a_{ik} = t_k$. Then

$$\sum_{i,k} a_{ik}\xi_i\xi_k = \sum_k \frac{t_k\xi_k^2}{\zeta_k} - \frac{1}{2}\sum_{i,k} \zeta_i\zeta_k a_{ik}\left(\frac{\xi_i}{\zeta_i} - \frac{\xi_k}{\zeta_k}\right)^2.$$

(In *a*), replace ξ_i by $\frac{\xi_i}{\zeta_i}$ and a_{ik} by $\zeta_i\zeta_k a_{ik}$.)

c) If there exist numbers $\zeta_1, \dots, \zeta_n > 0$ such that $\sum_i \zeta_i a_{ik} = 0$ $(k = 1, 2, \dots, n)$, and if $a_{ij} \leqslant 0$ for $i \neq j$, then the quadratic form $\sum_{i,k} a_{ik}\xi_i\xi_k$ is degenerate and positive. (Use *b*).)

d) Let $\sum_{i,j} q_{ij}\xi_i\xi_j$ be a quadratic form on $\mathbf{R}^n$ such that $q_{ij} \leqslant 0$ for $i \neq j$. Assume that there is no partition $I \cup J$ of $\{1, 2, \dots, n\}$ such that $q_{ij} = 0$ for $i \in I, j \in J$. Then the form is non-degenerate and positive if and only if there exist $\zeta_1 > 0, \dots, \zeta_n > 0$ such that $\sum_i \zeta_i q_{ik} = 0$ $(k = 1, \dots, n)$.

§ 4.

In the exercises below, (W, S) denotes a Coxeter system. We assume that S is *finite*; its cardinal is called the *rank* of (W, S). We identify W with a subgroup of **GL**(E) by means of σ (cf. nos. 3 and 4).

1) Let E^0 be the orthogonal complement of E with respect to the form B_M. Show that E^0 is the radical of the W-module E (*Algebra*, Chap. VIII, § 6, no. 2), and that E/E^0 is the direct sum of m absolutely simple, pairwise non-isomorphic modules, where m is the number of connected components of the graph of S.

2) *a*) Let Γ_w be the set of extremal generators of the cone $w(C)$ and let A be the union of the Γ_w for $w \in W$. Show that A, equipped with the set $\{\Gamma_w | w \in W\}$, is a building (Chap. IV, § 1, Exerc. 15). Show that the map j from the apartment A_0 associated to the Coxeter system (W, S) (Chap. IV, § 1, Exerc. 16) to A that transforms the point $wW^{(s)}$ of A_0 (for $w \in W$ and $s \in S$) to the generator $w(\mathbf{R}e_s)$, is an isomorphism from A_0 to A, compatible with the action of W. Show that, if $t = wsw^{-1}$, with $w \in W$ and $s \in S$, the image under j of the wall L_t defined by t (resp. of a half of A_0 defined by L_t) (*loc. cit.*) is the set of elements of A contained in the hyperplane (resp. the closed half-space) that is the transform by $\sigma^*(w)$ of the hyperplane $e_s = 0$ (resp. of one of the closed half-spaces $e_s \geqslant 0$ or $e_s \leqslant 0$).

b) Show that W is finite if and only if there exists an element $w_0 \in W$ such that $w_0(C) = -C$. This element w_0 is then unique and is the longest element of W (use Exerc. 22 of Chap. IV, § 1). Show that in that case $j(-a) = -j(a)$ for all $a \in A_0$ (cf. Exerc. 22 *c*) of Chap. IV, § 1).

c) Show that W is finite if and only if the cone U formed by taking the union of the cone closures $w(\overline{C})$ for $w \in W$ is equal to the whole of E^* (if W is finite, use *b*) and the convexity of U. If $U = E^*$, consider an element $w \in W$ such that $w(\overline{C}) \cap (-C) \neq \varnothing$ and show that $w(C) = -C$).

d) Let H be a finite subgroup of W. Show that there exists a subset X of S such that W_X is finite and contains a conjugate of H. (Argue by induction on Card(S). Let $x \in C$ and $\overline{x} = \sum_{h \in H} h(x)$. Show, by using *c*) above, that W is finite if $\overline{x} = 0$. If $\overline{x} \neq 0$, there exist $w \in W$ and $Y \subset S$, $Y \neq S$, such that $w(\overline{x})$ belongs to C_Y (in the notation of no. 6), and hence $H \subset w^{-1}W_Y w$; apply the induction hypothesis to Y.)

3) Assume that (W, S) is irreducible.

a) Show that the commutant of the W-module E reduces to the homotheties.

b) Show that the centre of W reduces to $\{1\}$ if W is infinite or if W is finite and the longest element w_0 (cf. Exerc. 2) is $\neq -1$. If W is finite and $w_0 = -1$, the centre of W is $\{1, w_0\}$.

c) Show that any element $w \neq 1$ of W such that $w\mathrm{S}w^{-1} = \mathrm{S}$ transforms C to $-\mathrm{C}$ (show that $w(e_s) = -e_{wsw^{-1}}$, first for some $s \in \mathrm{S}$, and then for all $s \in \mathrm{S}$). Deduce (Exerc. 2) that such an element exists only if W is finite and that it is then equal to w_0.

4) Assume that Card(S) = 3. If $s \in \mathrm{S}$, let $a(s) = m(u, v)$, where $\{u, v\} = \mathrm{S} - \{s\}$. Let $\mathrm{A} = \sum_{s \in \mathrm{S}} 1/a(s)$.

a) If $\mathrm{A} > 1$, show that $\mathrm{B_M}$ is non-degenerate and positive (in which case W is finite).

b) If $\mathrm{A} = 1$, show that $\mathrm{B_M}$ is degenerate and positive.

c) If $\mathrm{A} < 1$, show that $\mathrm{B_M}$ is non-degenerate and of signature $(2, 1)$ (cf. *Algebra*, Chap. IX, § 7, no. 2).

Show that, in case *a*), the order q of W is given by the formula $q = 4/(\mathrm{A} - 1)$ (use Exerc. 5 of § 3).

5) Let A be the subring of **R** generated by the numbers $2.\cos(\pi/m(s, s'))$. Show that A is a free **Z**-module of finite type, and that the matrices of the $\sigma(w)$ for $w \in \mathrm{W}$ have their coefficients in A. Deduce that the coefficients of the characteristic polynomials of the $\sigma(w)$ are algebraic integers.

¶ 6) *a*) Let m be an integer $\geqslant 2$, or $+\infty$. Show that $4\cos^2\frac{\pi}{m} \in \mathbf{Z}$ is equivalent to $m \in \{2, 3, 4, 6, +\infty\}$.

b) Let Γ be a *lattice* in E, i.e. a discrete subgroup of E of rank dim E. Show that, if Γ is stable under W, the integers $m(s, s')$ for $s \neq s'$ all belong to the set $\{2, 3, 4, 6, +\infty\}$. (Observe that $\mathrm{Tr}(\sigma(w)) \in \mathbf{Z}$ for all $w \in \mathrm{W}$; apply this result to $w = ss'$, and use *a*) above.)

c) Assume that $m(s, t) \in \{2, 3, 4, 6, , +\infty\}$ for $s \neq t \in \mathrm{S}$. A family $(x_s)_{s \in \mathrm{S}}$ of positive real numbers is called *radical* if it satisfies the following conditions:

$$m(s,t) = 3 \Longrightarrow x_s = x_t$$
$$m(s,t) = 4 \Longrightarrow x_s = \sqrt{2}.x_t \text{ or } x_t = \sqrt{2}.x_s$$
$$m(s,t) = 6 \Longrightarrow x_s = \sqrt{3}.x_t \text{ or } x_t = \sqrt{3}.x_s$$
$$m(s,t) = +\infty \Longrightarrow x_s = x_t \quad \text{ or } x_s = 2x_t \text{ or } x_t = 2x_s.$$

If $(x_s)_{s \in \mathrm{S}}$ is such a family, put $\alpha_s = x_s e_s$. Show that

$$\sigma_s(\alpha_t) = \alpha_t - n(s,t)\alpha_s, \quad \text{with } n(s,t) \in \mathbf{Z}.$$

Deduce that the lattice Γ with basis $(\alpha_s)_{s \in \mathrm{S}}$ is *stable* under W.

d) With the assumptions in *c*), suppose that the graph of (W, S) is a *forest*. Show that in that case there exists at least one radical family (x_s). (Argue by induction on Card(S); apply the induction hypothesis to $S - \{s_0\}$, where s_0 is a terminal vertex of the graph of S.)

e) With the assumptions in *c*), suppose that the graph of (W, S) is a *circuit*. Let n_4 (resp. n_6) be the number of arrows $\{s,t\}$ of this graph whose coefficient $m(s,t)$ is equal to 4 (resp. 6). Show that a radical family exists if and only if n_4 and n_6 are both *even*. If this condition is not satisfied, show that *no lattice* of E is stable under W (if $S = \{s_1, \ldots, s_n\}$, with s_i linked to s_{i+1} for $1 \leqslant i \leqslant n-1$, and s_n linked to s_1, put $c = s_1 \ldots s_n$ and show that $\mathrm{Tr}(\sigma(c))$ is not an integer).

7) Assume that (W, S) is irreducible and that B_M is positive.

a) Show that, for any subset T of S distinct from S, the group W_T is finite (use Th. 2 as well as Lemma 4 of §3, no. 5).

b) Show that, if Card(S) $\geqslant 3$, the $m(s, s')$ are all finite.

c) Assume that W is infinite. Show that, if $T \subset S, T \neq S$, the group $\sigma(W_T)$ leaves stable a lattice in $\mathbf{R}^T$. Deduce that, if Card(S) $\geqslant 3$, the $m(s,s'), s \neq s'$, all belong to the set $\{2, 3, 4, 6\}$ (use Exerc. 6).

8) Let $s \in S$ and $w \in W$. Show that, if $l(ws) > l(w)$, the element $w(e_s)$ is a linear combination with coefficients $\geqslant 0$ of the e_t for $t \in S$; show that, if $l(ws) < l(w)$, $w(e_s)$ is a linear combination with coefficients $\leqslant 0$ of the e_t. (Apply property (P_n) of no. 4 to w^{-1}, and argue by polarity.)

9) Show that the intersection of the subgroups of W of finite index reduces to the identity element (use Exerc. 5). Deduce that there exists a subgroup of W of finite index that contains no element of finite order other than the identity element. (Use Exerc. 2 *d*).)

¶ 10) Let G be a closed subgroup of $\mathbf{GL}(E)$ containing W. Assume that G is unimodular (*Integration*, Chap. VII, §1, no. 3). Let D be a half-line of E* contained in C, and let G_D be the stabiliser of D in G.

a) Let Δ be the set of elements $g \in G$ such that $g(D) \subset C$. Show that Δ is open, stable under right multiplication by G_D, and that the composite map $\Delta \to G \to W\backslash G$ is injective, $W\backslash G$ denoting the homogeneous space of right cosets of G with respect to W.

b) Let μ be a Haar measure on G. Show that, if $\mu(\Delta)$ is finite, the subgroup G_D is compact. (Let K be a compact neighbourhood of the identity element contained in Δ; show that there exist finitely many elements $h_i \in G_D$ such that every set of the form Kh, with $h \in G_D$, meets one of the Kh_i; deduce that G_D is contained in the union of the $K^{-1}.K.h_i$, and hence is compact.)

c) Let ν be a non-zero positive measure on $W\backslash G$ invariant under G. Show that, if $\nu(W\backslash G) < \infty$, then G_D is compact.

¶ 11) Let H be the subset of $\mathbf{R}^n$ consisting of the points $x = (x_0, \dots, x_{n-1})$ for which the form

$$\mathrm{B}(x) = -x_0^2 + x_1^2 + \dots + x_{n-1}^2$$

is < 0, and let **PH** be the image of H in the projective space $\mathbf{P}_{n-1}(\mathbf{R})$. Let G be the orthogonal group of the form B.

a) Show that **PH** is a homogeneous space of G, that the stabiliser of a point is compact, and that G acts properly on **PH**.

b) Let ω and Ω be the differential forms on H defined by the formulas

$$\omega = \sum_{i=0}^{n-1} (-1)^i x_i dx_0 \wedge \dots \wedge dx_{i-1} \wedge dx_{i+1} \wedge \dots \wedge dx_{n-1}$$

$$\Omega = \frac{\omega}{(-\mathrm{B}(x))^{n/2}}.$$

Show that Ω is the inverse image under the canonical projection $\pi : \mathrm{H} \to \mathbf{PH}$ of a differential form $\tilde{\Omega}$ on **PH**. Show that the positive measure ν associated to $\tilde{\Omega}$ (*Differentiable Varieties R*, 2nd part) is invariant under G, and that it is the only such measure, up to a scalar factor.

c) Let C be an open simplicial cone with vertex 0 in $\mathbf{R}^n$ (§ 1, no. 6). Assume that C is contained in H, and denote by **PC** the image of C under $\pi : \mathrm{H} \to \mathbf{PH}$. Show that, if $n \geqslant 3$, then $\nu(\mathbf{PC}) < \infty$ (identify **PH** with the subspace of $\mathbf{R}^{n-1}$ consisting of the $(x_1, \dots, x_{n-1})$ such that $\sum_{i=1}^{n-1} x_i^2 < 1$, and determine the measure corresponding to ν on this subspace). Show that **PC** is relatively compact in **PH** if and only if $\overline{\mathrm{C}}$ is contained in H.

¶ 12) Assume that the form $x.y = \mathrm{B_M}(x, y)$ is *non-degenerate* and that W is *infinite*. Identify E with its dual E* by means of $\mathrm{B_M}$; in particular, denote by (e_s^*) the basis of E dual to the basis (e_s), and by C the interior of the simplicial cone $\overline{\mathrm{C}}$ generated by the e_s^*. Let G be the orthogonal group of $\mathrm{B_M}$, and let μ be a Haar measure on G; the group G is unimodular and contains W.

a) Show that, if $\nu(\mathrm{W}\backslash\mathrm{G}) < \infty$ (where ν is a non-zero positive measure invariant under G), the form $\mathrm{B_M}$ is of signature $(n-1, 1)$, with

$$n = \dim(\mathrm{E}) = \mathrm{Card}(\mathrm{S}),$$

and that $x.x < 0$ for all $x \in \mathrm{C}$.

(Let $x \in \mathrm{C}$ be such that $x.x \neq 0$, and let L_x be the hyperplane orthogonal to x. Show, by using Exerc. 10, that the restriction of $\mathrm{B_M}$ to L_x is either positive or negative; show that the second case implies that $\mathrm{B_M}$ is of signature $(1, n-1)$ and that this is impossible. Deduce that $x.x \leqslant 0$ for all $x \in \mathrm{C}$, and hence $x.x < 0$ since C is open.)

b) Conversely, assume that B_M is of signature $(n-1,1)$ and $x.x<0$ for all $x \in C$ (in which case W, or (W, S), or the corresponding Coxeter graph, is said to be of *hyperbolic type*). Let H be the set of $x \in E$ such that $x.x<0$, and let H_+ be the connected component of H containing C. Show that H is the disjoint union of H_+ and $H_- = -H_+$, and that H_- is contained in the simplicial cone generated by $(e_s)_{s\in S}$ (use the fact that H_- is the polar of H_+). Show that H_+ and H_- are stable under W.

c) Retain the notation and assumptions of *b*). Let f be the linear form on E defined by $f(e_s)=1$ for all $s \in S$. If $x \in H$, put $\varphi(x)=f(x)^2/(x.x)$. If **PH** denotes the image of the cone H in the projective space **P**(E), the function φ defines a function $\tilde{\varphi}$ on **PH**. Show that the map

$$\tilde{\varphi}: \mathbf{PH} \to]-\infty, 0]$$

is proper. Deduce that, for all $x \in H_+$, the functions $w \mapsto \varphi(w.x)$ and $w \mapsto f(w.x)$ attain their maximum for a value $w_1 \in W$ (use the fact that G acts properly on **PH**, cf. Exerc. 11, and that W is discrete in G); show that these properties are equivalent to $w_1(x) \in \overline{C}$. Deduce that $\overline{C} \cap H_+$ is a *fundamental domain* for the action of W in H_+, and that the image of this fundamental domain in **PH** has finite measure for the invariant measure ν on **PH** (use Exerc. 11). Conclude that $\nu(W\backslash G) < \infty$. Show that $W\backslash G$ is compact if and only if $\overline{C}$ is contained in H_+, i.e. if $e_s^*.e_s^* < 0$ for all $s \in S$ (in which case W, or (W, S), or the corresponding Coxeter graph, is said to be of *compact hyperbolic type*).

¶ 13) Show that (W, S) is of hyperbolic type (cf. Exerc. 12) if and only if the following two conditions are satisfied:

(H_1) The form B_M is not positive.

(H_2) For any subset T of S distinct from S, the form $B_{M(T)}$ associated to the Coxeter system (W_T, T) is positive.

(If (W, S) is of hyperbolic type, we have seen that $e_s^*.e_s^* \leqslant 0$ for all $s \in S$, the notation being that of Exerc. 12. The restriction of B_M to the hyperplane $E(s)$ orthogonal to e_s^* is thus $\geqslant 0$; since $E(s)$ is generated by the e_t for $t \neq s$, (H_2) follows. Conversely, assume that (H_1) and (H_2) are satisfied; let $x = \sum_s a_s e_s$ be an element of E such that $x.x<0$; let x_+ (resp. x_-) be the sum of the $a_s e_s$ for which a_s is >0 (resp. $\leqslant 0$); show that either $x_+.x_+ < 0$ or $x_-.x_- < 0$. If V denotes the open simplicial cone generated by the e_s, and H the set of $x \in E$ such that $x.x<0$, deduce that there exists a connected component H_0 of H that meets V; by using (H_2), show that H_0 does not meet the walls of V, so $H_0 \subset V$. Deduce that the form $B_M(x,y) = x.y$ is non-degenerate of signature $(n-1,1)$, and that C is contained in $-H_0$, hence the fact that (W, S) is of hyperbolic type.)

14) Show that (W, S) is of compact hyperbolic type (Exerc. 12) if and only if the following two conditions are satisfied:

(H_1) The form B_M is not positive.

(HC) For any subset T of S distinct from S, the group W_T is finite (i.e. the form $B_{M(T)}$ is non-degenerate and positive).

(Use Exercs. 12 and 13.)

In particular, a Coxeter system of hyperbolic type of rank 3 is of compact hyperbolic type if and only if the $m(s, s')$ are all finite (cf. Exerc. 4).

¶ 15) *a) Show that the nine Coxeter graphs below[7] are of compact hyperbolic type, and that they are, up to isomorphism, the only graphs of rank 4 with this property (use the classification of Chap. VI, § 4):

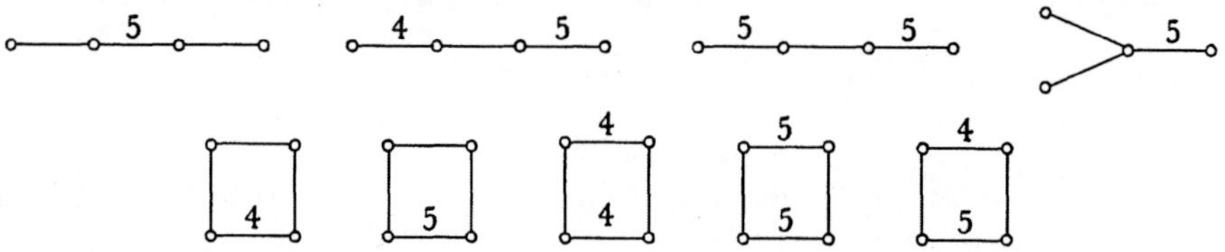

b) The same question for rank 5, the list consisting of the following five graphs:

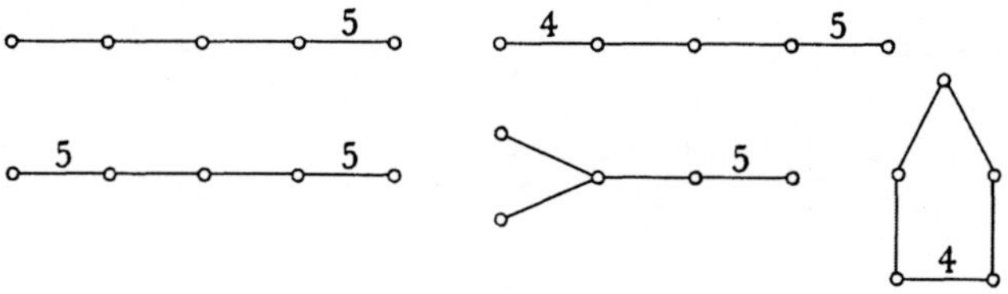

c) Show that there is no graph of compact hyperbolic type of rank $\geqslant 6$.*

16) *Show that any Coxeter graph of hyperbolic type of rank $\geqslant 4$ that has an edge with coefficient 6 is isomorphic to one of the following eleven graphs (which are non-compact and of rank 4):

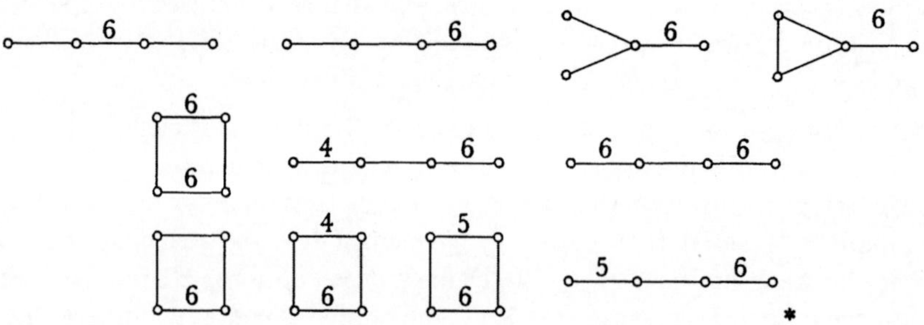

*

[7] In these graphs, any edge that has no label next to it is taken to have coefficient 3 (cf. Chap. IV, § 1, no. 9).

17) *Show that the hyperbolic Coxeter graphs of higher rank are the following three graphs (which are of rank 10):

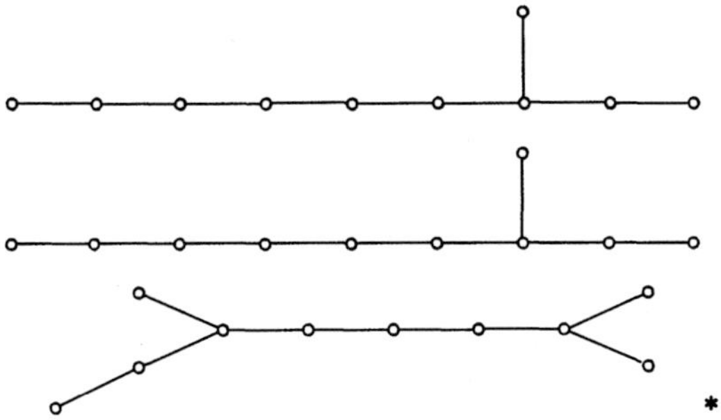

*

¶ 18) Assume that (W, S) is of hyperbolic type, and that W leaves stable a lattice Γ of E. Let G be the orthogonal group of $\mathrm{B_M}$, and let $\mathrm{G}(\Gamma)$ be the subgroup of elements $g \in \mathrm{G}$ such that $g\Gamma = \Gamma$. Show that $\mathrm{G}(\Gamma)$ is a discrete subgroup of G. Show that W is a subgroup of finite index of $\mathrm{G}(\Gamma)$ (use the fact that the measure of W\G is finite).

*If (W, S) is actually of compact hyperbolic type, show that the corresponding Coxeter graph is isomorphic to one of the following (use Exercs. 4, 6 and 15):

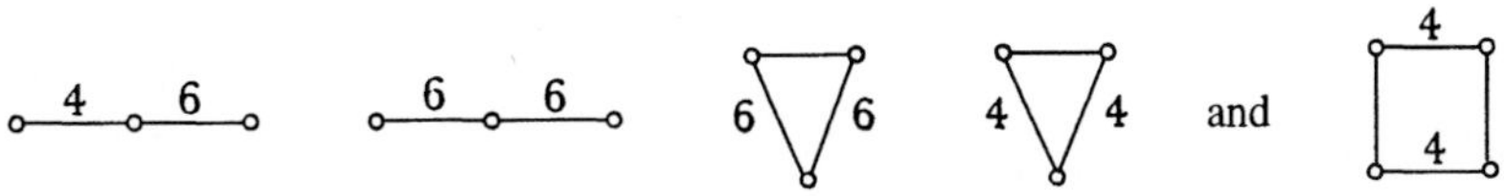

Show that all the groups corresponding to the graphs of Exerc. 16 (with the exception of the last four) leave stable a lattice (use the method of Exerc. 6).$_*$

19) Let (W, S) be the Coxeter system corresponding to the graph

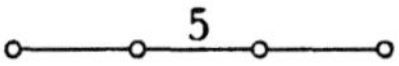

This is a system of compact hyperbolic type (cf. Exerc. 15). The coefficients of the form $\mathrm{B_M}$ with respect to the basis (e_s) belong to the subring A of the field $\mathbf{Q}(\sqrt{5})$ consisting of the elements of this field that are integers over $\mathbf{Z}$.

a) Let σ be the embedding of K into $\mathbf{R}$ that maps $\sqrt{5}$ to $-\sqrt{5}$. Show that the transform $\sigma(\mathrm{B_M})$ of the form $\mathrm{B_M}$ by σ is non-degenerate and positive.

b) Let G be the orthogonal group of $\mathrm{B_M}$, and let G_σ be that of $\sigma(\mathrm{B_M})$. Let $\mathrm{G_A}$ be the subgroup of G consisting of the elements whose matrices with respect to (e_s) have coefficients in A. Show that $\mathrm{G_A}$ can be identified with a discrete subgroup of $\mathrm{G} \times \mathrm{G}_\sigma$ and then, using *a*), show that $\mathrm{G_A}$ is a discrete subgroup of G.

c) Show that W is a subgroup of G_A of finite index.

d) Prove analogous results for the other graphs in Exerc. 15 (the field $\mathbf{Q}(\sqrt{5})$ sometimes being replaced by $\mathbf{Q}(\sqrt{2})$, with the exception of the graph

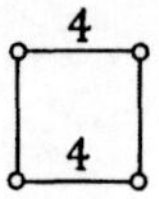

treated in Exerc. 18, and of the graph[8]

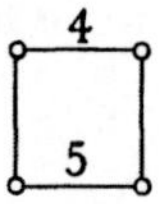

¶ 20) For every subset $\{s, s'\}$ of S such that $m(s, s') = \infty$, let $r(s, s')$ be a real number $\leqslant -1$. Equip E with the bilinear form B_r such that

$$B_r(e_s, e_{s'}) = B_M(e_s, e_{s'}) = -\cos\frac{\pi}{m(s,s')} \quad \text{if } m(s,s') \neq \infty$$

$$B_r(e_s, e_{s'}) = r(s, s') \quad \text{if } m(s,s') = \infty.$$

We define, as for B_M, the reflections σ_s with vector e_s, leaving the form B_r invariant.

a) Show that there exists a unique homomorphism $\sigma_r : W \to \mathbf{GL}(E)$ such that $\sigma_r(g_s)$ is equal to the reflection σ_s defined above.

b) Show that the assertions in Prop. 4, Th. 1, its Corollaries, and Lemma 1 remain true for σ_r.

§ 5.

1) Determine the algebra of symmetric invariants of a finite dihedral group (for its canonical representation of dimension 2, cf. § 4, no. 2).

2) Let A be a principal ring, E a free A-module of finite rank l, and G a finite subgroup of $\mathbf{GL}(E)$. Assume the following:

(i) If $q = \mathrm{Card}(G)$, the element $q.1$ of A is invertible.
(ii) G is generated by pseudo-reflections in E (i.e. by elements s such that $(s-1)(E)$ is a monogenic submodule of E, cf. § 2, Exerc. 1.)

[8] As E. Vinberg has shown, the group W corresponding to this last graph is not a subgroup of G of "arithmetic" type. The same situation arises for various other graphs of hyperbolic type (non-compact, this time), notably for the last four in Exerc. 16.

Let $\mathbf{S}(\mathrm{E})$ be the symmetric algebra of E, and let $\mathbf{S}(\mathrm{E})^{\mathrm{G}}$ be the subalgebra of $\mathbf{S}(\mathrm{E})$ consisting of the elements invariant under G. Show that, for any homomorphism from A into a field k, $\mathbf{S}(\mathrm{E})^{\mathrm{G}} \otimes k$ can be identified with $\mathbf{S}(\mathrm{E} \otimes k)^{\mathrm{G}}$. Deduce, by applying Th. 4, that $\mathbf{S}(\mathrm{E})^{\mathrm{G}}$ is a graded polynomial algebra over A.

¶ 3) Let K be a field of characteristic zero, V a vector space of finite dimension l over K, and G a subgroup of $\mathbf{GL}(\mathrm{V})$ generated by pseudo-reflections. Put $q = \mathrm{Card}(\mathrm{G})$; denote by S (resp. L) the symmetric algebra (resp. exterior algebra) of V. If $x \in \mathrm{V}$, denote by x (resp. x') its canonical image in S (resp. L).

a) Let $\mathrm{E} = \mathrm{S} \otimes \mathrm{L}$ be the tensor product of S and L. Show that there exists a unique derivation d on E such that $dx = x'$ and $dx' = 0$ for all $x \in \mathrm{V}$.

b) Let S^{G} be the algebra of symmetric invariants of G and let $\mathrm{P}_1, \ldots, \mathrm{P}_l$ be homogeneous elements of S^{G} such that $\mathrm{S}^{\mathrm{G}} = \mathrm{K}[\mathrm{P}_1, \ldots, \mathrm{P}_l]$. For every subset $\mathrm{I} = \{i_1, \ldots, i_r\}$ of $[1, l]$ with $i_1 < \cdots < i_r$, put

$$\omega_{\mathrm{I}} = d\mathrm{P}_{i_1} \ldots d\mathrm{P}_{i_r}.$$

Show that the ω_{I} are linearly independent over S, and that they belong to the subalgebra E^{G} consisting of the elements of E invariant under G. Deduce that, for all $\omega \in \mathrm{E}^{\mathrm{G}}$, there exist $a, c_{\mathrm{I}} \in \mathrm{S}^{\mathrm{G}}$, with $a \neq 0$, such that

$$a\omega = \sum_{\mathrm{I}} c_{\mathrm{I}} \omega_{\mathrm{I}}.$$

c) Show that every element of E^{G} contained in $\mathrm{S} \otimes \bigwedge^l \mathrm{V}$ is of the form $c.d\mathrm{P}_1 \ldots d\mathrm{P}_l$, with $c \in \mathrm{S}^{\mathrm{G}}$. (Apply Prop. 5.)

d) Show that the ω_{I} form a basis of the S^{G}-module E^{G}. (With the notation in *b*), multiply both sides of the relation $a\omega = \sum_{\mathrm{I}} c_{\mathrm{I}} \omega_{\mathrm{I}}$ by an element ω_{J}, and apply *c*); deduce that, if I is the complement of J, a divides c_{I}; hence[9] the fact that the ω_{I} generate E^{G}.)

e) Let S_n (resp. L_m) be the homogeneous component of S (resp. L) of degree n (resp. m). Put

$$\mathrm{E}_{n,m} = \mathrm{S}_n \otimes \mathrm{L}_m, \quad \mathrm{E}^{\mathrm{G}}_{n,m} = \mathrm{E}^{\mathrm{G}} \cap \mathrm{E}_{n,m}, \quad a_{n,m} = \dim \mathrm{E}^{\mathrm{G}}_{n,m},$$
$$a(\mathrm{X}, \mathrm{Y}) = \sum_{n,m \geqslant 0} a_{n,m} \mathrm{X}^n \mathrm{Y}^m.$$

By using *d*), prove the formula

$$a(\mathrm{X}, \mathrm{Y}) = \prod_{i=1}^{l} \frac{1 + \mathrm{Y}.\mathrm{X}^{p_i - 1}}{1 - \mathrm{X}^{p_i}},$$

where $p_i = \deg(\mathrm{P}_i)$.

[9] For more details, see L. SOLOMON, Invariants of finite reflection groups, *Nagoya Math. Journal*, v. XXII (1963), p. 57-64.

f) If $g \in \mathrm{G}$, let $\mathrm{Tr}_{n,m}(g)$ be the trace of the automorphism of $\mathrm{E}_{n,m}$ defined by g; put

$$\mathrm{Tr}(\mathrm{X},\mathrm{Y})(g) = \sum_{n,m \geqslant 0} \mathrm{Tr}_{n,m}(g)\mathrm{X}^n\mathrm{Y}^m.$$

Show that

$$\mathrm{Tr}(\mathrm{X},\mathrm{Y})(g) = \frac{\det(1+\mathrm{Y}g)}{\det(1-\mathrm{X}g)}.$$

g) Let $q = \mathrm{Card}(\mathrm{G})$. Show that

$$\frac{1}{q}\sum_{g \in \mathrm{G}} \mathrm{Tr}(\mathrm{X},\mathrm{Y})(g) = a(\mathrm{X},\mathrm{Y}),$$

i.e.

$$\frac{1}{q}\sum_{g \in \mathrm{G}} \frac{\det(1+\mathrm{Y}g)}{\det(1-\mathrm{X}g)} = \prod_{i=1}^{l} \frac{1+\mathrm{Y}.\mathrm{X}^{p_i-1}}{1-\mathrm{X}^{p_i}}.$$

(Use the following result: if G acts on a finite dimensional vector space E, the dimension of the space of elements of E invariant under G is equal to $\frac{1}{q}\sum_{g \in \mathrm{G}} \mathrm{Tr}_{\mathrm{E}}(g)$.)

What does this formula give for $\mathrm{Y} = 0$?

h) For any integer $p \geqslant 0$, let H_p be the set of elements $g \in \mathrm{G}$ that have 1 as an eigenvalue with multiplicity p. Let $h_p = \mathrm{Card}(\mathrm{H}_p)$. Prove the formula

$$\sum_{p=0}^{l} h_p \mathrm{T}^p = \prod_{i=1}^{l} (p_i - 1 + \mathrm{T}).$$

(In the formula in *g*) above, replace Y by $-1+\mathrm{T}(1-\mathrm{X})$ and then put $\mathrm{X} = 1$ in the result. If $g \in \mathrm{H}_p$, the term $\mathrm{Tr}(\mathrm{X},\mathrm{Y})(g)$ becomes T^p.)

¶ 4) *Let $\mathrm{G}_1 = \mathbf{SL}_3(\mathbf{F}_2)$.

a) Show that G_1 is a non-abelian simple group of order 168, containing 21 elements of order 2.

b) Show that the degrees of the irreducible complex representations of G_1 are 1, 3, 3, 6, 7, 8.

c) Let $\rho : \mathrm{G}_1 \to \mathbf{GL}_3(\mathbf{C})$ be an irreducible representation [10] of G_1 of degree 3. If $y \in \mathrm{G}_1$ is of order 2, show that $\mathrm{Tr}(\rho(y)) = -1$. Deduce that $-\rho(y)$ is a reflection.

d) Let G be the subgroup of $\mathbf{GL}_3(\mathbf{C})$ generated by the elements $-\rho(y)$, for y of order 2 in G_1. Show that G is isomorphic to $\mathrm{G}_1 \times \{1,-1\}$, and is thus of order 336.

---

[10] A detailed study of such a representation can be found in H. WEBER, *Lehrbuch der Algebra*, Bd. II, Abschn. 15.

e) Show that the characteristic degrees k_1, k_2, k_3 of the algebra of symmetric invariants of G are equal to 4, 6 and 14. (Use the relations $\prod_i k_i = 336$ and $\sum_i (k_i - 1) = 21$.)

f) Show that G is not a Coxeter group.$_*$

5) *Let K be a field and $S = K[X_1, \ldots, X_n]$ a graded polynomial algebra over K, generated by algebraically independent elements X_i, homogeneous of degrees > 0.

a) Let $Y_1, \ldots, Y_n$ be homogeneous elements of S of degrees > 0, and let $R = K[Y_1, \ldots, Y_n]$ be the subalgebra of S generated by these elements. Prove the equivalence of the following properties:

(i) $(Y_1, \ldots, Y_n)$ is an S-regular sequence.

(ii) S is integral over R.

(iii) The ideal of S generated by $Y_1, \ldots, Y_n$ is of finite codimension in S.

(iv) For any extension $\overline{K}$ of K, the system of equations $Y_i(x_1, \ldots, x_n) = 0$ $(1 \leqslant i \leqslant n,\ x_i \in \overline{K})$ has only the trivial solution $(0, \ldots, 0)$.

((i) $\Longleftrightarrow$ (iii) follows from a theorem of Macaulay (*Commutative Algebra*); (iii) $\Longleftrightarrow$ (iv) follows from the Zeros Theorem (*Commutative Algebra*, Chap. V, §3, no. 3, Prop. 2); (ii) $\Longleftrightarrow$ (iii) is easy.)

If these properties are satisfied, show that the Y_i are algebraically independent over K, and that S is a free R-module of rank equal to

$$\frac{\prod_i \deg(Y_i)}{\prod_i \deg(X_i)}.$$

b) Let G be a finite group of automorphisms of the graded algebra S, let S^G be its subalgebra of invariants, and let $Y_1, \ldots, Y_n$ be elements of S^G satisfying conditions (i),..., (iv) above. Show that $S^G = K[Y_1, \ldots, Y_n]$ if and only if

$$\mathrm{Card}(G) = \frac{\prod_i \deg(Y_i)}{\prod_i \deg(X_i)}.{}_*$$

¶ 6) *Let n be an integer $\geqslant 1$, q a power of a prime number, $K = \mathbf{F}_q$, $V = K^n$, $G = \mathbf{GL}(n, K)$ and $G_1 = \mathbf{SL}(n, K)$. Identify G with the group $\mathbf{GL}(V)$. Further, denote by S the algebra $\mathbf{S}(V) = K[X_1, \ldots, X_n]$ and R (resp. R_1) the subalgebra of S consisting of the elements invariant under G (resp. G_1).

a) Let $\mathbf{e} = (e_1, \ldots, e_n)$ be a sequence of integers $\geqslant 0$. Put

$$\mathrm{L}_{\mathbf{e}} = \det(\mathrm{X}_i^{q^{e_j}}).$$

This is an element of S.

Show that

$$g.\mathrm{L}_{\mathbf{e}} = \det(g)\mathrm{L}_{\mathbf{e}} \quad \text{for all } g \in \mathrm{G}.$$

(Remark that, if $g.\mathrm{X}_i = \sum_j a_{ij}\mathrm{X}_j$, then $g.\mathrm{X}_i^{q^e} = \sum_j a_{ij}\mathrm{X}_j^{q^e}$.) In particular, $\mathrm{L}_{\mathbf{e}}$ belongs to R_1.

b) Let $j \in [1, n]$. Put

$$\mathrm{Z}_j = \prod_{(a_{ij})} (\mathrm{X}_j + \sum_{i>j} a_{ij}\mathrm{X}_i),$$

the product being over all families $(a_{ij})_{j<i\leqslant n}$ of elements of K. Let

$$\mathrm{T} = \prod_{j=1}^{n} \mathrm{Z}_j.$$

Show that T divides all the $\mathrm{L}_{\mathbf{e}}$. Deduce that $\mathrm{T} = \mathrm{L}_{\mathbf{e}_n}$, where $\mathbf{e}_n = (0, 1, \ldots, n-1)$, and that T is invariant under G_1.

c) Denote by $\mathbf{e}_i$ $(1 \leqslant i \leqslant n-1)$ the sequence $(0, 1, \ldots, i-1, i+1, \ldots, n)$, and put $\mathrm{Y}_i = \mathrm{L}_{\mathbf{e}_i}/\mathrm{T}$, cf. *b*). Show that the Y_i belong to R and that $\deg(\mathrm{Y}_i) = q^n - q^i$.

d) Let $\mathrm{S}' = \mathrm{K}[\mathrm{X}_1, \ldots, \mathrm{X}_{n-1}]$, and let $\mathrm{T}', \mathrm{Y}'_1, \ldots, \mathrm{Y}'_{n-2}$ be the elements of S′ defined in the same way as $\mathrm{T}, \mathrm{Y}_1, \ldots, \mathrm{Y}_{n-1}$ (but replacing n by $n-1$). Let $f : \mathrm{S} \to \mathrm{S}'$ be the homomorphism defined by

$$f(\mathrm{X}_i) = \mathrm{X}_i \quad (1 \leqslant i \leqslant n-1), \quad f(\mathrm{X}_n) = 0.$$

Show that

$$f(\mathrm{T}) = 0, \quad f(\mathrm{Y}_1) = \mathrm{T}'^{q(q-1)}, \quad f(\mathrm{Y}_i) = \mathrm{Y}'^{q}_{i-1} \quad \textit{for} \quad 2 \leqslant i \leqslant n-1.$$

e) Show that the family $(\mathrm{T}, \mathrm{Y}_1, \ldots, \mathrm{Y}_{n-1})$ satisfies condition (iv) of Exerc. 5. (Let $x = (x_1, \ldots, x_n)$ be a zero of the system $(\mathrm{T}, \mathrm{Y}_1, \ldots, \mathrm{Y}_{n-1})$ in an extension $\overline{\mathrm{K}}$ of K. Since x is a zero of T, the x_i satisfy at least one non-trivial linear relation with coefficients in K. Transforming x by an element of G_1 if necessary, we can assume that $x_n = 0$. Conclude by applying *d*) and arguing by induction on n.)

f) Show that $\mathrm{R}_1 = \mathrm{K}[\mathrm{T}, \mathrm{Y}_1, \ldots, \mathrm{Y}_{n-1}]$, and that $\mathrm{T}, \mathrm{Y}_1, \ldots, \mathrm{Y}_{n-1}$ are algebraically independent ("Dickson's Theorem" – apply *e*) and Exerc. 5, remarking that the order of G_1 is equal to $\deg(\mathrm{T}) = \sum_i \deg(\mathrm{Y}_i)$).

g) Show that $\mathrm{R} = \mathrm{K}[\mathrm{T}^{q-1}, \mathrm{Y}_1, \ldots, \mathrm{Y}_{n-1}]$.$_*$

¶ 7) *Let R be a regular local ring (*Commutative Algebra*, Chap. VIII, §5, no. 1), with maximal ideal $\mathfrak{m}$ and residue field k. Let G be a finite group of automorphisms of R, and let $R' = R^G$ be the subring of R consisting of the elements invariant under G. This is a local ring with maximal ideal $\mathfrak{m}' = \mathfrak{m} \cap R'$. Assume the following:

(i) R' is noetherian and R is an R'-module of finite type.

(ii) The composite $R' \to R \to k$ is surjective.

Put $V = \mathfrak{m}/\mathfrak{m}^2$; this is a k-vector space. The action of G on R defines a homomorphism $\varepsilon : G \to \mathbf{GL}(V)$.

a) Let $\mathfrak{p}$ be a prime ideal of R of height 1 (*Commutative Algebra*, Chap. VII, §1, no. 6) and let $s \in G$ be such that $s(\mathfrak{p}) = \mathfrak{p}$ and that s acts trivially on $R/\mathfrak{p}$. Show that $\varepsilon(s)$ is a pseudo-reflection of V. (Remark that the image of $\mathfrak{p}$ in $\mathfrak{m}/\mathfrak{m}^2$ is of dimension 0 or 1.)

b) Show that, if R' is regular, the subgroup $\varepsilon(G)$ of $\mathbf{GL}(V)$ is generated by pseudo-reflections, (Let H be the subgroup of G generated by elements whose image under ε is a pseudo-reflection, and let R^H be the subring of R consisting of elements invariant under H. Show, using *a*), that no prime ideal of R' of height 1 is ramified in R^H; using the fact that R^H is integrally closed, deduce by means of the Purity Theorem[11] that $R' = R^H$, so $H = G$.)

c) Assume now that the order of G is coprime to the characteristic of k. Show that ε is injective.

Let $(\mathfrak{m}'_n)$ be the filtration of R' induced by the $\mathfrak{m}$-adic filtration $(\mathfrak{m}^n)$ of R, and let

$$i : \mathrm{gr}(R') \to \mathrm{gr}(R)$$

be the canonical homomorphism of the associated graded algebra of R' to that of R (*Commutative Algebra*, Chap. III, §2). Show that i is injective, and that its image is the subring $\mathrm{gr}(R)^G$ of $\mathrm{gr}(R)$ consisting of the elements invariant under G.

d) Retain the assumptions and notation of *c*), and assume further that $\varepsilon(G)$ is generated by pseudo-reflections. If $l = \dim V$, let $P_1, \ldots, P_l$ be algebraically independent homogeneous generators of the k-algebra $\mathrm{gr}(R)^G$ (such elements exist by Th. 4 and the fact that $\mathrm{gr}(R)$ can be identified with the symmetric algebra of V); let $p_1, \ldots, p_l$ be their degrees. By *c*), we can find $x_i \in \mathfrak{m}'_{p_i}$ such that $\mathrm{gr}(x_i) = P_i$. Show that the x_i generate the ideal $\mathfrak{m}'$ and deduce that R' is regular.*

¶ 8) *Let V be a finite dimensional vector space over a field K, let S be the symmetric algebra of V, and let G be a finite subgroup of $\mathbf{GL}(V)$. Assume

[11] Cf. M. AUSLANDER, On the purity of the branch locus, *Amer. J. of Math.*, v. LXXXIV (1962), p. 116-125.

that the algebra S^G of symmetric invariants of G is a graded polynomial algebra.

a) Let u be an element of the dual V^* of V, and let G_u be the subgroup of G consisting of the elements leaving u invariant. Show that G_u is generated by pseudo-reflections. (The linear form u extends to a homomorphism $f_u : S \to K$. If S_u denotes the local ring of S with respect to the kernel of f_u, the ring S_u is regular. Conclude by applying Exerc. 7 *b*) to G_u, considered as a group of automorphisms of S_u.)

In particular, G is generated by pseudo-reflections.

b) Let A be a subset of V^*, and let $G_A = \bigcap_{u \in A} G_u$. Show that G_A is generated by pseudo-reflections. (Extending the base field if necessary, we can assume that K is infinite. Show that in that case there exists an element v of the vector subspace of V^* generated by A such that $G_v = G_A$. Conclude by applying *a*) to v.)$_*$

9) Let V be a vector space of dimension 4 over a finite field K, of characteristic different from 2, and let Q be a non-degenerate quadratic form on V of index 2 (*Algebra*, Chap. IX, § 4, no. 2). Let $G = \mathbf{O}(Q)$ be the orthogonal group of this form; this is a finite group generated by reflections (*loc. cit.*, § 6, no. 4, Prop. 5).

a) Let E be a maximal totally isotropic subspace of V, and let G_E be the subgroup of G consisting of the elements g such that $g(x) = x$ for all $x \in E$. Show that G_E is isomorphic to the additive group of K, and contains no pseudo-reflection.

b) Show that the algebra of symmetric invariants of G is not a graded polynomial algebra (use the preceding exercise).

§ 6.

In the exercises below (with the exception of Exerc. 3), the assumptions and notation are those of § 6.

1) Assume that W is irreducible. Let c be a Coxeter transformation of W, let Γ be the subgroup of W generated by c, and let Δ be the set of unit vectors orthogonal to an element of $\mathfrak{H}$. Show that Γ has l orbits in Δ, and that each orbit has h elements. (Argue as in the proof of Prop. 33 of Chap. VI, § 1, no. 11.)

¶ 2) Assume that W is irreducible. Let C be a chamber relative to W, $(H_1, \ldots, H_l)$ its walls, and e_i a non-zero vector orthogonal to H_i. Assume that $e_1, \ldots, e_r$ (resp. $e_{r+1}, \ldots, e_l$) are pairwise orthogonal (cf. no. 2). For all $u \in \mathbf{Z}$, define H_u and s_u by $H_u = H_k$ if $u \equiv k \pmod{l}$ and $s_u = s_{H_u}$.

a) Show that the elements of $\mathfrak{H}$ are the $s_1 s_2 \ldots s_{u-1} \mathrm{H}_u$ for $u = 1, 2, \ldots, lh/2$.

b) Let $s' = s_1 \ldots s_r$ and $s'' = s_{r+1} \ldots s_l$, so that $c = s's''$ is the Coxeter transformation associated to the ordered chamber C. Let w_0 be the element of W that transforms C to −C (cf. § 4, Exerc. 2). Show that, if h is odd,

$$w_0 = \underbrace{s's''s' \ldots s''s'}_{h \text{ terms}} = \underbrace{s''s's'' \ldots s's''}_{h \text{ terms}} = s''c^{(h-1)/2} = c^{(h-1)/2}s'.$$

c) Put $\mathrm{S} = \{s_1, \ldots, s_l\}$. The pair (W, S) is a Coxeter system. If $w \in \mathrm{W}$, denote by $l_{\mathrm{S}}(w)$ the length of w with respect to S (Chap. IV, § 1, no. 1). Show that

$$l_{\mathrm{S}}(s') = r, \quad l_{\mathrm{S}}(s'') = l - r, \quad l_{\mathrm{S}}(c) = l.$$

Deduce that, with the assumptions in *b*),

$$l_{\mathrm{S}}(w_0) \leqslant r + \frac{h-1}{2} l \quad \text{and} \quad l_{\mathrm{S}}(w_0) \leqslant (l - r) + \frac{h-1}{2} l.$$

Show on the other hand that $l_{\mathrm{S}}(w_0) = \mathrm{Card}(\mathfrak{H}) = hl/2$ (use Exerc. 22 of Chap. IV, § 1). Deduce that $r = l/2$ and that $(s_1, s_2, \ldots, s_{lh/2})$ is a reduced decomposition of w_0.

d) Show that, if h is even, $(s_1, \ldots, s_{lh/2})$ is a reduced decomposition of $w_0 = c^{h/2}$. (Same method.)

¶ 3) Let K be a commutative ring, E a free K-module with basis $(e_1, \ldots, e_l)$, and $f_1, \ldots, f_l$ elements of the dual of E. Put $a_{ij} = f_i(e_j)$. If $1 \leqslant i \leqslant l$, let s_i be the pseudo-reflection s_{e_i, f_i} (§ 2, Exerc. 1). Then

$$s_i(e_j) = e_j - a_{ij} e_i.$$

Put $c = s_1 \ldots s_l$, and $z_i = c(e_i)$.

a) For $1 \leqslant i, k \leqslant l$, put

$$y_i^k = s_1 \ldots s_k(e_i) \quad \text{and} \quad y_i = s_1 \ldots s_{i-1}(e_i) = y_i^{i-1}.$$

Thus $y_i^0 = e_i$ and $y_i^l = z_i$.

Show that

$$y_i^{k-1} - y_i^k = a_{ki} y_k.$$

Deduce the formulas

$$e_i = y_i + \sum_{k<i} a_{ki} y_k$$

$$z_i = y_i - \sum_{k \geqslant i} a_{ki} y_k.$$

b) Let C be the matrix of c with respect to the basis (e_i). Let $\mathrm{U} = (u_{ij})$ and $\mathrm{V} = (v_{ij})$ be the matrices defined by

$$u_{ij} = \begin{cases} a_{ij} & \text{if } i < j \\ 0 & \text{otherwise,} \end{cases} \qquad v_{ij} = \begin{cases} 0 & \text{if } i < j \\ a_{ij} & \text{otherwise.} \end{cases}$$

The matrix $\mathrm{I} + \mathrm{U}$ is invertible with determinant 1. Show that

$$\mathrm{C} = (\mathrm{I} - \mathrm{V})(\mathrm{I} + \mathrm{U})^{-1}.$$

Deduce that

$$\det(\lambda\mathrm{I} - \mathrm{C}) = \det((\lambda - 1)\mathrm{I} + \mathrm{V} + \lambda\mathrm{U}),$$

in other words

$$\det(\lambda\mathrm{I} - \mathrm{C}) = \begin{vmatrix} (\lambda-1)+a_{11} & \lambda a_{12} & \lambda a_{13} & \cdots & \lambda a_{1l} \\ a_{21} & \lambda(\lambda-1)+a_{22} & \lambda a_{23} & \cdots & \lambda a_{2l} \\ a_{31} & a_{32} & (\lambda-1)+a_{33} & \cdots & \lambda a_{3l} \\ \vdots & \vdots & \vdots & \ddots & \vdots \\ a_{l1} & a_{l2} & a_{l3} & \cdots & (\lambda-1)+a_{ll} \end{vmatrix}.$$

c) Let $\Gamma = (\mathrm{I}, \mathrm{S})$ be the graph whose set of vertices is $\mathrm{I} = [1, l]$ and whose set S of arrows is the set of subsets $\{i, j\}$ of I with 2 elements such that $a_{ij} \neq 0$ or $a_{ji} \neq 0$. If $\alpha = \{i, j\}$ belongs to S, denote by σ_α the transposition of i and j (considered as an element of the symmetric group $\mathrm{S_I}$), and put $a_\alpha = -a_{ij}a_{ji}$.

Let $\mathfrak{B}$ be the set of subsets of S consisting of the arrows whose vertices are disjoint. If $\mathrm{X} \in \mathfrak{B}$, denote by C(X) the set of $i \in \mathrm{I}$ that are not vertices of any arrow of X, and put $\sigma_\mathrm{X} = \prod_{\alpha \in \mathrm{X}} \sigma_\alpha$, $a_\mathrm{X} = \prod_{\alpha \in \mathrm{X}} a_\alpha$.

Let $\sigma \in \mathrm{S_I}$, and let d_σ be the term corresponding to σ in the expansion of the determinant of $(\lambda - 1)\mathrm{I} + \mathrm{V} + \lambda\mathrm{U}$. Show that, if σ is of the form σ_X, with $\mathrm{X} \in \mathfrak{B}$, then

$$d_\sigma = a_\mathrm{X}\lambda^{\mathrm{Card(X)}} \prod_{i \in \mathrm{C(X)}} (\lambda - 1 + a_{ii}).$$

Assume now that Γ is a *forest* (Chap. IV, Appendix, no. 3). Show that, if $\sigma \in \mathrm{S}_l$ is not of the form σ_X with $\mathrm{X} \in \mathfrak{B}$, then $d_\sigma = 0$. Deduce the formula

$$\det(\lambda - c) = \sum_{\mathrm{X} \in \mathfrak{B}} a_\mathrm{X}\lambda^{\mathrm{Card(X)}} \prod_{i \in \mathrm{C(X)}} (\lambda - 1 + a_{ii}).$$

d) Consider the polynomial

$$\mathrm{P(X)} = \begin{vmatrix} \mathrm{X} & a_{12} & \cdots & a_{1l} \\ a_{21} & \mathrm{X} & \cdots & a_{2l} \\ \vdots & \vdots & \ddots & \vdots \\ a_{l1} & a_{l2} & \cdots & \mathrm{X} \end{vmatrix}.$$

To the assumptions in *c*), we add that $a_{ii} = 1$ for all i. Show that in that case

$$\det(\lambda^2 - c) = \lambda^l \mathrm{P}(\lambda + \lambda^{-1}).$$

4) With the assumptions and notation of no. 1, denote by n_{ij} the order of $s_{H_i} s_{H_j}$, and put $a_{ij} = -2\cos\frac{\pi}{n_{ij}}$. Then $a_{ii} = 2$ and $a_{ij} \leqslant 0$ if $i \neq j$, cf. § 3. Show[12], by using the method of the preceding exercise, that

$$\begin{vmatrix} X & a_{12} & \dots & a_{1l} \\ a_{21} & X & \dots & a_{2l} \\ \vdots & \vdots & \ddots & \vdots \\ a_{l1} & a_{l2} & \dots & X \end{vmatrix} = \prod_{i=1}^{l} (X - 2\cos(\pi m_i/h)),$$

where $m_1, \dots, m_l$ are the exponents of W.

[12]For more details, see: H. S. M. COXETER, The product of the generators of a finite group generated by reflections, *Duke Math. Journal.*, v. XVIII (1951), p. 765-782.

CHAPTER VI
Root Systems

§ 1. ROOT SYSTEMS

In this paragraph, k denotes a field of characteristic zero. From no. 3 onwards, we assume that $k = \mathbf{R}$.

1. DEFINITION OF A ROOT SYSTEM

Lemma 1. Let V *be a vector space over* k*,* R *a finite subset of* V *generating* V*. For any* $\alpha \in \mathrm{R}$ *such that* $\alpha \neq 0$*, there exists at most one reflection* s *of* V *such that* $s(\alpha) = -\alpha$ *and* $s(\mathrm{R}) = \mathrm{R}$*.*

Let G be the group of automorphisms of V leaving R stable. Since R generates V, G is isomorphic to a subgroup of the symmetric group of R, and hence is finite. Let s, s' be reflections of V such that $s(\alpha) = s'(\alpha) = -\alpha$, $s(\mathrm{R}) = \mathrm{R}$, $s'(\mathrm{R}) = \mathrm{R}$. Then $t = ss'$ belongs to G, and hence is of finite order m. On the other hand,

$$t(\alpha) = \alpha \ \text{ and } \ t(x) \equiv x \text{ mod. } k\alpha \ \text{ for all } x \in \mathrm{V}.$$

Hence, there exists a linear form f on V such that

$$t(x) = x + f(x)\alpha \ \text{ for all } x \in \mathrm{V}$$

and $f(\alpha) = 0$. By induction on n, it follows that

$$t^n(x) = x + nf(x)\alpha \text{ for all } x \in \mathrm{V}.$$

Taking n equal to m, we see that $mf(x) = 0$ for all $x \in \mathrm{V}$, so $f = 0$, $t = 1$ and $s = s'$.

DEFINITION 1. *Let* V *be a vector space over* k*, and* R *a subset of* V*. Then* R *is said to be a root system in* V *if the following conditions are satisfied:*

($\mathrm{RS_I}$) R *is finite, does not contain* 0*, and generates* V*.*

($\mathrm{RS_{II}}$) *For all* $\alpha \in \mathrm{R}$*, there exists an element* $\alpha\check{}$ *of the dual* V^* *of* V *such that* $\langle \alpha, \alpha\check{} \rangle = 2$ *and that the reflection* $s_{\alpha,\alpha\check{}}$ *(*cf. Chap. V, § 2*) leaves* R *stable.*

(RS_{III}) *For all* $\alpha \in R$, $\alpha\check{}(R) \subseteq \mathbf{Z}$.

By Lemma 1, the reflection $s_{\alpha,\alpha\check{}}$ (and hence also the linear form $\alpha\check{}$) is determined uniquely by α, so (RS_{III}) makes sense. We put $s_{\alpha,\alpha\check{}} = s_\alpha$. Then $s_\alpha(x) = x - \langle \alpha\check{}, x\rangle\alpha$ for all $x \in V$.

The elements of R are called the *roots* (of the system considered). The dimension of V is called the *rank* of the system.

The automorphisms of V that leave R stable are called the automorphisms of R. They form a finite group denoted by A(R). The subgroup of A(R) generated by the s_α is called the *Weyl group* of R and is denoted by W(R), or simply by W.

Remark. 1) Let k' be an extension of k. Identify V canonically with a subset of $V \otimes k'$ and V^* with a subset of $V^* \otimes k' = (V \otimes k')^*$. Then, R is a root system in $V \otimes k'$, and the $\alpha\check{}$ are the same as before.

Lemma 2. Let R *be a root system in* V. *Let* $(x|y)$ *be a symmetric bilinear form on* V, *non-degenerate and invariant under* W(R). *Identify* V *with* V^* *by means of this form. If* $\alpha \in R$, *then* α *is non-isotropic and*

$$\alpha\check{} = \frac{2\alpha}{(\alpha|\alpha)}.$$

This follows from formula (4) of Chap. V, § 2, no. 3.

PROPOSITION 1. *Let* $V_{\mathbf{Q}}$ *(resp.* $V^*_{\mathbf{Q}}$*) be the* **Q***-vector subspace of* V *(resp.* V^**) generated by the* α *(resp. the* $\alpha\check{}$*). Then* $V_{\mathbf{Q}}$ *(resp.* $V^*_{\mathbf{Q}}$*) is a* **Q***-structure on* V *(resp.* V^**)* (*Algebra,* Chap. II, § 8, no. 1). *The restriction to* $V_{\mathbf{Q}} \times V^*_{\mathbf{Q}}$ *of the canonical bilinear form on* $V \times V^*$ *gives an identification of each of the spaces* $V_{\mathbf{Q}}, V^*_{\mathbf{Q}}$ *with the dual of the other. The set* R *is a root system in* $V_{\mathbf{Q}}$.

If $k = \mathbf{R}$, there exists a scalar product on V invariant under W(R) (*Integration,* Chap. VII, § 3, no. 1, Prop. 1); Lemma 2 now shows that the $\alpha\check{}$ generate V^*. By *Remark* 1, the $\alpha\check{}$ again generate V^* if $k = \mathbf{Q}$. We now go to the general case. Put $E = V_{\mathbf{Q}}$. By (RS_{III}), each $\alpha\check{}$ maps E to $\mathbf{Q}$, and so defines an element $\tilde{\alpha}$ of E^*. It is immediate that R is a root system in E, and that the element corresponding to α in E^* is $\tilde{\alpha}$. By what we said above, the $\tilde{\alpha}$ generate the vector space E^*. Consider the canonical homomorphism $i : E \otimes_{\mathbf{Q}} k \to V$, and its transpose ${}^t i : V^* \to E^* \otimes_{\mathbf{Q}} k$. Since R generates V, ${}^t i$ is injective; but the image of ${}^t i$ contains the $\tilde{\alpha}$, so ${}^t i$ is surjective. From this we conclude finally that i and ${}^t i$ are isomorphisms. We can therefore identify V with $E \otimes k$, V^* with $E^* \otimes k$, $\alpha\check{}$ with $\tilde{\alpha}$, and $V^*_{\mathbf{Q}}$ with E^*. Thus, $V_{\mathbf{Q}}$ (resp. $V^*_{\mathbf{Q}}$) is a **Q**-structure on V (resp. V^*). The restriction to $V_{\mathbf{Q}} \times V^*_{\mathbf{Q}}$ of the canonical bilinear form on $V \times V^*$ can be identified with the canonical bilinear form on $E \times E^*$, hence the proposition.

Remarks. 2) Proposition 1 reduces the study of root systems to the case $k = \mathbf{Q}$. *Remark* 1 reduces it further to the study of root systems in the real vector space $V_{\mathbf{R}} = V_{\mathbf{Q}} \otimes_{\mathbf{Q}} \mathbf{R}$. The Weyl groups associated to these different systems are canonically identified.

3) Since the $\alpha^{\vee}$ generate V^*, the group $W(R)$, considered as a subgroup of $\mathbf{GL}(V_{\mathbf{R}})$, is *essential* (Chap. V, § 3, no. 7). Moreover, the Cor. of Th. 1 of Chap. V, § 3, no. 2 shows that the only reflections belonging to $W(R)$ are the s_α.

PROPOSITION 2. *The* $\alpha^{\vee}$ *form a root system in* V^*, *and* $\alpha^{\vee\vee} = \alpha$ *for all* $\alpha \in R$.

The $\alpha^{\vee}$ satisfy (RS_I) by Prop. 1. Since $s_{\alpha,\alpha^{\vee}}$ is an automorphism of the vector space V equipped with the subset R, ${}^t(s_{\alpha,\alpha^{\vee}})^{-1}$ leaves the set $R^{\vee}$ of the $\alpha^{\vee}$ stable; but ${}^t(s_{\alpha,\alpha^{\vee}})^{-1} = s_{\alpha^{\vee},\alpha}$, which proves that $R^{\vee}$ satisfies (RS_{II}) and that $\alpha^{\vee\vee} = \alpha$. Finally, $\langle \alpha^{\vee}, \beta \rangle \in \mathbf{Z}$ for all $\alpha^{\vee} \in R^{\vee}$ and $\beta \in R$, so $R^{\vee}$ satisfies (RS_{III}).

The set $R^{\vee}$ is called the *inverse root system of* R. The map $\alpha \mapsto \alpha^{\vee}$ is a bijection from R to $R^{\vee}$, called the *canonical bijection from* R *to* $R^{\vee}$. Note that, if α, β are elements of R such that $\alpha + \beta \in R$, then $(\alpha + \beta)^{\vee} \neq \alpha^{\vee} + \beta^{\vee}$ in general.

Since $s_\alpha(\alpha) = -\alpha$, axiom (RS_{II}) shows that $-R = R$. Evidently $(-\alpha)^{\vee} = -\alpha^{\vee}$ and $-1 \in A(R)$ (but it is not always true that $-1 \in W(R)$).

The equality ${}^t(s_{\alpha,\alpha^{\vee}})^{-1} = s_{\alpha^{\vee},\alpha}$ shows that the map $u \mapsto {}^t u^{-1}$ is an isomorphism from the group $W(R)$ to the group $W(R^{\vee})$. We identify these two groups by means of this isomorphism; in other words, we consider $W(R)$ as acting both in V and in V^*. Similarly for $A(R)$.

PROPOSITION 3. *For* $x, y \in V$, *put*

$$(x|y) = \sum_{\alpha \in R} \langle \alpha^{\vee}, x \rangle \langle \alpha^{\vee}, y \rangle.$$

Then $(x|y)$ *is a non-degenerate symmetric bilinear form on* V, *invariant under* $A(R)$. *For* $x, y \in V_{\mathbf{Q}}$ *we have* $(x|y) \in \mathbf{Q}$. *The canonical extension of* $(x|y)$ *to*

$$V_{\mathbf{R}} = V_{\mathbf{Q}} \otimes_{\mathbf{Q}} \mathbf{R}$$

is non-degenerate and positive.

It is clear that $(x|y)$ is a symmetric bilinear form on V. If $g \in A(R)$,

$$(g(x)|g(y)) = \sum_{\alpha \in R} \langle {}^t g(\alpha^{\vee}), x \rangle \langle {}^t g(\alpha^{\vee}), y \rangle = (x|y)$$

since $({}^t g)(R^{\vee}) = R^{\vee}$. If $x, y \in V_{\mathbf{Q}}$, then $(x|y) \in \mathbf{Q}$ by (RS_{III}). If $z \in V_{\mathbf{R}}$, then $(z|z) = \sum_{\alpha \in R} \langle \alpha^{\vee}, z \rangle^2 \geqslant 0$, and $(z|z) > 0$ if $z \neq 0$ by Prop. 1, so the canonical extension of $(x|y)$ to $V_{\mathbf{R}}$ is positive and non-degenerate. The restriction of $(x|y)$ to $V_{\mathbf{Q}}$ is thus non-degenerate, and hence the form $(x|y)$ on V is non-degenerate.

PROPOSITION 4. (i) *Let* X *be a subset of* R, *let* V_X *be the vector subspace of* V *generated by* X, *and let* V'_X *be the vector subspace of* V^* *generated by the* $\alpha\check{}$, *where* $\alpha \in X$. *Then* V *is the direct sum of* V_X *and the orthogonal complement of* V'_X, V^* *is the direct sum of* V'_X *and the orthogonal complement of* V_X, *and* V'_X *is identified with the dual of* V_X.

(ii) $R \cap V_X$ *is a root system in* V_X, *and the canonical bijection from* $R \cap V_X$ *to its inverse root system is identified with the restriction of the map* $\alpha \mapsto \alpha\check{}$ *to* $R \cap V_X$.

By *Remark* 2, we can assume that $k = \mathbf{R}$. Identify V with V^* by means of the symmetric bilinear form of Prop. 3. We have $\alpha\check{} = \frac{2\alpha}{(\alpha|\alpha)}$ for all $\alpha \in R$ (Lemma 2). Every vector subspace of V is non-isotropic, and the proposition is now clear.

COROLLARY. *Let* V_1 *be a vector subspace of* V, *and let* V_2 *be the vector subspace generated by* $R \cap V_1$. *Then* $R \cap V_1$ *is a root system in* V_2.

This follows from (ii) applied to $X = R \cap V_1$.

For $\alpha, \beta \in R$, put

$$\langle \alpha, \beta\check{} \rangle = n(\alpha, \beta). \tag{1}$$

Then

$$n(\alpha, \alpha) = 2 \tag{2}$$

$$n(-\alpha, \beta) = n(\alpha, -\beta) = -n(\alpha, \beta). \tag{3}$$

By (RS_{III}),

$$n(\alpha, \beta) \in \mathbf{Z}. \tag{4}$$

By the definition of $n(\alpha, \beta)$,

$$s_\beta(\alpha) = \alpha - n(\alpha, \beta)\beta. \tag{5}$$

Formula (1) and Prop. 2 imply that

$$n(\alpha, \beta) = n(\beta\check{}, \alpha\check{}). \tag{6}$$

Let $(x|y)$ be a symmetric bilinear form on V, non-degenerate and invariant under W(R) (Prop. 3). By Lemma 2,

$$n(\alpha, \beta) = \frac{2(\alpha|\beta)}{(\beta|\beta)}. \tag{7}$$

It follows that

$$n(\alpha, \beta) = 0 \Longleftrightarrow n(\beta, \alpha) = 0 \Longleftrightarrow (\alpha|\beta) = 0 \Longleftrightarrow s_\alpha \text{ and } s_\beta \text{ commute.} \tag{8}$$

$$\text{If } (\alpha|\beta) \neq 0, \text{ then } \frac{n(\beta, \alpha)}{n(\alpha, \beta)} = \frac{(\beta|\beta)}{(\alpha|\alpha)}. \tag{9}$$

2. DIRECT SUM OF ROOT SYSTEMS

Let V be a vector space over k that is the direct sum of a family $(\mathrm{V}_i)_{1\leqslant i\leqslant r}$ of vector spaces. Identify V^* with the direct sum of the V_i^*. For all i, let R_i be a root system in V_i. Then $\mathrm{R} = \bigcup_i \mathrm{R}_i$ is a root system in V whose inverse system is $\mathrm{R}^\vee = \bigcup_i \mathrm{R}_i^\vee$; the canonical bijection from R to $\mathrm{R}^\vee$ extends, for all i, the canonical bijection from R_i to $\mathrm{R}_i^\vee$. The set R is called the *direct sum of the root systems* R_i. Let $\alpha \in \mathrm{R}_i$. If $j \neq i$, the kernel of $\alpha^\vee$ contains V_j, so s_α induces the identity on V_j; on the other hand, $k\alpha \subseteq \mathrm{V}_i$, so s_α leaves V_i stable. These remarks show that W(R) *can be identified with* $\prod_{i=1}^{r} \mathrm{W}(\mathrm{R}_i)$.

A root system R is said to be *irreducible* if $\mathrm{R} \neq \varnothing$ and if R is not the direct sum of two non-empty root systems.

PROPOSITION 5. *Let* V *be a vector space over* k *that is the direct sum of vector spaces* $\mathrm{V}_1, \ldots, \mathrm{V}_r$. *Let* R *be a root system in* V. *Put* $\mathrm{R}_i = \mathrm{R} \cap \mathrm{V}_i$. *The following three conditions are equivalent:*

(i) *the* V_i *are stable under* W(R);
(ii) $\mathrm{R} \subseteq \mathrm{V}_1 \cup \mathrm{V}_2 \cup \cdots \cup \mathrm{V}_r$;
(iii) *for all* i, R_i *is a root system in* V_i, *and* R *is the direct sum of the* R_i.

(iii) $\Longrightarrow$ (i): this follows from what we said at the beginning of this number.

(i) $\Longrightarrow$ (ii): assume that the V_i are stable under W(R). Let $\alpha \in \mathrm{R}$ and let H be the kernel of $\alpha^\vee$. By Prop. 3 of Chap. V, § 2, no. 2, each V_i is the sum of a subspace of H and a subspace of $k\alpha$. Hence one of the V_i contains $k\alpha$, so $\alpha \in \mathrm{V}_1 \cup \mathrm{V}_2 \cup \cdots \cup \mathrm{V}_r$.

(ii) $\Longrightarrow$ (iii): if condition (ii) is satisfied, R_i generates V_i for all i, so R_i is a root system in V_i (Prop. 4). It is clear that R is the direct sum of the R_i.

COROLLARY. *Let* R *be a root system in* V. *The following conditions are equivalent:*

(i) R *is irreducible;*
(ii) *the* W(R)*-module* V *is simple;*
(iii) *the* W(R)*-module* V *is absolutely simple.*

(ii) $\Longleftrightarrow$ (i): this follows from Prop. 5 and Maschke's Theorem (Chap. V, Appendix, Prop. 2).

(iii) $\Longleftrightarrow$ (ii): this follows from Prop. 1 of Chap. V, § 2, no. 1.

PROPOSITION 6. *Every root system* R *in* V *is the direct sum of a family* $(\mathrm{R}_i)_{i\in \mathrm{I}}$ *of irreducible root systems that is unique up to a bijection of the index set.*

The existence of the R_i is proved by induction on Card R: if R is non-empty and not irreducible, R is the direct sum of two root systems R', R'' such that Card R′ < Card R, Card R″ < Card R, and the induction hypothesis applies to R′ and R″. To prove uniqueness, it suffices to prove that, if R is the direct sum of R′ and R″, every R_i is necessarily contained either in R′ or in R″. Let V', V'', V'_i, V''_i be the vector subspaces of V generated by $R', R'', R' \cap R_i, R'' \cap R_i$. Since the sum $V' + V''$ is direct, the sum $V'_i + V''_i$ is direct. Since $R_i \subseteq R' \cup R''$, R_i is the direct sum of the root systems $R' \cap R_i$ and $R'' \cap R_i$; hence either $R' \cap R_i = \varnothing$ or $R'' \cap R_i = \varnothing$, which proves the assertion.

The R_i are called the *irreducible components* of R. For any non-zero scalars λ_i, the union of the $\lambda_i R_i$ is a root system in V, whose inverse system is the union of the $\lambda_i^{-1} R_i\check{}$, and whose Weyl group is W(R).

PROPOSITION 7. *Let* R *be a root system in* V, (R_i) *the family of its irreducible components,* V_i *the vector subspace of* V *generated by* R_i, B *the invariant symmetric bilinear form on* V *defined in Prop. 3, and* B′ *a symmetric bilinear form on* V *invariant under* W(R). *Then the* V_i *are pairwise orthogonal with respect to* B′, *and, for all i, the restrictions of* B *and* B′ *to* V_i *are proportional.*

If $v_i \in V_i$, $v_j \in V_j$, $i \neq j$, and if $w \in W(R_j)$, then

$$B'(v_i, w(v_j)) = B'(v_i, v_j),$$

which shows that $w(v_j) - v_j$ is orthogonal to v_i with respect to B′. Since V_j is irreducible for $W(R_j)$, it is generated by the $w(v_j) - v_j$, and it is therefore orthogonal to V_i.

The fact that the restrictions of B and B′ to each of the V_i are proportional follows from Prop. 1 of Chap. V, § 2, no. 1.

Remark. Choose a scalar product on $V_{\mathbf{R}}$ invariant under W(R). It is then possible to speak of the *length* of a root and the *angle* between two roots. Prop. 7 shows that this angle is independent of the choice of scalar product, as is the ratio of the lengths of two roots, provided they belong to the *same* irreducible component of R.

3. RELATION BETWEEN TWO ROOTS

Recall that *we assume from now on that* $k = \mathbf{R}$. (We leave to the reader the task of extending the definitions and results to the general case, by using the method indicated in *Remark* 2 of no. 1.)

Throughout the following, R *denotes a root system in a vector space* V; *and* V *is equipped with a scalar product* $(x, y) \mapsto (x|y)$ *invariant under* W(R), cf. Prop. 3.

Let $\alpha, \beta \in R$. By formula (7) of no. 1,

$$n(\alpha, \beta) n(\beta, \alpha) = 4 \cos^2 (\widehat{\alpha, \beta}) \leqslant 4. \tag{10}$$

Thus, the integer $n(\alpha,\beta)n(\beta,\alpha)$ must take one of the values $0,1,2,3,4$. In view of Chap. V, § 2, no. 5, Cor. of Prop. 6, and of the footnote on the page of Chap. V, § 4, no. 8, we see that the only possibilities are the following, up to interchanging α and β:

1)	$n(\alpha,\beta) = n(\beta,\alpha) = 0$;	$\widehat{(\alpha,\beta)} = \frac{\pi}{2}$;	$s_\alpha s_\beta$ of order 2;
2)	$n(\alpha,\beta) = n(\beta,\alpha) = 1$;	$\widehat{(\alpha,\beta)} = \frac{\pi}{3}$; $\parallel \alpha \parallel = \parallel \beta \parallel$;	$s_\alpha s_\beta$ of order 3;
3)	$n(\alpha,\beta) = n(\beta,\alpha) = -1$;	$\widehat{(\alpha,\beta)} = \frac{2\pi}{3}$; $\parallel \alpha \parallel = \parallel \beta \parallel$;	$s_\alpha s_\beta$ of order 3;
4)	$n(\alpha,\beta) = 1,\ n(\beta,\alpha) = 2$;	$\widehat{(\alpha,\beta)} = \frac{\pi}{4}$; $\parallel \beta \parallel = \sqrt{2} \parallel \alpha \parallel$;	$s_\alpha s_\beta$ of order 4;
5)	$n(\alpha,\beta) = -1,\ n(\beta,\alpha) = -2$;	$\widehat{(\alpha,\beta)} = \frac{3\pi}{4}$; $\parallel \beta \parallel = \sqrt{2} \parallel \alpha \parallel$;	$s_\alpha s_\beta$ of order 4;
6)	$n(\alpha,\beta) = 1,\ n(\beta,\alpha) = 3$;	$\widehat{(\alpha,\beta)} = \frac{\pi}{6}$; $\parallel \beta \parallel = \sqrt{3} \parallel \alpha \parallel$;	$s_\alpha s_\beta$ of order 6;
7)	$n(\alpha,\beta) = -1,\ n(\beta,\alpha) = -3$;	$\widehat{(\alpha,\beta)} = \frac{5\pi}{6}$; $\parallel \beta \parallel = \sqrt{3} \parallel \alpha \parallel$;	$s_\alpha s_\beta$ of order 6;
8)	$n(\alpha,\beta) = n(\beta,\alpha) = 2$;	$\alpha = \beta$;	
9)	$n(\alpha,\beta) = n(\beta,\alpha) = -2$;	$\alpha = -\beta$;	
10)	$n(\alpha,\beta) = 1,\ n(\beta,\alpha) = 4$;	$\beta = 2\alpha$;	
11)	$n(\alpha,\beta) = -1,\ n(\beta,\alpha) = -4$;	$\beta = -2\alpha$.	

In particular:

PROPOSITION 8. (i) *If two roots are proportional, the factor of proportionality can only be* $\pm 1, \pm\frac{1}{2}, \pm 2$.

(ii) *If* α *and* β *are two non-proportional roots, and if* $\parallel \alpha \parallel \leqslant \parallel \beta \parallel$, *then* $n(\alpha,\beta)$ *takes one of the values* $0, 1, -1$.

If a root $\alpha \in \mathrm{R}$ is such that $\frac{1}{2}\alpha \notin \mathrm{R}$, then α is called an *indivisible* root.

THEOREM 1. *Let* α, β *be two roots.*

(i) *If* $n(\alpha,\beta) > 0$, $\alpha - \beta$ *is a root unless* $\alpha = \beta$.

(ii) *If* $n(\alpha,\beta) < 0$, $\alpha + \beta$ *is a root unless* $\alpha = -\beta$.

If $n(\alpha,\beta) > 0$, the possibilities, by the list above, are the following:

1) $n(\alpha,\beta) = 1$; then $\alpha - \beta - s_\beta(\alpha) \in \mathrm{R}$;
2) $n(\beta,\alpha) = 1$; then $\beta - \alpha = s_\alpha(\beta) \in \mathrm{R}$, so $\alpha - \beta \in \mathrm{R}$;
3) $\beta = \alpha$.

This proves (i), and (ii) follows by changing β to $-\beta$.

COROLLARY. *Let* α *and* β *be two roots.*

(i) *If* $(\alpha|\beta) > 0$, $\alpha - \beta$ *is a root unless* $\alpha = \beta$.
(ii) *If* $(\alpha|\beta) < 0$, $\alpha + \beta$ *is a root unless* $\alpha = -\beta$.
(iii) *If* $\alpha - \beta \notin \mathrm{R} \cup \{0\}$ *and* $\alpha + \beta \notin \mathrm{R} \cup \{0\}$, *then* $(\alpha|\beta) = 0$.

Assertions (i) and (ii) follow from Th. 1 and formula (7) of no. 1. Assertion (iii) follows from (i) and (ii).

It is possible that $\alpha + \beta \in \mathrm{R}$, $(\alpha|\beta) = 0$ (cf. Plate X, System B_2). When $\alpha - \beta \notin \mathrm{R} \cup \{0\}$ and $\alpha + \beta \notin \mathrm{R} \cup \{0\}$, α and β are said to be *strongly orthogonal.*

PROPOSITION 9. *Let* α *and* β *be two non-proportional roots.*

(i) *The set* I *of integers* j *such that* $\beta + j\alpha$ *is a root is an interval* $[-q, p]$ *in* $\mathbf{Z}$ *containing* 0.

(ii) *Let* S *be the set of* $\beta + j\alpha$ *for* $j \in \mathrm{I}$. *Then,*

$$s_\alpha(\mathrm{S}) = \mathrm{S} \quad \text{and} \quad s_\alpha(\beta + p\alpha) = \beta - q\alpha.$$

(iii) $p - q = -n(\beta, \alpha)$.

Clearly, $0 \in \mathrm{I}$. Let p (resp. $-q$) be the largest (resp. smallest) element of I. If not all the integers in $[-q, p]$ belong to I, there exist two integers r, s in $[-q, p]$ with the following properties: $s > r + 1, s \in \mathrm{I}, r \in \mathrm{I}, r + k \notin \mathrm{I}$ for $1 \leqslant k \leqslant s - r - 1$. With the notation of the Cor. of Th. 1, $(\alpha|\beta + s\alpha) \leqslant 0, (\alpha|\beta + r\alpha) \geqslant 0$, which is absurd because

$$(\alpha|\beta + s\alpha) \leqslant 0 > (\alpha|\beta + r\alpha).$$

This proves (i).

We have $s_\alpha(\beta + j\alpha) = \beta - n(\beta, \alpha)\alpha - j\alpha = \beta + j'\alpha$ with $j' = -j - n(\beta, \alpha)$. Thus $s_\alpha(\mathrm{S}) \subseteq \mathrm{S}$ and consequently $s_\alpha(\mathrm{S}) = \mathrm{S}$. Now $j \mapsto -j - n(\beta, \alpha)$ is a decreasing bijection from I to I. It follows that, $j' = -q$ when $j = p$, so that $-q = -p - n(\beta, \alpha)$. This proves (ii) and (iii).

The set S is called the *α-chain of roots* defined by β, $\beta - q\alpha$ is its *origin,* $\beta + p\alpha$ is its *end,* and $p + q$ is its *length.*

COROLLARY. *Let* S *be an* α*-chain of roots, and* γ *the origin of* S. *The length of* S *is* $-n(\gamma, \alpha)$; *it is equal to* $0, 1, 2$ *or* 3.

The first assertion follows from Prop. 9, (iii), applied to $\beta = \gamma$, and using the fact that $q = 0$.

On the other hand, since γ is not proportional to α, the list given at the beginning of this no. shows that $|n(\gamma, \alpha)| \leqslant 3$, hence the corollary.

Remark. We retain the notation above. Then:

1) If the length of S is 0, then $(\alpha|\gamma) = 0$.

2) If the length of S is 1, then $n(\gamma,\alpha) = -1$, and there are three cases:

$$n(\alpha,\gamma) = -1, \quad (\alpha|\alpha) = (\gamma|\gamma), \quad (\alpha|\gamma) = -\tfrac{1}{2}(\alpha|\alpha), \quad (\widehat{\alpha,\gamma}) = \tfrac{2\pi}{3}$$
$$n(\alpha,\gamma) = -2, \quad (\alpha|\alpha) = 2(\gamma|\gamma), \quad (\alpha|\gamma) = -\tfrac{1}{2}(\alpha|\alpha), \quad (\widehat{\alpha,\gamma}) = \tfrac{3\pi}{4}$$
$$n(\alpha,\gamma) = -3, \quad (\alpha|\alpha) = 3(\gamma|\gamma), \quad (\alpha|\gamma) = -\tfrac{1}{2}(\alpha|\alpha), \quad (\widehat{\alpha,\gamma}) = \tfrac{5\pi}{6}$$

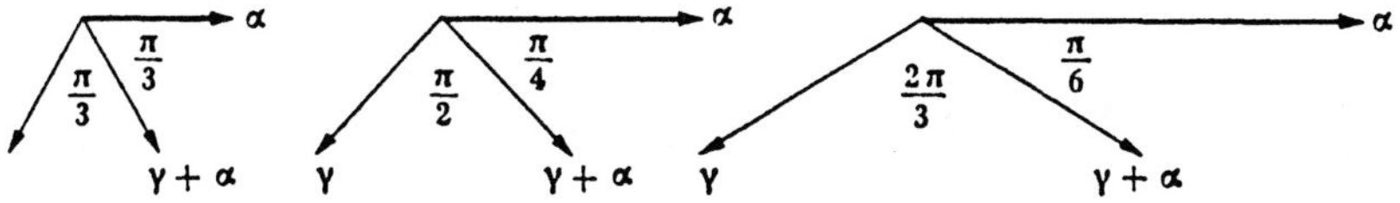

3) If the length of S is 2, then $n(\gamma,\alpha) = -2$, so

$$n(\alpha,\gamma) = -1,\ (\alpha|\alpha) = \frac{1}{2}(\gamma|\gamma),\ (\alpha|\gamma) = -(\alpha|\alpha),\ (\widehat{\alpha,\gamma}) = \frac{3\pi}{4}.$$

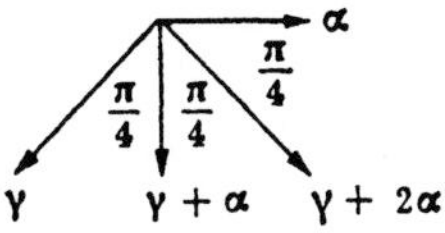

4) If the length of S is 3, then $n(\gamma,\alpha) = -3$, so

$$n(\alpha,\gamma) = -1,\ (\alpha|\alpha) = \frac{1}{3}(\gamma|\gamma),\ (\alpha|\gamma) = -\frac{3}{2}(\alpha|\alpha),\ (\widehat{\alpha,\gamma}) = \frac{5\pi}{6}.$$

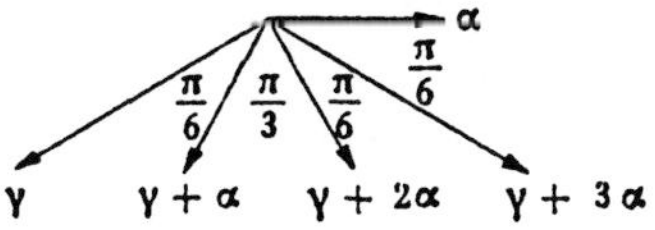

We shall see (Plate X, Systems A_2, B_2, G_2) that all these cases are actually realised.

PROPOSITION 10. *Let α,β be two non-proportional roots such that $\beta+\alpha$ is a root. Let p, q be the integers in Prop. 9. Then*

$$\frac{(\beta+\alpha|\beta+\alpha)}{(\beta|\beta)} = \frac{q+1}{p}.$$

Let S be the α-chain defined by β, γ its origin; its length l is $\geqslant 1$ since $\beta+\alpha$ is a root. The following cases are possible:

1) $l = 1$; then $\beta = \gamma, q = 0, p = 1, (\beta+\alpha|\beta+\alpha) = (\beta|\beta)$.
2) $l = 2$, $\beta = \gamma$; then $q = 0, p = 2, (\beta+\alpha|\beta+\alpha) = \frac{1}{2}(\beta|\beta)$.
3) $l = 2$, $\beta = \gamma+\alpha$; then $q = 1, p = 1, (\beta+\alpha|\beta+\alpha) = 2(\beta|\beta)$.

4) $l = 3$, $\beta = \gamma$; then $q = 0, p = 3, (\beta + \alpha|\beta + \alpha) = \frac{1}{3}(\beta|\beta)$.
5) $l = 3$, $\beta = \gamma + \alpha$; then $q = 1, p = 2, (\beta + \alpha|\beta + \alpha) = (\beta|\beta)$.
6) $l = 3$, $\beta = \gamma + 2\alpha$; then $q = 2, p = 1, (\beta + \alpha|\beta + \alpha) = 3(\beta|\beta)$.

In each case, the formula to be proved is satisfied.

PROPOSITION 11. *Assume that* R *is irreducible. Let* α *and* β *be two roots such that* $\| \alpha \| = \| \beta \|$. *There exists* $g \in \mathrm{W(R)}$ *such that* $g(\alpha) = \beta$.

The transforms of α by W(R) generate V (no. 2, Cor. of Prop. 5). Hence there exists $g \in \mathrm{W(R)}$ such that $(g(\alpha)|\beta) \neq 0$. We assume from now on that $(\alpha|\beta) \neq 0$. By formula (9) of no. 1, $n(\alpha, \beta) = n(\beta, \alpha)$. Replacing β if necessary by $s_\beta(\beta) = -\beta$, we can assume that $n(\alpha, \beta) > 0$. Then, by the list at the beginning of no. 3, either $\alpha = \beta$ (in which case the proposition is clear), or $n(\alpha, \beta) = n(\beta, \alpha) = 1$; in that case

$$s_\alpha s_\beta s_\alpha(\beta) = s_\alpha s_\beta(\beta - \alpha) = s_\alpha(-\beta - \alpha + \beta) = \alpha.$$

4. REDUCED ROOT SYSTEMS

A root system is said to be *reduced* if every root of the system is indivisible (no. 3).

PROPOSITION 12. *Assume that* R *is irreducible and reduced.*

(i) *The ratio* $\frac{(\beta|\beta)}{(\alpha|\alpha)}$ *for* $\alpha \in \mathrm{R}, \beta \in \mathrm{R}$ *must take one of the values* $1, 2, \frac{1}{2}, 3, \frac{1}{3}$.

(ii) *The set of the* $(\alpha|\alpha)$ *for* $\alpha \in \mathrm{R}$ *has at most two elements.*

Since R is irreducible, the transforms of a root by W(R) generate V (no. 2, Cor. of Prop. 5). Hence, for any roots α, β, there exists a root β' such that $(\alpha|\beta') \neq 0$ and $(\beta'|\beta') = (\beta|\beta)$. By formula (9) of no. 1 and the list of no. 3, $\frac{(\beta'|\beta')}{(\alpha|\alpha)}$ takes one of the values $1, 2, \frac{1}{2}, 3, \frac{1}{3}$ (recall that the system is assumed to be reduced). By multiplying $(x|y)$ by a suitable scalar, we can assume that $(\alpha|\alpha) = 1$ for certain roots and that the other possible values of $(\beta|\beta)$ for $\beta \in \mathrm{R}$ are 2 and 3. The values 2 and 3 cannot both be attained, since in that case there would exist $\beta \in \mathrm{R}, \gamma \in \mathrm{R}$ such that $\frac{(\gamma|\gamma)}{(\beta|\beta)} = \frac{3}{2}$, contrary to what we have seen above.

PROPOSITION 13. *Assume that* R *is irreducible, non-reduced and of rank* $\geqslant 2$.

(i) *The set* R_0 *of indivisible roots is a root system in* V*; this system is irreducible and reduced; and* $\mathrm{W(R_0)} = \mathrm{W(R)}$.

(ii) *Let* A *be the set of roots* α *for which* $(\alpha|\alpha)$ *takes the smallest value* λ. *Then any two non-proportional elements of* A *are orthogonal.*

(iii) *Let* B *be the set of* $\beta \in \mathrm{R}$ *such that* $(\beta|\beta) = 2\lambda$. *Then* $\mathrm{B} \neq \varnothing$, $\mathrm{R_0} = \mathrm{A} \cup \mathrm{B}$, $\mathrm{R} = \mathrm{A} \cup \mathrm{B} \cup 2\mathrm{A}$.

If $\alpha \in \mathrm{R} - \mathrm{R}_0$, then $\frac{1}{2}\alpha \in \mathrm{R}$, but $\frac{1}{2}\left(\frac{1}{2}\alpha\right) \notin \mathrm{R}$ (Prop. 8), so $\frac{1}{2}\alpha \in \mathrm{R}_0$. This proves that R_0 satisfies $(\mathrm{RS_I})$. It is clear that, for all $\alpha \in \mathrm{R}$, $s_{\alpha,\alpha^\vee}(\mathrm{R}_0) = \mathrm{R}_0$, so R_0 satisfies $(\mathrm{RS_{II}})$ and $(\mathrm{RS_{III}})$. Since $\alpha \in \mathrm{R} - \mathrm{R}_0$ implies that $\frac{1}{2}\alpha \in \mathrm{R}_0$ and since $s_\alpha = s_{\alpha/2}$, we have $\mathrm{W(R)} = \mathrm{W(R_0)}$. Thus R_0 is irreducible (Cor. of Prop. 5), and it is evidently reduced.

Since R is not reduced, there exists $\alpha \in \mathrm{R}_0$ such that $2\alpha \in \mathrm{R}$. Since R_0 is irreducible and $\dim \mathrm{V} \geqslant 2$, α cannot be proportional or orthogonal to every root. Let $\beta \in \mathrm{R}_0$ be such that $n(\beta, \alpha) \neq 0$ and β is not proportional to α. Changing β to $-\beta$ if necessary, we can assume that $n(\beta, \alpha) > 0$. Now $\frac{1}{2}n(\beta, \alpha) = n(\beta, 2\alpha) \in \mathbf{Z}$, so $n(\beta, \alpha) \in 2\mathbf{Z}$. From the list in no. 3, $n(\beta, \alpha) = 2$, $(\beta|\beta) = 2(\alpha|\alpha)$. Since R_0 is reduced, Prop. 12 shows that, for all $\gamma \in \mathrm{R}_0$, either $(\gamma|\gamma) = (\alpha|\alpha)$ or $(\gamma|\gamma) = 2(\alpha|\alpha)$. Also, the above shows that, for all $\gamma \in \mathrm{R} - \mathrm{R}_0$, the vector $\frac{1}{2}\gamma$ is an element of R_0 such that $\left(\frac{1}{2}\gamma|\frac{1}{2}\gamma\right) = (\alpha|\alpha)$. Thus, $\lambda = (\alpha|\alpha)$, $\mathrm{B} \neq \varnothing$, $\mathrm{R}_0 = \mathrm{A} \cup \mathrm{B}$, and $\mathrm{R} \subseteq \mathrm{A} \cup \mathrm{B} \cup 2\mathrm{A}$; on the other hand, if $\gamma \in \mathrm{A}$, there exists $g \in \mathrm{W(R)}$ such that $\gamma = g(\alpha)$ (Prop. 11), so $2\gamma = g(2\alpha) \in \mathrm{R}$; thus $2\mathrm{A} \subseteq \mathrm{R}$ and $\mathrm{R} = \mathrm{A} \cup \mathrm{B} \cup 2\mathrm{A}$. Finally, let γ, γ' be two non-proportional elements of A. Then

$$n(2\gamma, \gamma') = 2n(\gamma, \gamma') = 4n(\gamma, 2\gamma') \in 4\mathbf{Z}, \quad \text{and} \quad |n(\gamma, \gamma')| \leqslant 1$$

since γ and γ' have the same length, so $n(\gamma, \gamma') = 0$ and $(\gamma|\gamma') = 0$.

PROPOSITION 14. *Assume that* R *is irreducible and reduced, and that* $(\alpha|\alpha)$ *takes the values* λ *and* 2λ *for* $\alpha \in \mathrm{R}$. *Let* A *be the set of roots* α *such that* $(\alpha|\alpha) = \lambda$. *Assume that any two non-proportional elements of* A *are orthogonal. Then* $\mathrm{R}_1 = \mathrm{R} \cup 2\mathrm{A}$ *is an irreducible non-reduced root system and* R *is the set of indivisible roots of* R_1.

It is clear that R_1 satisfies $(\mathrm{RS_I})$ and $(\mathrm{RS_{III}})$. We show that, if $\alpha, \beta \in \mathrm{R}_1$, then $\langle \alpha^\vee, \beta \rangle \in \mathbf{Z}$. This is clear if $\alpha \in \mathrm{R}$. Since $(2\alpha)^\vee = \frac{1}{2}\alpha^\vee$ for $\alpha \in \mathrm{A}$, it is also immediate if $\alpha, \beta \in 2\mathrm{A}$. Finally, assume that $\beta \in \mathrm{R}$ and that $\alpha = 2\gamma$ with $\gamma \in \mathrm{A}$.

1) If $\gamma = \pm\beta$, then $\langle \alpha^\vee, \beta \rangle = \pm\frac{1}{2}\langle \gamma^\vee, \gamma \rangle = \pm 1$.

2) If γ is not proportional to β and if $\beta \in \mathrm{A}$, the assumption on A implies that $\langle \gamma^\vee, \beta \rangle = 0$, so $\langle \alpha^\vee, \beta \rangle = 0$.

3) If $\beta \in \mathrm{R} - \mathrm{A}$, then $(\beta|\beta) = 2\lambda = 2(\gamma|\gamma)$, so $\langle \beta, \gamma^\vee \rangle$ is equal to 0, 2 or -2 by the list in no. 3. Thus $\langle \beta, \alpha^\vee \rangle = \frac{1}{2}\langle \beta, \gamma^\vee \rangle \in \mathbf{Z}$.

Thus R_1 is a root system in V, and the other assertions are clear.

5. CHAMBERS AND BASES OF ROOT SYSTEMS

For all $\alpha \in \mathrm{R}$, let L_α be the hyperplane of V consisting of the points invariant under s_α. The chambers in V determined by the set of the L_α (Chap. V, § 1, no. 3) are called the *chambers* of R. The bijection $\mathrm{V} \to \mathrm{V}^*$ defined by the scalar product $(x|y)$ takes α to $\frac{2\alpha^\vee}{(\alpha^\vee|\alpha^\vee)}$ for $\alpha \in \mathrm{R}$, hence L_α to $\mathrm{L}_{\alpha^\vee}$, and hence the chambers of R to those of $\mathrm{R}^\vee$. If C is a chamber of R, the corresponding chamber of $R^\vee$ is denoted by $C^\vee$. By Prop. 7 of no. 2, $C^\vee$ depends only on C and not on the choice of $(x|y)$.

THEOREM 2. (i) *The group* W(R) *acts simply-transitively on the set of chambers.*

(ii) *Let* C *be a chamber. Then* $\overline{C}$ *is a fundamental domain for* W(R).

(iii) C *is an open simplicial cone* (Chap. V, § 1, no. 6).

(iv) *Let* $L_1, L_2, \ldots, L_l$ *be the walls of* C. *For all* i, *there exists a unique indivisible root* α_i *such that* $L_i = L_{\alpha_i}$ *and such that* α_i *is on the same side of* L_i *as* C.

(v) *The set* $B(C) = \{\alpha_1, \ldots, \alpha_l\}$ *is a basis of* V.

(vi) C *is the set of* $x \in V$ *such that* $\langle \alpha_i^\vee, x\rangle > 0$ *for all* i *(or, equivalently, the set of* $x \in V$ *such that* $(x|\alpha_i) > 0$ *for all* i*).*

(vii) *Let* S *be the set of the* s_{α_i}. *The pair* (W(R), S) *is a Coxeter system* (Chap. IV, § 1, no. 3).

Assertions (i) and (vii) follow from Chap. V, § 3, no. 2, Th. 1. Assertion (ii) follows from Chap. V, § 3, no. 3, Th. 2. Assertion (iv) is clear. The root α_i is orthogonal to L_i, and $\alpha_i^\vee$ is identified with $2\alpha_i/(\alpha_i|\alpha_i)$. Since W(R) is essential (no. 1, *Remark* 3), assertions (iii), (v) and (vi) follow from Chap. V, § 3, no. 9, Prop. 7.

Remarks. 1) Assertion (vii) shows in particular that W(R) is *generated* by the reflections s_{α_i}.

2) If $x, y \in C$, then $(x|y) > 0$ (Chap. V, § 3, no. 5, Lemma 6), in other words the angle $\widehat{(x,y)}$ is *acute*.

3) Let $m(\alpha,\beta)$ be the order of $s_\alpha s_\beta$ $(\alpha, \beta \in B(C))$. The matrix $(m(\alpha,\beta))$ is identified with the *Coxeter matrix* (Chap. IV, § 1, no. 9) of (W, S). If $\alpha \neq \beta$, Prop. 3 of Chap. V, § 3, no. 4 shows that the angle $\widehat{(\alpha,\beta)}$ is equal to $\pi - \frac{\pi}{m(\alpha,\beta)}$; in particular, this angle is either obtuse or equal to π, and $(\alpha|\beta) \leqslant 0$. By using the list in no. 3, it follows that $m(\alpha,\beta)$ *is equal to* 2, 3, 4 *or* 6.

DEFINITION 2. *A subset* B *of* R *is called a basis of* R *if there exists a chamber* C *of* R *such that* B = B(C). *If* C *is a chamber,* B(C) *is called the basis of* R *defined by* C.

Remarks. 4) Assertion (vi) of Th. 2 shows that the map $C \mapsto B(C)$ is a *bijection* from the set of chambers to the set of bases. Consequently, W(R) acts *simply-transitively* on the set of bases.

5) Let C be a chamber of R, and let B be the corresponding basis. If $\alpha \in B$, put $\varphi(\alpha) = \alpha^\vee$ if $2\alpha \notin R$ and $\varphi(\alpha) = \frac{1}{2}\alpha^\vee$ if $2\alpha \in R$. Then $\varphi(B)$ *is the basis of* $R^\vee$ *defined by* $C^\vee$; this follows from the fact that the walls of $C^\vee$ are the $L_{\alpha^\vee}$, for $\alpha \in B$.

DEFINITION 3. *Let* B *be a basis of* R. *The Cartan matrix of* R *(relative to* B*) is the matrix* $(n(\alpha,\beta))_{\alpha,\beta\in\mathrm{B}}$.

For all $\alpha \in \mathrm{B}$, $n(\alpha,\alpha) = 2$. For $\alpha, \beta \in \mathrm{B}$,

$$n(\alpha,\beta) = 2\frac{(\alpha|\beta)}{(\beta|\beta)} = -2\frac{\| \alpha \|}{\| \beta \|}\cos\frac{\pi}{m(\alpha,\beta)}, \tag{11}$$

where $m(\alpha,\beta)$ denotes as above the order of $s_\alpha s_\beta$. If $\alpha \neq \beta$, $n(\alpha,\beta) = 0$, $-1, -2$ or -3 (cf. no. 3).

Remarks. 6) The Cartan matrix $(n(\alpha,\beta))$ should not be confused with the Coxeter matrix $(m(\alpha,\beta))$. Note in particular that the Cartan matrix is not necessarily symmetric.

7) *Canonical indexing.* If B and B′ are two bases of R, there exists a unique element $w \in \mathrm{W}$ such that $w(\mathrm{B}) = \mathrm{B}'$. We have

$$n(w(\alpha), w(\beta)) = n(\alpha,\beta) \quad\text{and}\quad m(w(\alpha), w(\beta)) = m(\alpha,\beta)$$

for $\alpha, \beta \in \mathrm{B}$. Consequently, the Cartan and Coxeter matrices associated to B can be obtained from those associated to B′ by composition with the bijection

$$\alpha \mapsto w(\alpha)$$

from B to B′.

The Cartan and Coxeter matrices can actually be defined *canonically* in the following way. Let X be the set of pairs (B, α), where B is a basis of R and $\alpha \in \mathrm{B}$. The group W acts in an obvious way on X and each orbit of W on X meets each of the sets $\{\mathrm{B}\} \times \mathrm{B}$ in exactly one point. If I is the set of these orbits, each basis B admits a *canonical indexing* $(\alpha_i)_{i\in\mathrm{I}}$. Moreover, there exists a unique matrix $\mathrm{N} = (n_{ij})$ (resp. $\mathrm{M} = (m_{ij})$), of type $\mathrm{I} \times \mathrm{I}$, such that for any basis B, the Cartan (resp. Coxeter) matrix associated to B can be obtained from N (resp. M) by composing with the canonical indexing of B; it is called the *canonical Cartan matrix* (resp. *Coxeter matrix*) of R.

PROPOSITION 15. *Let* B *be a basis of* R *and* α *an indivisible root. There exist* $\beta \in \mathrm{B}$ *and* $w \in \mathrm{W(R)}$ *such that* $\alpha = w(\beta)$.

Let C be the chamber such that $\mathrm{B} = \mathrm{B(C)}$. The hyperplane L_α is a wall of a chamber C′ of R, and there exists an element of W(R) that transforms C′ to C. We are therefore reduced to the case where L_α is a wall of C. Then α is proportional to an element β of R. Since α and β are indivisible, $\alpha = \pm\beta$. If $\alpha = -\beta$, then $\alpha = s_\beta(\beta)$, hence the proposition.

COROLLARY. *Let* R_1 *and* R_2 *be two reduced root systems in vector spaces* V_1 *and* V_2*, and let* B_1 *and* B_2 *be bases of* R_1 *and* R_2. *Let* $f : \mathrm{B}_1 \to \mathrm{B}_2$ *be a bijection that transforms the Cartan matrix of* R_1 *to that of* R_2. *Then there* *exists an isomorphism* $\mathrm{F} : \mathrm{V}_1 \to \mathrm{V}_2$ *that transforms* R_1 *to* R_2 *and* α *to* $f(\alpha)$ *for all* $\alpha \in \mathrm{B}_1$.

Let F be the isomorphism from V_1 to V_2 that takes α to $f(\alpha)$ for all $\alpha \in \mathrm{B}_1$. Then F transforms s_α to $s_{f(\alpha)}$, hence $\mathrm{W}(\mathrm{R}_1)$ to $\mathrm{W}(\mathrm{R}_2)$ (Th. 2), and hence R_1 to R_2 (Prop. 15).

PROPOSITION 16. *Let* B *be a basis of* R, *and* G *the subgroup of* A(R) *consisting of the elements leaving* B *stable. Then* W(R) *is a normal subgroup of* A(R) *and* A(R) *is the semi-direct product of* G *and* W(R).

If $\alpha \in \mathrm{R}$ and $t \in \mathrm{A}(\mathrm{R})$, then $ts_\alpha t^{-1} = s_{t(\alpha)}$; since W(R) is generated by the s_α, we see that W(R) is a normal subgroup of A(R). By transport of structure, A(R) transforms a basis of R to a basis of R. Since W(R) acts simply-transitively on the set of bases, every element of A(R) can be written uniquely in the form $g_1 g_2$, where $g_1 \in \mathrm{W}(\mathrm{R})$ and $g_2 \in \mathrm{G}$.

Remarks. 8) Let $\mathrm{R}_1, \dots, \mathrm{R}_p$ be root systems in vector spaces $\mathrm{V}_1, \dots, \mathrm{V}_p$, R the direct sum of the R_i in $\mathrm{V} = \prod_i \mathrm{V}_i$, C_i a chamber of R_i, and $\mathrm{B}_i = \mathrm{B}(\mathrm{C}_i)$. It is immediate that $\mathrm{C} = \prod_i \mathrm{C}_i$ is a chamber of R and that $\mathrm{B}(\mathrm{C}) = \bigcup_i \mathrm{B}_i$. It follows from Th. 2 that all the chambers and bases of R are obtained in this way.

6. POSITIVE ROOTS

Let C be a chamber of R, and let $\mathrm{B}(\mathrm{C}) = \{\alpha_1, \dots, \alpha_l\}$ be the corresponding basis of R. The *order relation on* V (resp. V^*) *defined by* C is the order relation campatible with the vector space structure of V (resp. V^*) for which the elements $\geqslant 0$ are the linear combinations of the α_i (resp. the $\alpha_i^{\vee}$) with coefficients $\geqslant 0$. An element that is positive for one of these relations is said to be *positive for* C, or *positive for the basis* B(C). These order relations are also defined by $\mathrm{C}^{\vee}$, as one sees by identifying V with V^* by using a scalar product invariant under W(R). In view of Th. 2, no. 5, an element of V^* is $\geqslant 0$ if and only if its values on C are $\geqslant 0$. An element x of V is $\geqslant 0$ if and only if its values on $\mathrm{C}^{\vee}$ are $\geqslant 0$, or, equivalently, if $(x|y) \geqslant 0$ for all $y \in \mathrm{C}$.

The elements of $\overline{\mathrm{C}}$ are $\geqslant 0$ for C by Lemma 6 of Chap. V, § 3, no. 5. But the set of elements $\geqslant 0$ for C is in general distinct from $\overline{\mathrm{C}}$ (cf. Plate X, Systems $\mathrm{A}_2, \mathrm{B}_2, \mathrm{G}_2$).

THEOREM 3. *Every root is a linear combination with integer coefficients of the same sign of elements of* B(C). *In particular, every root is either positive or negative for* C.

If $\alpha \in \mathrm{R}$, the kernel L_α of α does not meet $\mathrm{C}^{\vee}$, so α is either > 0 on the whole of $\mathrm{C}^{\vee}$ or < 0 on the whole of $\mathrm{C}^{\vee}$, hence the second assertion. It remains to show that α is contained in the *subgroup* P of V generated by B(C); we can assume that α is indivisible. Now the group P is clearly stable under the s_γ, for $\gamma \in \mathrm{B(C)}$, hence also under W(R) by Th. 2. Since α is of the form $w(\beta)$, with $w \in \mathrm{W(R)}$ and $\beta \in \mathrm{B(C)}$ (cf. Prop. 15), we have $\alpha \in \mathrm{P}$. Q.E.D.

Denote by $\mathrm{R}_+(\mathrm{C})$ the set of roots that are positive for C. Thus,

$$\mathrm{R} = \mathrm{R}_+(\mathrm{C}) \cup (-\mathrm{R}_+(\mathrm{C}))$$

is a partition of R.

COROLLARY. *Let γ be a linear combination of roots with integer coefficients, and α an indivisible root. If γ is proportional to α, then $\gamma \in \mathbf{Z}\alpha$.*

By Prop. 15 of no. 5, C can be chosen so that $\alpha \in \mathrm{B(C)}$. By Th. 3,

$$\gamma = \sum_{\beta \in \mathrm{B(C)}} n_\beta \beta \quad \text{with} \quad n_\beta \in \mathbf{Z}.$$

Thus, if γ is proportional to α, then $\gamma = n_\alpha \alpha$, which proves the corollary.

Now let S be the set of reflections s_α for $\alpha \in \mathrm{B(C)}$ and let T be the union of the conjugates of S under W. For $\alpha \in \mathrm{B(C)}$ and $w \in \mathrm{W}$, the element $t = w s_\alpha w^{-1}$ of T is the orthogonal reflection s_β associated to the root $\beta = w(\alpha)$; conversely, for any indivisible root β, there exists an element $w \in \mathrm{W}$ such that $\alpha = w^{-1}(\beta) \in \mathrm{B(C)}$ (Prop. 15) and $s_\beta = w s_\alpha w^{-1} \in \mathrm{T}$. It follows that a *bijection* ψ from the set of indivisible roots to $\{\pm 1\} \times \mathrm{T}$ is obtained by associating to an indivisible root β the pair (ε, s_β), where $\varepsilon = +1$ if β is positive and $\varepsilon = -1$ if β is negative.

On the other hand, (W, S) is a Coxeter system (Th. 2) and the results of Chap. IV, § 1, no. 4 can be applied. We have seen that, if w is an element of W of length (with respect to S) equal to q, there exists a subset T_w of T, with q elements, such that, if $w = s_1 \dots s_q$ with $s_i \in \mathrm{S}$ and if

$$t_i = s_1 \dots s_{i-1} s_i s_{i-1} \dots s_1$$

(for $1 \leqslant i \leqslant q$), then $\mathrm{T}_w = \{t_1, \dots, t_q\}$. Recall that we have also defined in no. 4 of § 1 a number $\eta(w,t)$ (for $w \in \mathrm{W}$ and $t \in \mathrm{T}$) equal to $+1$ if $t \notin \mathrm{T}_w$ and to -1 if $t \in \mathrm{T}_w$. Finally, recall that, if we define a map U_w from the set $\{\pm 1\} \times \mathrm{T}$ to itself by the formula

$$\mathrm{U}_w(\varepsilon, t) = (\varepsilon \eta(w^{-1}, t), w t w^{-1}),$$

the map $w \mapsto \mathrm{U}_w$ is a *homomorphism* from W to the group of permutations of the set $\{\pm 1\} \times \mathrm{T}$ (Chap. IV, § 1, no. 4, Lemma 1).

PROPOSITION 17. *Assume that* R *is reduced and let $w \in \mathrm{W}$ and $\alpha \in \mathrm{R}$.*

(i) *We have $\psi(w(\alpha)) = \mathrm{U}_w(\psi(\alpha))$.*
(ii) *Assume that α is positive. The root $w(\alpha)$ is negative if and only if*

$$\eta(w^{-1}, s_\alpha) = -1,$$

in other words if $s_\alpha \in \mathrm{T}_{w^{-1}}$.

(iii) *We have* $\eta(w, s_\alpha) = -1$ *if and only if the chambers* C *and* $w(\mathrm{C})$ *are on opposite sides of the hyperplane* L_α. *In other words, the set* T_w *consists of the reflections with respect to the walls separating* C *and* $w(\mathrm{C})$.

Let $\beta \in \mathrm{B(C)}$ and put $s = s_\beta$. Clearly $\mathrm{T}_s = \{s\}$ and consequently

$$\mathrm{U}_s(\varepsilon, t) = \begin{cases} (\varepsilon, sts^{-1}) & \text{if } t \neq s \\ (-\varepsilon, s) & \text{if } t = s. \end{cases} \tag{12}$$

On the other hand, let $\rho = \sum_{\gamma \in \mathrm{B(C)}} n_\gamma(\rho)\gamma$ be a positive root. Put

$$s(\rho) = \sum_{\gamma \in \mathrm{B(C)}} n_\gamma(s(\rho))\gamma.$$

If $\rho \neq \beta$, there exists an element $\gamma \in \mathrm{B(C)}$ with $\gamma \neq \beta$, such that $n_\gamma(\rho) > 0$, and we have $n_\gamma(s(\rho)) = n_\gamma(\rho) > 0$ (no. 1, formula (5)). Hence $s(\rho)$ is positive. We deduce immediately that

$$\psi(s(\varepsilon.\rho)) = \begin{cases} (\varepsilon, ss_\rho s^{-1}) & \text{if } \rho \neq \beta \\ (-\varepsilon, s) & \text{if } \rho = \beta. \end{cases} \tag{13}$$

Comparison of (12) and (13) now shows that $\mathrm{U}_s(\psi(\gamma)) = \psi(s(\gamma))$ for all roots γ and all $s \in \mathrm{S}$. Since S generates W, (i) follows.

On the other hand, saying that $w(\alpha)$ is negative is equivalent to saying that

$$\psi(w(\alpha)) = (-1, ws_\alpha w^{-1}),$$

or, by (i), that $\mathrm{U}_w(\psi(\alpha)) = (-1, ws_\alpha w^{-1})$. If in addition α is positive, then $\psi(\alpha) = (+1, s_\alpha)$ and $\mathrm{U}_w(\psi(\alpha)) = (\eta(w^{-1}, s_\alpha), ws_\alpha w^{-1})$, hence (ii).

Finally, by (ii), $\eta(w, s_\alpha) = -1$ if and only if one of the roots α and $w^{-1}(\alpha)$ is positive and the other negative. This is equivalent to saying that $(\alpha|x).(w^{-1}(\alpha)|x) = (\alpha|x).(\alpha|w(x)) < 0$ for all $x \in \mathrm{C}$, hence the first assertion in (iii). The second assertion in (iii) follows immediately.

COROLLARY 1. *Let* $\beta \in \mathrm{B(C)}$. *The reflection* s_β *permutes the positive roots not proportional to* β.

We reduce immediately to the case in which R is reduced. In that case, our assertion follows from (ii) and the fact that $\mathrm{T}_{s_\beta} = s_\beta$.

COROLLARY 2. *Assume that* R *is reduced. Let* $w \in \mathrm{W}$, *let* q *be the length of* w *with respect to* S (Chap. IV, § 1, no. 1), *and let* $w = s_1 \dots s_q$ *be a reduced decomposition of* w. *Let* $\alpha_1, \dots, \alpha_q$ *be the elements of* B(C) *corresponding to* $s_1, \dots, s_q$. *Put*

$$\theta_i = s_q s_{q-1} \dots s_{i+1}(\alpha_i), \qquad i = 1, \dots, q.$$

The roots θ_i *are* > 0, *pairwise distinct,* $w(\theta_i) < 0$, *and every root* $\alpha > 0$ *such that* $w(\alpha) < 0$ *is equal to one of the* θ_i.

Let X be the set of $\alpha > 0$ such that $w(\alpha) < 0$. By (ii),

$$\mathrm{Card}(X) = \mathrm{Card}(T_{w^{-1}}) = l(w^{-1}) = l(w) = q.$$

On the other hand, if $\alpha \in X$ it is clear that there exists $i \in [1, q]$ such that

$$s_{i+1} \dots s_q(\alpha) > 0 \quad \text{and} \quad s_i s_{i+1} \dots s_q(\alpha) < 0.$$

By Cor. 1, this implies that $s_i s_{i+1} \dots s_q(\alpha) = \alpha_i$ and hence that $\alpha = \theta_i$. The set X is thus contained in the set of θ_i. Since $\mathrm{Card}(X) = q$, this is possible only if X is equal to the set of θ_i and these are pairwise distinct. Hence the corollary.

COROLLARY 3. *Assume that* R *is reduced. There exists a unique longest element* w_0 *in* W. *Its length is equal to the number of positive roots and* w_0 *transforms the chamber* C *to* $-$C. *We have* $w_0^2 = 1$ *and* $l(ww_0) = l(w_0) - l(w)$ *for all* $w \in W$.

It is clear that $-$C is a chamber. Hence there exists an element w_0 of W that transforms C to $-$C. Then $w_0(\alpha) < 0$ for all positive roots α and the first two assertions of Cor. 3 are immediate consequences of Cor. 2. We have $w_0^2(C) = C$, so $w_0^2 = 1$. Finally, if $w \in W$, the length $l(w)$ (resp. $l(ww_0)$) is equal, by Prop. 17 (iii), to the number of walls separating C and $w(C)$ (resp. $ww_0(C) = -w(C)$). Since $w(C)$ and $-w(C)$ are on opposite sides of every wall, the sum $l(w) + l(ww_0)$ is equal to the total number of walls, that is to $l(w_0)$.

PROPOSITION 18. *Let* $x \in V$. *The following three properties are equivalent:*

(i) $x \in \overline{C}$;

(ii) $x \geqslant s_\alpha(x)$ *for all* $\alpha \in B(C)$ *(with respect to the order relation defined by* C*)*;

(iii) $x \geqslant w(x)$ *for all* $w \in W$.

Since $s_\alpha(x) = x - \langle x, \alpha\check{}\rangle\alpha$ and since $\overline{C}$ is the set of elements $x \in V$ such that $\langle x, \alpha\check{}\rangle \geqslant 0$ for all $\alpha \in B(C)$, the equivalence of (i) and (ii) is obvious. On the other hand, it is clear that (iii) $\Longrightarrow$ (ii). We show that (i) $\Longrightarrow$ (iii). Let $x \in \overline{C}$, and let $w \in W$. We argue by induction on the length $l(w)$ of w. The case $l(w) = 0$ is trivial. If $l(w) \geqslant 1$, w can be written in the form $w = w's_\alpha$, with $\alpha \in B(C)$ and $l(w') = l(w) - 1$. Then

$$x - w(x) = x - w'(x) + w'(x - s_\alpha(x)).$$

The induction hypothesis shows that $x - w'(x)$ is positive. On the other hand,

$$w'(x - s_\alpha(x)) = w(s_\alpha(x) - x) = -\langle x, \alpha\check{}\rangle w(\alpha).$$

Now $s_\alpha \in T_{w^{-1}}$, and Prop. 17 (ii) shows that $w(\alpha) < 0$. Hence the result.

COROLLARY. *An element* $x \in \mathrm{C}$ *if and only if* $x > w(x)$ *for all* $w \in \mathrm{W}$ *such that* $w \neq 1$.

PROPOSITION 19. *Let* $(\beta_i)_{1 \leqslant i \leqslant n}$ *be a sequnce of positive roots for the chamber* C *such that* $\beta_1 + \beta_2 + \cdots + \beta_n$ *is a root. Then there exists a permutation* $\pi \in \mathfrak{S}_n$ *such that, for all* $i \in \{1, 2, \dots, n\}$, $\beta_{\pi(1)} + \beta_{\pi(2)} + \cdots + \beta_{\pi(\mathrm{i})}$ *is a root.*

We argue by induction on n, the proposition being clear for $n \leqslant 2$. Put $\beta = \beta_1 + \cdots + \beta_n$. Then $\sum_{i=1}^{n} (\beta|\beta_i) = (\beta|\beta) > 0$, so there exists an index k such that $(\beta|\beta_k) > 0$. If $\beta = \beta_k$, then $n = 1$ since $\beta_i > 0$ for all i. Otherwise $\beta - \beta_k$ is a root (no. 3, Cor. of Th. 1); it then suffices to apply the induction hypothesis to $\beta - \beta_k = \sum_{i \neq k} \beta_i$.

COROLLARY 1. *Let* $\alpha \in \mathrm{R}_+(\mathrm{C})$. *Then* $\alpha \in \mathrm{B}(\mathrm{C})$ *if and only if* α *is the sum of two positive roots.*

If α is the sum of two positive roots, Th. 3 shows that $\alpha \in \mathrm{B}(\mathrm{C})$. If $\alpha \notin \mathrm{B}(\mathrm{C})$, Th. 3 shows that $\alpha = \sum_{k=1}^{n} \beta_k$ with $\beta_k \in \mathrm{B}(\mathrm{C})$ for all k and $n \geqslant 2$. Permuting the β_k if necessary, we can assume that $\sum_{k=1}^{n-1}$ is a root (Prop. 19), and hence that α is the sum of the positive roots $\sum_{k=1}^{n-1} \beta_k$ and β_n.

COROLLARY 2. *Let* φ *be a map from* R *to a abelian group* Γ *having the following properties:*

1) $\varphi(-\alpha) = -\varphi(\alpha)$ *for* $\alpha \in \mathrm{R}$;

2) if $\alpha \in \mathrm{R}$, $\beta \in \mathrm{R}$ *are such that* $\alpha + \beta \in \mathrm{R}$, *then* $\varphi(\alpha+\beta) = \varphi(\alpha) + \varphi(\beta)$.

Let Q *be the subgroup of* V *generated by* R. *Then* φ *extends to a homomorphism from* Q *to* Γ.

Let B be a basis of R. Let ψ be the unique homomorphism from Q to Γ that coincides with φ on B. It suffices to show that $\psi(\alpha) = \varphi(\alpha)$ when α is a positive root relative to B. We have $\alpha = \beta_1 + \cdots + \beta_m$ with $\beta_i \in \mathrm{B}$ for all i, and $\beta_1 + \cdots + \beta_h \in \mathrm{R}$ for all h (Prop. 19). We show that $\psi(\alpha) = \varphi(\alpha)$ by induction on m. This is clear if $m = 1$. The induction hypothesis gives

$$\psi(\beta_1 + \cdots + \beta_{m-1}) = \varphi(\beta_1 + \cdots + \beta_{m-1}),$$

and we have $\psi(\beta_m) = \varphi(\beta_m)$, hence $\psi(\alpha) = \varphi(\alpha)$, which proves the corollary.

For any root $\alpha = \sum_{\beta \in \mathrm{B}(\mathrm{C})} n_\beta \beta$ in R, denote by $\mathrm{Y}(\alpha)$ the set of $\beta \in \mathrm{B}(\mathrm{C})$ such that $n_\beta \neq 0$. Moreover, observe that B(C) can be identified with the set of vertices of the *graph* of the Coxeter system formed by W(R) and the s_{α_i} (cf. Chap. IV, § 1, no. 9 and Chap. V, § 3, no. 2).

COROLLARY 3. *a) Let* $\alpha \in \mathrm{R}$. *Then* $\mathrm{Y}(\alpha)$ *is a connected subset of* $\mathrm{B(C)}$ (Chap. IV, Appendix).

b) Let Y *be a non-empty connected subset of* B(C). *Then* $\sum_{\beta \in \mathrm{Y}} \beta$ *belongs to* R.

To prove *a*), we can assume that α is positive. We argue by induction on $\mathrm{Card}(\mathrm{Y}(\alpha))$, the assertion being trivial if $\mathrm{Card}(\mathrm{Y}(\alpha)) = 1$. By Prop. 19, there exists $\beta \in \mathrm{B(C)}$ such that $\alpha - \beta \in \mathrm{R}$. Let p be the largest integer $\geqslant 0$ such that $\gamma = \alpha - p\beta \in \mathrm{R}$. Since $\gamma - \beta \notin \mathrm{R}$ and $\gamma + p\beta \in \mathrm{R}$, $(\gamma|\beta) \neq 0$ (Prop. 9); thus β is linked to at least one element of $\mathrm{Y}(\gamma)$. But $\mathrm{Y}(\alpha) = \mathrm{Y}(\gamma) \cup \{\beta\}$, and $\mathrm{Y}(\gamma)$ is connected by the induction hypothesis. Thus $\mathrm{Y}(\alpha)$ is connected, which proves *a*).

Now let Y be a non-empty connected subset of B(C); we show by induction on Card(Y) that $\sum_{\beta \in \mathrm{Y}} \beta$ is a root. The case in which $\mathrm{Card(Y)} \leqslant 1$ is trivial. Assume that $\mathrm{Card(Y)} \geqslant 2$. Since X is a forest (Chap. V, § 4, no. 8, Prop. 8), Y is a *tree* and has a terminal vertex β (Chap. IV, Appendix). The set $\mathrm{Y} - \{\beta\}$ is connected, and one of its element is linked to β. By the induction hypothesis, $\alpha = \sum_{\gamma \in \mathrm{Y} - \{\beta\}} \gamma \in \mathrm{R}$, and since $(\alpha|\beta) < 0$, it follows that $\alpha + \beta \in \mathrm{R}$ (Th. 1). Q.E.D.

7. CLOSED SETS OF ROOTS

DEFINITION 4. *Let* P *be a subset of* R.

(i) P *is said to be closed if the conditions* $\alpha \in \mathrm{P}, \beta \in \mathrm{P}, \alpha + \beta \in \mathrm{R}$ *imply* $\alpha + \beta \in \mathrm{P}$.

(ii) P *is said to be parabolic if* P *is closed and if* $\mathrm{P} \cup (-\mathrm{P}) = \mathrm{R}$.

(iii) P *is said to be symmetric if* $\mathrm{P} = -\mathrm{P}$.

Lemma 3. Let C *be a chamber of* R *and* P *a closed subset of* R *containing* $\mathrm{R}_+(\mathrm{C})$ *(in the notation of no. 6). Let* $\Sigma = \mathrm{B(C)} \cap (-\mathrm{P})$, *and let* Q *be the set of roots that are linear combinations of elements of* Σ *with non-positive integer coefficient. Then,* $\mathrm{P} = \mathrm{R}_+(\mathrm{C}) \cup \mathrm{Q}$.

It is enough to show that $\mathrm{P} \cap (-\mathrm{R}_+(\mathrm{C})) = \mathrm{Q}$. Let $-\alpha \in \mathrm{Q}$. Then α is the sum of n elements of Σ. We show, by induction on n, that $-\alpha \in \mathrm{P}$. This is clear if $n = 1$. If $n > 1$, then by Prop. 19 of no. 6 we can write $\alpha = \beta + \gamma$ with $\gamma \in \Sigma$ and β the sum of $n - 1$ elements of Σ. By the induction hypothesis, $-\beta \in \mathrm{P}$; since $-\gamma \in \mathrm{P}$ and since P is closed, $-\alpha \in \mathrm{P}$. Thus, $\mathrm{Q} \subseteq \mathrm{P} \cap (-\mathrm{R}_+(\mathrm{C}))$. Conversely, let $-\alpha \in \mathrm{P} \cap (-\mathrm{R}_+(\mathrm{C}))$. Then α is the sum of p elements of B(C). We show, by induction on p, that $-\alpha \in \mathrm{Q}$. This is clear if $p = 1$. If $p > 1$, then by Prop. 19, we can write $\alpha = \beta + \gamma$ with $\gamma \in \mathrm{B(C)}$ and β a root that is the sum of $p - 1$ elements of B(C). Since $-\gamma = \beta + (-\alpha)$ and since P is closed, $-\gamma \in \mathrm{P}$, hence $\gamma \in \Sigma$. Moreover,

$-\beta = \gamma + (-\alpha)$ so $-\beta \in \mathrm{P}$ since P is closed. By the induction hypothesis, $-\beta \in \mathrm{Q}$, so $-\alpha = -\beta - \gamma \in \mathrm{Q}$. Thus, $\mathrm{P} \cap (-\mathrm{R}_+(\mathrm{C})) \subseteq \mathrm{Q}$.

PROPOSITION 20. *Let* P *be a subset of* R. *The following conditions are equivalent:*

(i) P *is parabolic;*

(ii) P *is closed and there exists a chamber* C *of* R *such that* $\mathrm{P} \supseteq \mathrm{R}_+(\mathrm{C})$;

(iii) *there exist a chamber* C *of* R *and a subset* Σ *of* B(C) *such that* P *is the union of* $\mathrm{R}_+(\mathrm{C})$ *and the set* Q *of roots that are linear combinations of elements of* Σ *with non-positive integer coefficients.*

(ii) $\Longrightarrow$ (iii): this follows from Lemma 3.

(iii) $\Longrightarrow$ (i): we adopt the assumptions and notation of (iii). It is clear that $\mathrm{P} \cup (-\mathrm{P}) = \mathrm{R}$. We show that, if $\alpha, \beta \in \mathrm{P}$ are such that $\alpha + \beta \in \mathrm{R}$, then $\alpha + \beta \in \mathrm{P}$. This is obvious if the root $\alpha + \beta$ is positive. Assume that $\alpha + \beta$ is negative. Then $\alpha + \beta = \sum_{\gamma \in \mathrm{B}(\mathrm{C})} n_\gamma \gamma$, with $n_\gamma \leqslant 0$. But the coefficient of every element γ of $\mathrm{B}(\mathrm{C}) - \Sigma$ in α or β is $\geqslant 0$; hence $n_\gamma = 0$ if $\gamma \in \mathrm{B}(\mathrm{C}) - \Sigma$, so $\alpha + \beta \in \mathrm{Q} \subseteq \mathrm{P}$.

(i) $\Longrightarrow$ (ii): assume that P is parabolic. Let C be a chamber such that $\mathrm{Card}(\mathrm{P} \cap \mathrm{R}_+(\mathrm{C}))$ is as large as possible. Let $\alpha \in \mathrm{B}(\mathrm{C})$ and assume that $\alpha \notin \mathrm{P}$, so that $-\alpha \in \mathrm{P}$. For all $\beta \in \mathrm{P} \cap \mathrm{R}_+(\mathrm{C})$, β is not proportional to α (for the hypothesis $\beta = 2\alpha$ would imply that $\alpha = 2\alpha + (-\alpha) \in \mathrm{P}$ since P is closed). Thus $s_\alpha(\beta) \in \mathrm{R}_+(\mathrm{C})$ (no. 6, Cor. 1 of Prop. 17). If we put $\mathrm{C}' = s_\alpha(\mathrm{C})$, then $\beta = s_\alpha(s_\alpha(\beta)) \in s_\alpha(\mathrm{R}_+(\mathrm{C})) = \mathrm{R}_+(\mathrm{C}')$, so $-\alpha \in \mathrm{P} \cap \mathrm{R}_+(\mathrm{C}')$ and hence $\mathrm{Card}(\mathrm{P} \cap \mathrm{R}_+(\mathrm{C}')) > \mathrm{Card}(\mathrm{P} \cap \mathrm{R}_+(\mathrm{C}))$. This is absurd, since $\alpha \notin \mathrm{P}$. Thus $\mathrm{B}(\mathrm{C}) \subseteq \mathrm{P}$, and consequently $\mathrm{R}_+(\mathrm{C}) \subseteq \mathrm{P}$ by Prop. 19 and the fact that P is closed.

COROLLARY 1. *Let* P *be a subset of* R. *The following conditions are equivalent:*

(i) *there exists a chamber* C *such that* $\mathrm{P} = \mathrm{R}_+(\mathrm{C})$;

(ii) P *is closed and* $\{\mathrm{P}, -\mathrm{P}\}$ *is a partition of* R.

The chamber C *such that* $\mathrm{P} = \mathrm{R}_+(\mathrm{C})$ *is then unique.*

If $\mathrm{P} = \mathrm{R}_+(\mathrm{C})$, $\mathrm{C}^\vee$ is the set of $x^* \in \mathrm{V}^*$ such that $\langle x^*, x \rangle > 0$ for all $x \in \mathrm{P}$, hence the uniqueness of C.

COROLLARY 2. *Assume that* V *is equipped with the structure of an ordered vector space such that, for this structure, every root of* R *is either positive or negative. Let* P *be the set of positive roots for this structure. Then there exists a unique chamber* C *of* R *such that* $\mathrm{P} = \mathrm{R}_+(\mathrm{C})$.

Indeed, P satisfies condition (ii) of Cor. 1.

This corollary applies in particular when the order being considered is total, the condition on R then being automatically satisfied. Recall that such an order can be obtained, for example, by choosing a basis $(e_i)_{1\leqslant i\leqslant n}$ of V and taking the *lexicographic* order on V, so $x = \sum_i \xi_i e_i$ is $\geqslant 0$ if all the ξ_i are 0, or if $\xi_i > 0$ for the smallest index i such that $\xi_i \neq 0$.

COROLLARY 3. *A subset* B *of* R *is a basis of* R *if and only if the following conditions are satisfied:*

(i) *the elements of* B *are linearly independent;*

(ii) *every root of* R *is a linear combination of elements of* B *in which the coefficients are either all positive or all negative;*

(iii) *every root of* B *is indivisible.*

We already know that the conditions are necessary (no. 5, Th. 2, and no. 6, Th. 3). Assume that conditions (i), (ii), (iii) are satisfied. Let P be the set of roots that are linear combinations of elements of B with coefficients $\geqslant 0$. Since P satisfies condition (ii) of Cor. 1, there exists a chamber C such that $P = R_+(C)$; let $B' = B(C)$, and let X and X′ be the convex cones generated by B and B′. Then

$$B \subseteq P \subseteq X \quad \text{and} \quad B' \subseteq P \subseteq X',$$

which shows that X and X′ are both generated by P, and hence coincide. But the half-lines generated by the elements of B (resp. by B′) are the extreme generators of X (resp. X′); since such a half-line contains only one indivisible root, $B = B'$.

COROLLARY 4. *Let* B *be a basis of* R, B′ *a subset of* B, V′ *the vector subspace of* V *generated by* B′, *and* $R' = R \cap V'$. *Then* B′ *is a basis of the root system* B′.

This follows immediately from Cor. 3 and the Cor. of Prop. 4.

We call R′ the root system *generated* by B′.

COROLLARY 5. *Let* B *be a basis of* R, $A_1, A_2, \ldots, A_r$ *pairwise orthogonal subsets of* B, *and* $A = A_1 \cup A_2 \cup \cdots \cup A_r$. *Then every root* α *that is a linear combination of elements of* A *is actually a linear combination of elements of one of the* A_i. *In particular, if* R *is irreducible, there is no partition of* B *into pairwise orthogonal subsets.*

Let $E_1, \ldots, E_r, E$ be the vector subspaces of V generated by $A_1, \ldots, A_r, A$, respectively. By Cor. 4, we can assume that $E = V$. Then, by Th. 2 (vii) of no. 5, the E_i are stable under W(R), so R is the union of the $R \cap E_i$ (no. 2, Prop. 5).

COROLLARY 6. *We adopt the hypotheses and notation of Prop. 20. Let* V_1 *be the vector subspace of* V *generated by* Σ. *Then* $P \cap (-P) = Q \cup (-Q) = V_1 \cap R$ *is a root system in* V_1 *with basis* Σ.

We have $P \cap (-P) = (R_+(C) \cup Q) \cap ((-R_+(C)) \cup (-Q)) = Q \cup (-Q)$. Th. 3 proves that $Q \cup (-Q) = V_1 \cap R$. Finally, Σ is a basis of the root system $V_1 \cap R$ by Cor. 4.

PROPOSITION 21. *Let* C *(resp.* C′*) be a chamber of* R, Σ *(resp.* Σ'*) a subset of* B(C) *(resp.* B(C′)*),* Q *(resp.* Q′*) the set of linear combinations of elements of* Σ *(resp.* Σ'*) with negative integer coefficients, and* $P = Q \cup R_+(C)$ *(resp.* $P' = Q' \cup R_+(C')$*). If there exists an element of the Weyl group transforming* P *to* P′*, then there exists an element of the Weyl group transforming* C *to* C′ *and* Σ *to* Σ'.

We reduce immediately to the case $P = P'$. Let V_1 be the vector subspace of V generated by $P \cap (-P)$. Then Σ and Σ' are bases of the root system $R_1 = P \cap (-P)$ in V_1 (Cor. 6 of Prop. 20). Hence there exists $g_1 \in W(R_1)$ such that $g_1(\Sigma) = \Sigma'$. It is clear that g_1 is induced by an element g of W(R) that is a product of the symmetries s_σ with $\sigma \in \Sigma$. Let $\gamma = \sum_{\beta \in B(C)} c_\beta \beta$ be an element of $P - R_1$. Then $c_\beta > 0$ for at least one $\beta \in B(C) - \Sigma$. Moreover, if $\sigma \in \Sigma$, then $s_\sigma(\gamma) - \gamma \in V_1$, so $s_\sigma(\gamma)$ has at least one coordinate > 0 with respect to B(C) (no. 1, formula (5)), hence $s_\sigma(\gamma) \in R_+(C)$ and finally $s_\sigma(\gamma) \in P - R_1$. It follows that $P - R_1$ is stable under the s_σ, $\sigma \in \Sigma$, and hence under g, so $g(P) = P$. We are thus reduced to proving the proposition when $P = P'$ and $\Sigma = \Sigma'$. In this case, $Q = Q'$, so $R_+(C) = P - Q = P - Q'$ $= R_+(C')$, and hence $C = C'$ (Cor. 1 of Prop. 20).

COROLLARY. *Let* P, P′ *be two parabolic subsets of* R *transformed into each other by an element of the Weyl group. If there exists a chamber* C *of* R *such that* $R_+(C) \subseteq P$ *and* $R_+(C) \subseteq P'$*, then* $P = P'$.

This follows from Lemma 3 and Prop. 21 since the only element of W(R) transforming C to C is 1, cf. no. 5, Th. 2.

PROPOSITION 22. *Let* P *be a closed subset of* R *such that* $P \cap (-P) = \varnothing$. *Then there exists a chamber* C *of* R *such that* $P \subseteq R_+(C)$.

1) In view of the Cor. of Th. 1, no. 3, the assumptions $\alpha \in P$, $\beta \in P$, $(\alpha|\beta) < 0$ imply that $\alpha + \beta \in P$.

2) We show that no sum $\alpha_1 + \cdots + \alpha_q$ $(q \geqslant 1)$ of elements of P is zero. We proceed by induction on q. The assertion being clear for $q = 1$, assume that $q \geqslant 2$. If $\alpha_1 + \cdots + \alpha_q = 0$, then

$$-\alpha_1 = \alpha_2 + \cdots + \alpha_q,$$

so $(-\alpha_1|\alpha_2 + \cdots + \alpha_q) > 0$, hence there exists $j \in [2, q]$ such that $(\alpha_1|\alpha_j) < 0$. By part 1) of the proof, $\alpha_1 + \alpha_j \in P$, and the relation $(\alpha_1 + \alpha_j) + \sum_{i \neq 1, j} \alpha_i = 0$ contradicts the induction hypothesis.

3) We show that there exists a non-zero element γ in V such that $(\gamma|\alpha) \geqslant 0$ for all $\alpha \in \mathrm{P}$. If not, the result of 1) would show that an infinite sequence $\alpha_1, \alpha_2, \ldots$ of elements of P could be found such that

$$\beta_i = \alpha_1 + \cdots + \alpha_i \in \mathrm{P}$$

for all i; there would exist two distinct integers i, j such that $\beta_i = \beta_j$, which would contradict the result of 2).

4) To prove the proposition, it is enough (Cor. 2 of Prop. 20) to show that there exists a basis $(\alpha_k)_{1 \leqslant k \leqslant l}$ of V such that, for the lexicographic order defined by this basis, every element of P is > 0. We proceed by induction on $l = \dim \mathrm{V}$, and assume that the proposition is established for all dimensions $< l$. Let $\gamma \in \mathrm{V}$ be such that $\gamma \neq 0$ and $(\gamma|\alpha) \geqslant 0$ for all $\alpha \in \mathrm{P}$ (cf. 3)). Let L be the hyperplane orthogonal to γ, and V' the subspace of L generated by $\mathrm{R} \cap \mathrm{L}$. Then $\mathrm{R} \cap \mathrm{L}$ is a root system in V' and $\mathrm{P} \cap \mathrm{L}$ is closed in $\mathrm{R} \cap \mathrm{L}$. By the induction hypothesis, there exists a basis $(\beta_1, \ldots, \beta_{l'})$ of V' such that the elements of $\mathrm{P} \cap \mathrm{L}$ are > 0 for the lexicographic order defined by this basis. Then any basis of V whose first $l' + 1$ elements are $\gamma, \beta_1, \ldots, \beta_{l'}$ and whose remaining elements are in L has the required property.

PROPOSITION 23. *Let* P *be a subset of* R *and* V_1 *(resp.* Γ*) the vector subspace (resp. the subgroup) of* V *generated by* P*. The following conditions are equivalent:*

(i) P *is closed and symmetric;*
(ii) P *is closed, and* P *is a root system in* V_1*;*
(iii) $\Gamma \cap \mathrm{R} = \mathrm{P}$.

Assume that these conditions are satisfied. For any $\alpha \in \mathrm{P}$*, let* $\alpha_1^{\vee}$ *be the restriction of* $\alpha^{\vee}$ *to* V_1*. Then the map* $\alpha \mapsto \alpha_1^{\vee}$ *is the canonical bijection from the root system* P *to* $\mathrm{P}^{\vee}$*.*

(iii) $\Longrightarrow$ (i): clear.

(i) $\Longrightarrow$ (ii): assume that P is closed and symmetric. First, P satisfies $(\mathrm{RS_I})$ in V_1. We show that, if $\alpha, \beta \in \mathrm{P}$, then $s_\alpha(\beta) \in \mathrm{P}$. This is clear if α and β are proportional. Otherwise, $s_\alpha(\beta) = \beta - n(\beta,\alpha)\alpha$ and $\beta - p\alpha \in \mathrm{R}$ for all rational integers p between 0 and $n(\beta, \alpha)$ (Prop. 9, no. 3), so

$$\beta - n(\beta, \alpha)\alpha \in \mathrm{P}$$

since P is closed and symmetric. Thus, $s_{\alpha,\alpha_1^{\vee}}(\mathrm{P}) = \mathrm{P}$, and P satisfies $(\mathrm{RS_{II}})$. It is clear that P satisfies $(\mathrm{RS_{III}})$. Thus, P satisfies (ii), and we have proved the last assertion of the proposition at the same time.

(ii) $\Longrightarrow$ (iii): we show that, if condition (ii) is satisfied, then $\Gamma \cap \mathrm{R} = \mathrm{P}$. It is clear that $\mathrm{P} \subseteq \Gamma \cap \mathrm{R}$. Let $\beta \in \Gamma \cap \mathrm{R}$. Since $\beta \in \Gamma$ and $\mathrm{P} = -\mathrm{P}$, $\beta = \alpha_1 + \alpha_2 + \cdots + \alpha_k$ with $\alpha_1, \ldots, \alpha_k \in \mathrm{P}$. We shall prove that $\beta \in \mathrm{P}$. This is clear if $k = 1$. We argue by induction on k. We have

$$0 < (\beta|\beta) = \sum_{i=1}^{k} (\beta|\alpha_i),$$

so $(\beta|\alpha_i) > 0$ for some index i. If $\beta = \alpha_i$, then $\beta \in \mathrm{P}$. Otherwise, $\beta - \alpha_i \in \mathrm{R}$ (Cor. of Th. 1, no. 3), so $\beta - \alpha_i \in \mathrm{P}$ by the induction hypothesis, hence $\beta \in \mathrm{P}$ since P is closed.

The conditions of Prop. 23 can be realised with $\mathrm{V}_1 = \mathrm{V}$ and yet $\mathrm{P} \neq \mathrm{R}$. For example, this is the case when R is a system of type G_2 and P a system of type A_2; cf. Plate X.

PROPOSITION 24. *Let* R' *be the intersection of* R *with a vector subspace of* V, *so that* R' *is a root system in the vector subspace* V' *that it generates* (cf. Cor. of Prop. 4, no. 1). *Let* B' *be a basis of* R'.

(i) *There exists a basis of* R *containing* B'.

(ii) R' *is the set of elements of* R *that are linear combinations of elements of* B'.

Assertion (ii) is clear. We prove (i). Let $(\varepsilon_1, \varepsilon_2, \dots, \varepsilon_l)$ be a basis of V such that $\mathrm{B}' = (\varepsilon_{p+1}, \varepsilon_{p+2}, \dots, \varepsilon_l)$. The lexicographic order on V corresponding to this basis defines a chamber C of R. It is clear that every element of B' is minimal in $\mathrm{R}_+(\mathrm{C})$. Thus $\mathrm{B}' \subseteq \mathrm{B}(\mathrm{C})$.

8. HIGHEST ROOT

PROPOSITION 25. *Assume that* R *is irreducible. Let* C *be a chamber of* R, *and let* $\mathrm{B}(\mathrm{C}) = \{\alpha_1, \dots, \alpha_l\}$ *be the corresponding basis.*

(i) *There exists a root* $\tilde{\alpha} = \sum_{i=1}^{l} n_i\alpha_i$ *such that, for every root* $\sum_{i=1}^{l} p_i\alpha_i$, *we have* $n_1 \geqslant p_1, n_2 \geqslant p_2, \dots, n_l \geqslant p_l$. *In other words,* R *has a largest element for the ordering defined by* C.

(ii) *We have* $\tilde{\alpha} \in \overline{\mathrm{C}}$.

(iii) *We have* $(\tilde{\alpha}\,|\,\tilde{\alpha}) \geqslant (\alpha\,|\,\alpha)$ *for every root* α.

(iv) *For every positive root* α' *not proportional to* $\tilde{\alpha}$, *we have* $n(\alpha', \tilde{\alpha}) = 0$ *or* 1.

1) Let $\alpha = \sum_{i=1}^{l} n_i\alpha_i$, $\beta = \sum_{i=1}^{l} p_i\alpha_i$ be two maximal roots for the ordering defined by C. We shall prove that $\alpha = \beta$, which will establish (i).

2) If $(\alpha\,|\alpha_i) < 0$ for some index i, it follows that either $\alpha + \alpha_i \in \mathrm{R}$ or $\alpha = -\alpha_i$ (Cor. of Th. 1, no. 3), and both possibilities are absurd by the maximality of α. Thus $(\alpha\,|\,\alpha_i) \geqslant 0$ for all i.

3) If $\alpha < 0$, then $\alpha < -\alpha$, which is absurd. Thus $n_i \geqslant 0$ for all i. Let J be the set of i such that $n_i > 0$, and J′ the complement of J in $\{1, 2, \dots, l\}$. Then $\mathrm{J} \neq \varnothing$. If J′ were non-empty, there would exist an $i \in \mathrm{J}$ and an $i' \in \mathrm{J}'$ such that $(\alpha_i\,|\,\alpha_{i'}) < 0$ (Cor. 5 of Prop. 20, no. 7); we would then have

$$(\alpha \,|\, \alpha_{i'}) = \sum_{i \in \mathrm{I}} n_i (\alpha_i \,|\, \alpha_{i'}) < 0$$

since $(\alpha_j \,|\, \alpha_k) \leqslant 0$ whenever j and k are distinct, which would contradict 2). Thus $\mathrm{J}' = \varnothing$ and $n_i > 0$ for all i.

4) We have $(\beta \,|\, \alpha_i) \geqslant 0$ for all i by 2). We cannot have $(\beta \,|\, \alpha_i) = 0$ for all i since $\beta \neq 0$. We deduce from 3) that

$$(\beta \,|\, \alpha) = \sum_i n_i (\beta \,|\, \alpha_i) > 0.$$

If $\gamma = \alpha - \beta \in \mathrm{R}$, either $\alpha > \beta$ or $\beta > \alpha$ (Th. 3, no. 6), which contradicts the maximality of α and β. Thus $\alpha = \beta$ (Cor. of Th. 1, no. 3).

5) By 2), $\tilde{\alpha} \in \overline{\mathrm{C}}$. We shall prove that $(\alpha' \,|\, \alpha') \leqslant (\tilde{\alpha} \,|\, \tilde{\alpha})$ for every $\alpha' \in \mathrm{R}$. Since $\overline{\mathrm{C}}$ is a fundamental domain for $\mathrm{W(R)}$, we can assume that $\alpha' \in \overline{\mathrm{C}}$. We have $\tilde{\alpha} - \alpha' \geqslant 0$, so $(\tilde{\alpha} - \alpha' \,|\, x) \geqslant 0$ for all $x \in \overline{\mathrm{C}}$. In particular $(\tilde{\alpha} - \alpha' \,|\, \tilde{\alpha}) \geqslant 0$ and $(\tilde{\alpha} - \alpha' \,|\, \alpha') \geqslant 0$, hence $(\tilde{\alpha} \,|\, \tilde{\alpha}) \geqslant (\alpha' \,|\, \tilde{\alpha}) \geqslant (\alpha' \,|\, \alpha')$. Thus $n(\alpha', \tilde{\alpha})$ must be equal to 0, 1 or -1 if α' is not proportional to $\tilde{\alpha}$. If $\alpha' \geqslant 0$, then $(\tilde{\alpha} \,|\, \alpha') \geqslant 0$ by 2), so $n(\alpha', \tilde{\alpha}) \geqslant 0$ and $n(\alpha', \tilde{\alpha})$ must be either 0 or 1. Q.E.D.

Remark. The root

$$\tilde{\alpha} = \sum_i n_i \alpha_i$$

in (i) is said to be the *highest root* of R (with respect to C). Note that, by (i), we have $n_i \geqslant 1$ for all i.

9. WEIGHTS, RADICAL WEIGHTS

Let $l = \dim \mathrm{V}$. Denote by $\mathrm{Q(R)}$ the subgroup of V generated by R; the elements of $\mathrm{Q(R)}$ are called the *radical weights* of R. By Th. 3 of no. 6, $\mathrm{Q(R)}$ is a discrete subgroup of V of rank l, and every basis of R is a basis of $\mathrm{Q(R)}$.

Similarly, the group $\mathrm{Q(R\check{})}$ is a discrete subgroup of V^* of rank l.

PROPOSITION 26. *The set of* $x \in \mathrm{V}$ *such that* $\langle x, y^* \rangle \in \mathbf{Z}$ *for all* $y^* \in \mathrm{Q(R\check{})}$ *(or, equivalently, for all* $y^* \in \mathrm{R\check{}}$*) is a discrete subgroup* G *of* V *containing* $\mathrm{Q(R)}$. *If* B' *is a basis of* $\mathrm{R\check{}}$, *the basis of* V *dual to* B' *is a basis of* G.

Let $x \in \mathrm{V}$. The following three properties are equivalent:

(i) $\langle x, y^* \rangle \in \mathbf{Z}$ for all $y^* \in \mathrm{Q(R\check{})}$;
(ii) $\langle x, y^* \rangle \in \mathbf{Z}$ for all $y^* \in \mathrm{B}'$;
(iii) the coordinates of x with respect to the dual basis of B' are in $\mathbf{Z}$.

We deduce from this that the basis dual to B' is a basis of G. On the other hand, $(\mathrm{RS_{III}})$ proves that $\mathrm{R} \subseteq \mathrm{G}$, so $\mathrm{Q(R)} \subseteq \mathrm{G}$.

The group G of Prop. 26 is denoted by $\mathrm{P(R)}$, and its elements are called the *weights* of R. We can also consider the group $\mathrm{P(R\check{})}$ of weights of $\mathrm{R\check{}}$.

By *Algebra*, Chap. VII, 2nd edn., § 4, no. 8,

$$\mathrm{P(R)/Q(R)}, \quad \mathrm{P(R^{\check{}})/Q(R^{\check{}})}$$

are finite groups in duality over $\mathbf{Q}/\mathbf{Z}$, and hence are isomorphic. The common order of these two groups is called the *connection index* of R (or of $R^{\check{}}$).

If R is a direct sum of root systems R_i, the group Q(R) (resp. P(R)) is identified canonically with the direct sum of the $Q(R_i)$ (resp. $P(R_i)$).

PROPOSITION 27. *Let* R_1 *be a subset of* R, Q_1 *the subgroup of* Q(R) *generated by* R_1, *and* W_1 *the subgroup of* W(R) *generated by the* s_α $(\alpha \in R_1)$. *If* $p \in P(R)$ *and* $w \in W_1$, *then* $p - w(p) \in Q_1$.

If $w = s_\alpha$ with $\alpha \in R_1$, then

$$p - w(p) = \langle p, \alpha^{\check{}} \rangle \alpha \in \mathbf{Z}\alpha \subseteq Q_1.$$

If $w = s_{\alpha_1} s_{\alpha_2} \ldots s_{\alpha_r}$, with $\alpha_1, \ldots, \alpha_r \in R_1$, it is still true that $p - w(p) \in Q_1$, as we see by induction on r.

The group A(R) leaves P(R) and Q(R) invariant, and hence acts on the quotient P(R)/Q(R). By Prop. 27, the group W(R) acts trivially on P(R)/Q(R). Passing to the quotient, we see that *the quotient group* A(R)/W(R) (cf. Prop. 16, no. 5) *acts canonically on* P(R)/Q(R).

10. FUNDAMENTAL WEIGHTS, DOMINANT WEIGHTS

Assume that R is *reduced*. Let C be a chamber of R, and let B be the corresponding basis of R. Since R is reduced, $B^{\check{}} = \{\alpha^{\check{}}\}_{\alpha \in B}$ is a basis of $R^{\check{}}$. The *dual basis* $(\varpi_\alpha)_{\alpha \in B}$ of $B^{\check{}}$ is thus a basis of the group of weights; its elements are called the *fundamental weights* (relative to B, or to C); if the elements of B are denoted by $(\alpha_1, \ldots, \alpha_l)$, the corresponding fundamental weights are denoted by $(\varpi_1, \ldots, \varpi_l)$.

Let $x \in V$. Then, $x \in C$ if and only if $\langle x, \alpha^{\check{}} \rangle > 0$ for all $\alpha \in B$. It follows that C is the set of linear combinations of the ϖ_α with coefficients $\geqslant 0$.

The entries $n(\alpha, \beta) = \langle \alpha, \beta^{\check{}} \rangle$ of the Cartan matrix are, for fixed α, the coordinates of α with respect to the basis $(\varpi_\beta)_{\beta \in B}$:

$$\alpha = \sum_{\beta \in B} n(\alpha, \beta) \varpi_\beta. \tag{14}$$

The Cartan matrix is thus the transpose of the matrix of the canonical injection

$$Q(R) \to P(R)$$

with respect to the bases B and $(\varpi_\alpha)_{\alpha \in B}$ of the $\mathbf{Z}$-modules Q(R) and P(R).

A weight ϖ is said to be *dominant* if it belongs to $\overline{C}$, in other words if its coordinates with respect to $(\varpi_\alpha)_{\alpha \in B}$ are integers $\geqslant 0$, or equivalently if $g(\varpi) \leqslant \varpi$ for all $g \in W(R)$ (no. 6, Prop. 18). Since $\overline{C}$ is a fundamental domain for W(R) (Th. 2), there exists, for any weight ϖ, a unique weight ϖ' such that ϖ' is a transform of ϖ by W(R).

We have

$$\langle\varpi_\alpha, \beta\check{}\rangle = (\varpi_\alpha \,|\, \frac{2\beta}{(\beta\,|\,\beta)}) = \delta_{\alpha\beta}$$

for $\alpha, \beta \in \mathrm{B}$ ($\delta_{\alpha\beta}$ denoting the Kronecker symbol), hence

$$s_\beta(\varpi_\alpha) = \varpi_\alpha - \delta_{\alpha\beta}\beta \quad \text{and} \quad (\varpi_\alpha \,|\, \beta) = \frac{1}{2}(\beta\,|\,\beta)\delta_{\alpha\beta}.$$

In other words, ϖ_α *is orthogonal to* β *for* $\beta \neq \alpha$, *and its orthogonal projection onto* $\mathbf{R}\alpha$ *is* $\frac{1}{2}\alpha$. Since $\varpi_\alpha \in \overline{\mathrm{C}}$, $(\varpi_\alpha \,|\, \varpi_\beta) \geqslant 0$ for $\alpha, \beta \in \mathrm{B}$, i.e. the angle $(\widehat{\varpi_\alpha, \varpi_\beta})$ is acute or a right angle. The dominant weights are the $\varpi \in \mathrm{V}$ such that $2(\varpi \,|\, \alpha)/(\alpha \,|\, \alpha)$ is an integer $\geqslant 0$ for all $\alpha \in \mathrm{B}$.

PROPOSITION 28. *Let* B *be a basis of* R, B′ *a subset of* B, V′ *the vector subspace of* V *generated by* B′, $\mathrm{R}' = \mathrm{R} \cap \mathrm{V}'$ *(which is a root system in* V′*),* $\mathrm{R}'\check{}$ *the inverse root system (which is identified with the canonical image of* R′ *in* $\mathrm{R}\check{}$*),* V_1 *the orthogonal complement of* $\mathrm{R}'\check{}$ *in* V*, and* p *the projection of* V *onto* V′ *parallel to* V_1*. Then,* $\mathrm{Q}(\mathrm{R}') = \mathrm{Q}(\mathrm{R}) \cap \mathrm{V}'$, $\mathrm{P}(\mathrm{R}') = p(\mathrm{P}(\mathrm{R}))$*. The set of dominant weights of* R′ *is the image under* p *of the set of dominant weights of* R.

Indeed, Q(R) is the subgroup of V with basis B, Q(R′) is the subgroup of V′ with basis B′ (no. 7, Cor. 4 of Prop. 20) from which $\mathrm{Q}(\mathrm{R}') = \mathrm{Q}(\mathrm{R}) \cap \mathrm{V}'$ is immediate. If $\varpi \in \mathrm{P}(\mathrm{R})$ and $\alpha \in \mathrm{R}'$, $\langle p(\varpi), \alpha\check{}\rangle = \langle \varpi, \alpha\check{}\rangle \in \mathbf{Z}$, so $p(\varpi) \in \mathrm{P}(\mathrm{R}')$, and hence $p(\mathrm{P}(\mathrm{R})) \subseteq \mathrm{P}(\mathrm{R}')$. If $\varpi' \in \mathrm{P}(\mathrm{R}')$, ϖ' extends to a linear form ϖ on V^* vanishing on $(\mathrm{B}-\mathrm{B}')\check{}$; we have $\langle \varpi, \alpha\check{}\rangle \in \mathbf{Z}$ for all $\alpha \in \mathrm{B}$, so $\varpi \in \mathrm{P}(\mathrm{R})$, and $\varpi' = p(\varpi)$; hence $\mathrm{P}(\mathrm{R}') \subseteq p(\mathrm{P}(\mathrm{R}))$. Thus $\mathrm{P}(\mathrm{R}') = p(\mathrm{P}(\mathrm{R}))$, and the assertion about dominant weights is proved in the same way.

PROPOSITION 29. *Let* ρ *be half the sum of the roots* > 0.

(i) $\rho = \sum_{\alpha \in \mathrm{B}} \varpi_\alpha$*; this is an element of* C.

(ii) $s_\alpha(\rho) = \rho - \alpha$ *for all* $\alpha \in \mathrm{B}$.

(iii) $(2\rho \,|\, \alpha) = (\alpha \,|\, \alpha)$ *for all* $\alpha \in \mathrm{B}$.

Since R is reduced, $s_\alpha(\mathrm{R}_+(\mathrm{C}) - \{\alpha\}) = \mathrm{R}_+(\mathrm{C}) - \{\alpha\}$ and $s_\alpha(\alpha) = -\alpha$ for $\alpha \in \mathrm{B}$ (no. 6, Cor. 1 of Prop. 17), so $s_\alpha(2\rho) = 2\rho - 2\alpha$. Since $s_\alpha(\rho) = \rho - \langle \rho, \alpha\check{}\rangle$, we see that

$$\langle \rho, \alpha\check{}\rangle = 1 = \langle \sum_{\beta \in \mathrm{B}} \varpi_\beta, \alpha\check{}\rangle.$$

Hence, $\rho = \sum_\beta \varpi_\beta$, and consequently $\rho \in \mathrm{C}$. Finally, (iii) is equivalent to $\langle \rho, \alpha\check{}\rangle = 1$.

COROLLARY. *Let σ be half the sum of the elements > 0 of* $R^\vee$ *(for* $B^\vee$*). For all $\alpha \in V$, the sum of the coordinates of α with respect to the basis* B *is $\langle \alpha, \sigma \rangle$. If $\alpha \in R$, this sum is equal to $\frac{1}{2} \sum_{\beta \in R_+(C)} n(\alpha, \beta)$.*

Interchanging the roles of R and $R^\vee$ above, we have $\langle \alpha, \sigma \rangle = 1$ for all $\alpha \in B$, hence the corollary.

11. COXETER TRANSFORMATION

Let C be a chamber of R, let $\{\alpha_1, \dots, \alpha_l\}$ be the corresponding basis of R, and let $c = s_{\alpha_1} \dots s_{\alpha_l}$. The element c of W is called the *Coxeter transformation* of W defined by C and the bijection $i \mapsto \alpha_i$ (Chap. V, § 6, no. 1). Its order h is called the *Coxeter number* of W (or of R).

PROPOSITION 30. *Assume that* R *is irreducible. Let m be an integer between* 1 *and $h - 1$ and prime to h. Then $\exp(\frac{2i\pi m}{h})$ is an eigenvalue of c of multiplicity* 1.

In particular, m is an *exponent* of W, cf. Chap. V, § 6, no. 2.

We first prove a lemma:

Lemma 4. For all $w \in W$, the characteristic polynomial of w has integer coefficients.

We know (no. 6, Th. 3) that $\{\alpha_1, \dots, \alpha_l\}$ is a basis of the subgroup Q(R) of V generated by R. Since w leaves Q(R) stable, its matrix with respect to $\{\alpha_1, \dots, \alpha_l\}$ has integer entries; hence its characteristic polynomial has integer coefficients.

Let P be the characteristic polynomial of c. The above lemma shows that the coefficients of P are integers. By Chap. V, § 6, no. 2, Cor. 2 of Prop. 3, the primitive hth root of unity $z = \exp(\frac{2i\pi}{h})$ is a simple root of P. Every *conjugate* of z over $\mathbf{Q}$ is therefore also a simple root of P. But we know (*Algebra*, Chap. V) that the primitive hth roots of unity are conjugate over $\mathbf{Q}$. They are thus all simple roots of P, which proves the proposition.

PROPOSITION 31. *Assume that* R *is irreducible and reduced, and let $\beta = n_1\alpha_1 + \dots + n_l\alpha_l$ be the highest root of* R (cf. no. 8). *Then $n_1 + \dots + n_l = h - 1$.*

Let R_+ be the set of positive roots relative to C. Then (no. 10, Cor. of Prop. 29):

$$n_1 + \dots + n_l = \frac{1}{2} \sum_{\alpha \in R_+} n(\beta, \alpha)$$

$$= 1 + \frac{1}{2} \sum_{\alpha \in R_+, \alpha \neq \beta} n(\beta, \alpha) = 1 + \sum_{\alpha \in R_+, \alpha \neq \beta} \frac{(\alpha \mid \beta)}{(\alpha \mid \alpha)}.$$

By no. 8, Prop. 25 (iv), for all $\alpha \in R_+$ and $\alpha \neq \beta$, $n(\alpha, \beta) = 0$ or 1, so $n(\alpha, \beta)^2 = n(\alpha, \beta)$, that is $\frac{4(\alpha \mid \beta)^2}{(\beta \mid \beta)^2} = \frac{2(\alpha \mid \beta)}{(\beta \mid \beta)}$. Hence:

$$n_1 + \cdots + n_l + 1 = 2 + 2 \sum_{\alpha \in \mathrm{R}_+, \alpha \neq \beta} \frac{(\alpha \,|\, \beta)^2}{(\alpha \,|\, \alpha)(\beta \,|\, \beta)}$$
$$= 2 \sum_{\alpha \in \mathrm{R}_+} \frac{(\alpha \,|\, \beta)^2}{(\alpha \,|\, \alpha)(\beta \,|\, \beta)} = (\beta \,|\, \beta)^{-1} \sum_{\alpha \in \mathrm{R}} (\frac{\alpha}{\| \alpha \|} \,|\, \beta)^2.$$

By Chap. V, § 6, no. 2, Cor. of Th. 1,

$$\sum_{\alpha \in \mathrm{R}} (\frac{\alpha}{\| \alpha \|} \,|\, \beta)^2 = h(\beta \,|\, \beta)$$

so $n_1 + \cdots + n_l + 1 = h$.

PROPOSITION 32. *Assume that* R *is irreducible, and that all roots have the same length. Let* $\alpha \in \mathrm{R}$. *The number of elements of* R *not orthogonal to* α *is* $4h - 6$.

Let R′ be the set of roots not proportional to and not orthogonal to α. By Chap. V, § 6, no. 2, Cor. of Th. 1,

$$(\alpha \,|\, \alpha)^2 + (\alpha \,|\, -\alpha)^2 + \sum_{\beta \in \mathrm{R}'} (\alpha \,|\, \beta)^2 = h(\alpha \,|\, \alpha)^2,$$

that is

$$\sum_{\beta \in \mathrm{R}'} (\alpha \,|\, \beta)^2 = (h-2)(\alpha \,|\, \alpha)^2.$$

If $\beta \in \mathrm{R}'$, then $(\alpha \,|\, \beta) = \pm \frac{1}{2}(\alpha \,|\, \alpha)$ by the list in no. 3. Hence

$$\frac{1}{4} \mathrm{Card}\, \mathrm{R}' = h - 2, \quad \mathrm{Card}\, \mathrm{R}' = 4h - 8,$$

and the number of roots not orthogonal to α is $\mathrm{Card}\, \mathrm{R}' + 2 = 4h - 6$.

PROPOSITION 33. *Assume that* R *is irreducible and reduced. Put* $s_{\alpha_i} = s_i$, *and let* Γ *be the subgroup of* W *generated by* $c = s_1 \ldots s_l$.

(i) *Let* $\theta_i = s_l s_{l-1} \ldots s_{i+1}(\alpha_i)$ $(i = 1, \ldots, l)$. *Then,* $\theta_i > 0, c(\theta_i) < 0$.

(ii) *If* α *is a root* > 0 *such that* $c(\alpha) < 0$, *then* α *is equal to one of the* θ_i.

(iii) *The family* $(\theta_i)_{1 \leqslant i \leqslant l}$ *is a basis of* Q(R).

(iv) *Let* Ω_i *be the orbit of* θ_i *under* Γ. *The sets* Ω_i *are pairwise disjoint, they are all the orbits of* Γ *on* R, *and each has* h *elements.*

Observe first that $(s_1, \ldots, s_l)$ is a *reduced decomposition* of c (Chap. IV, § 1, no. 1) with respect to the set S of the s_i. Indeed, otherwise there would exist a subset $\mathrm{X} = \mathrm{S} - \{j\}$ of $l - 1$ elements of S such that $c \in \mathrm{W_X}$, which would contradict Cor. 2 of Prop. 7 of Chap. IV, § 1, no. 8.

Applying Cor. 2 of Prop. 17 of no. 6 to c gives assertions (i) and (ii).

Let Q_i be the subgroup of Q(R) generated by the α_j, $j > i$. It is immediate that Q_i is stable under the s_j, $j > i$, and that $s_j(\alpha_i) = \alpha_i$ mod. Q_i for $j > i$. Hence:

$$\theta_i = s_l \ldots s_{i+1}(\alpha_i) = \alpha_i \text{ mod. } \mathrm{Q}_i.$$

In other words, there exist integers c_{ij} such that

$$\theta_i = \alpha_i + \sum_{j>i} c_{ij}\alpha_j.$$

Part (iii) follows immediately.

Finally, let α be a root. The element $\sum_{k=0}^{h-1} c^k(\alpha)$ is invariant under c, and hence zero (Chap. V, § 6, no. 2). The $c^k(\alpha)$ cannot therefore all have the same sign, and there exists a k such that $c^k(\alpha) > 0$ and $c^{k+1}(\alpha) < 0$. By (ii), $c^k(\alpha)$ is one of the θ_i. Thus every orbit of Γ on R is one of the Ω_i. Extend $(x \mid y)$ to a hermitian form on $\mathrm{V} \otimes \mathbf{C}$. Each orbit of Γ in R has at most h elements, and there are at most l distinct orbits, by the above remarks. Now (Chap. V, § 6, no. 2, Theorem 2, ii)), the cardinal of R is equal to hl, which immediately implies (iv).

12. CANONICAL BILINEAR FORM

We have seen (no. 1, Prop. 3) that the symmetric bilinear form

$$(x, y) \mapsto \mathrm{B_R}(x, y) = \sum_{\alpha \in \mathrm{R}} \langle \alpha\check{}, x\rangle\langle \alpha\check{}, y\rangle$$

on V is non-degenerate and invariant under A(R). Interchanging the roles of R and R$\check{}$, it follows that the symmetric bilinear form $(x^*, y^*) \mapsto \mathrm{B_{R\check{}}}(x^*, y^*) = \sum_{\alpha \in \mathrm{R}} \langle \alpha, x^*\rangle\langle \alpha, y^*\rangle$ on V^* is non-degenerate and invariant under A(R).

The inverse form of $\mathrm{B_{R\check{}}}$ (resp. $\mathrm{B_R}$) on V (resp. V^*) will be called the *canonical bilinear form* on V (resp. V^*) and denoted by Φ_R (resp. $\Phi_{\mathrm{R}\check{}}$). It is non-degenerate and invariant under A(R). Let σ be the isomorphism from V to V^* defined by $\mathrm{B_{R\check{}}}$. Then, for $x \in \mathrm{V}$ and $y \in \mathrm{V}$:

$$\Phi_\mathrm{R}(x, y) = \mathrm{B_{R\check{}}}(\sigma(x), \sigma(y)) = \sum_{\alpha \in \mathrm{R}} \langle \alpha, \sigma(x)\rangle\langle \alpha, \sigma(y)\rangle.$$

But $\langle \alpha, \sigma(x)\rangle = \mathrm{B_{R\check{}}}(\sigma(\alpha), \sigma(x)) = \Phi_\mathrm{R}(\alpha, x)$. Hence,

$$\Phi_\mathrm{R}(x, y) = \sum_{\alpha \in \mathrm{R}} \Phi_\mathrm{R}(\alpha, x)\Phi(\alpha, y). \tag{16}$$

In view of Prop. 7 of no. 2, Φ_R is the only non-zero symmetric bilinear form invariant under W(R) which satisfies the identity (16).

For $\beta \in \mathrm{R}$, (16) gives

$$\Phi_\mathrm{R}(\beta, \beta) = \sum_{\alpha \in \mathrm{R}} \Phi_\mathrm{R}(\alpha, \beta)^2 = \frac{1}{4}\Phi_\mathrm{R}(\beta, \beta)^2 \sum_{\alpha \in \mathrm{R}} n(\alpha, \beta)^2,$$

hence

$$4\Phi_\mathrm{R}(\beta, \beta)^{-1} = \sum_{\alpha \in \mathrm{R}} n(\alpha, \beta)^2. \tag{17}$$

Moreover, by Lemma 2 of no. 1, we have, for $x, y \in \mathrm{V}$:

$$\begin{aligned}\mathrm{B_R}(x,y) &= \sum_{\alpha\in\mathrm{R}} \Phi_\mathrm{R}\left(\frac{2\alpha}{\Phi_\mathrm{R}(\alpha,\alpha)},x\right)\left(\frac{2\alpha}{\Phi_\mathrm{R}(\alpha,\alpha)},y\right)\\ &= 4\sum_{\alpha\in\mathrm{R}} \Phi_\mathrm{R}(\alpha,x)\Phi_\mathrm{R}(\alpha,y)\Phi_\mathrm{R}(\alpha,\alpha)^{-2}.\end{aligned}$$

It follows that, if R is *irreducible*, there exists a constant $\gamma(\mathrm{R}) > 0$ such that

$$\sum_{\alpha\in\mathrm{R}} \Phi_\mathrm{R}(\alpha,x)\Phi_\mathrm{R}(\alpha,y)\Phi_\mathrm{R}(\alpha,\alpha)^{-2} = \gamma(\mathrm{R})\Phi_\mathrm{R}(x,y). \tag{18}$$

By the definition of $\gamma(\mathrm{R})$, we have $\mathrm{B_R}(x,y) = 4\gamma(\mathrm{R})\Phi_\mathrm{R}(x,y)$, so

$$\Phi_{\mathrm{R}^\vee}(x^*,y^*) = (4\gamma(\mathrm{R}))^{-1}\mathrm{B}_{\mathrm{R}^\vee}(x^*,y^*)$$

for $x^*, y^* \in \mathrm{V}^*$. This proves that $\gamma(\mathrm{R}) = \gamma(\mathrm{R}^\vee)$. On the other hand, for $\beta\in\mathrm{R}$,

$$\begin{aligned}\Phi_{\mathrm{R}^\vee}(\beta^\vee,\beta^\vee) &= (4\gamma(\mathrm{R}))^{-1}\sum_{\alpha\in\mathrm{R}}\langle\beta^\vee,\alpha\rangle^2\\ &= \gamma(\mathrm{R})^{-1}\sum_{\alpha\in\mathrm{R}}\frac{\Phi_\mathrm{R}(\alpha,\beta)^2}{\Phi_\mathrm{R}(\beta,\beta)^2}\end{aligned}$$

so, by (16),

$$\Phi_{\mathrm{R}^\vee}(\beta^\vee,\beta^\vee) = \gamma(\mathrm{R})^{-1}\Phi_\mathrm{R}(\beta,\beta)^{-2}\Phi_\mathrm{R}(\beta,\beta)$$

or finally

$$\Phi_\mathrm{R}(\beta,\beta)\Phi_{\mathrm{R}^\vee}(\beta^\vee,\beta^\vee) = \gamma(\mathrm{R})^{-1}. \tag{19}$$

Further, if all the roots of R have the same length λ for Φ_R, (16) and (18) show that

$$\gamma(\mathrm{R}) = \lambda^{-4}. \tag{20}$$

Moreover, if h is the Coxeter number of W, the Cor. of Th. 1 of Chap. V, § 6, no. 2 shows that:

$$h\Phi_\mathrm{R}(x,x) = \sum_{\alpha\in\mathrm{R}}\left(x,\frac{\alpha}{\lambda}\right)^2 \quad \text{for all } x\in\mathrm{V}.$$

Comparing with (16), we deduce that

$$\lambda = h^{-1/2} \quad\text{or}\quad \gamma(\mathrm{R}) = h^2. \tag{21}$$

Finally, formula (19) shows that the roots of $\mathrm{R}^\vee$ have length λ for $\Phi_{\mathrm{R}^\vee}$.

§ 2. AFFINE WEYL GROUP

In this paragraph (except in no. 5), we denote by R a reduced root system in a real vector space V. We denote by W the Weyl group of R; we identify it with a group of automorphisms of the dual V^* of V (§ 1, no. 1), and we provide V^* with a scalar product invariant under W. Let E be the affine space underlying V^*; for $v\in\mathrm{V}^*$, we denote by $t(v)$ the translation of E by the vector v. Finally, we denote by P (resp. Q) the group of translations $t(v)$ whose vector v belongs to the group of weights $\mathrm{P}(\mathrm{R}^\vee)$ (resp. to the group of radical weights $\mathrm{Q}(\mathrm{R}^\vee)$) of the inverse root system $\mathrm{R}^\vee$ of R.

1. AFFINE WEYL GROUP

For $\alpha \in \mathrm{R}$ and $k \in \mathbf{Z}$, let $\mathrm{L}_{\alpha,k}$ be the hyperplane of E defined by:

$$\mathrm{L}_{\alpha,k} = \{x \in \mathrm{E} \,|\, \langle \alpha, x \rangle = k\}$$

and let $s_{\alpha,k}$ be the orthogonal reflection with respect to $\mathrm{L}_{\alpha,k}$. Then

$$s_{\alpha,k}(x) = x - (\langle \alpha, x \rangle - k)\alpha\check{} = s_{\alpha,0}(x) + k\alpha\check{}$$

for all $x \in \mathrm{E}$. In other words,

$$s_{\alpha,k} = t(k\alpha\check{}) \circ s_\alpha \tag{1}$$

where s_α is the orthogonal reflection with respect to the hyperplane $\mathrm{L}_\alpha = \mathrm{L}_{\alpha,0}$, i.e. the reflection associated to the root α.

Formula (1) shows that $s_{\alpha,k}$ does not depend on the choice of scalar product.

DEFINITION 1. *The group of affine transformations of* E *generated by the reflections* $s_{\alpha,k}$ *for* $\alpha \in \mathrm{R}$ *and* $k \in \mathbf{Z}$ *is called the affine Weyl group of the root system* R *and denoted by* $\mathrm{W}_a(\mathrm{R})$ *(or simply by* W_a*).*

PROPOSITION 1. *The group* W_a *is the semi-direct product of* W *by* Q.

Since W is generated by the reflections s_α, it is contained in W_a. On the other hand, $t(\alpha\check{}) = s_{\alpha,1} \circ s_\alpha$ if $\alpha \in \mathrm{R}$, which shows that $\mathrm{Q} \subseteq \mathrm{W}_a$.

Since W leaves $\mathrm{Q}(\mathrm{R}\check{})$ stable (§ 1, no. 9), the group G of affine transformations generated by W and Q is the semi-direct product of W by Q. Now $\mathrm{G} \subseteq \mathrm{W}_a$ from above and $s_{\alpha,k} \in \mathrm{G}$ for all $\alpha \in \mathrm{R}$ and $k \in \mathbf{Z}$ by (1). It follows that $\mathrm{W}_a = \mathrm{G}$.

PROPOSITION 2. *The group* W_a*, with the discrete topology, acts properly on* E *and permutes the hyperplanes* $\mathrm{L}_{\alpha,k}$ *(for* $\alpha \in \mathrm{R}$ *and* $k \in \mathbf{Z}$*).*

Since $\mathrm{Q}(\mathrm{R}\check{})$ is a discrete subgroup of V^*, the group Q acts properly on E. Hence, so does $\mathrm{W}_a = \mathrm{W.Q}$, since W is finite. Moreover, for $\alpha, \beta \in \mathrm{R}$ and $k \in \mathbf{Z}$:

$$s_\beta(\mathrm{L}_{\alpha,k}) = \mathrm{L}_{\gamma,k} \quad \text{with} \quad \gamma = s_\beta(\alpha) \in \mathrm{R},$$
$$t(\beta\check{})(\mathrm{L}_{\alpha,k}) = \mathrm{L}_{\alpha,k+n(\alpha,\beta)},$$

where $n(\alpha,\beta) = \langle \beta\check{}, \alpha \rangle$ is an integer, hence the second assertion.

We can thus apply the results of Chapter V, § 3 to W_a acting on E. To avoid any confusion with the chambers of the Weyl group W in V^*, we shall call the chambers determined by the system of hyperplanes $\mathrm{L}_{\alpha,k}$ (for $\alpha \in \mathrm{R}$ and $k \in \mathbf{Z}$) in E *alcoves. The group* W_a *thus acts simply transitively on the set of alcoves and the closure of an alcove is a fundamental domain for* W_a *acting on* E (Chap. V, § 3, no. 2, Th. 1 and no. 3, Th. 2). It is clear that the Weyl group W is identified with the canonical image $\mathrm{U}(\mathrm{W}_a)$ of W_a in the orthogonal group of V* (cf. Chap. V, § 3, no. 6). It follows that W_a is *essential* (Chap. V, § 3, no. 7) and that W_a is *irreducible* if and only if the root system R is (§ 1, no. 2, Cor. of Prop. 5). If R is irreducible, every alcove is an open simplex (Chap. V, § 3, no. 9, Prop. 8). In the general case, the canonical product decomposition of the affine space E (Chap. V, § 3, no. 8) corresponds to the decomposition of R into irreducible components. In particular, the alcoves are products of open simplexes.

Note also that the Cor. of Th. 1 of Chap. V, § 3, no. 2 shows that the $s_{\alpha,k}$ are the only reflections in W_a.

2. WEIGHTS AND SPECIAL WEIGHTS

PROPOSITION 3. *The special points* (Chap. V, § 3, no. 10, Def. 1) *of* W_a *are the weights of* $R^\vee$.

Let $x_0 \in E$ and let $\alpha \in R$. The hyperplane L parallel to $\operatorname{Ker}\alpha$ and passing through x_0 has equation $\langle\alpha, x\rangle = \langle\alpha, x_0\rangle$. To be equal to some $L_{\beta,k}$, it is necessary on the one hand that α and β are proportional, and so, since R is reduced, that $\beta = \pm\alpha$, and on the other hand that $\langle\alpha, x_0\rangle$ is an integer. It follows immediately that x_0 is a special point of W_a if and only if $\langle\alpha, x_0\rangle \in \mathbf{Z}$ for all $\alpha \in R$, in other words, if and only if $x_0 \in P(R^\vee)$ (§ 1, no. 9).

COROLLARY. (i) *If* $\overline{\omega} \in P(R^\vee)$, *there exists an alcove* C *such that* $\overline{\omega}$ *is an extremal point of* $\overline{C}$.

(ii) *If* C *is an alcove,* $\overline{C} \cap Q(R^\vee)$ *reduces to a single point and this is an extremal point of* $\overline{C}$.

This follows from Prop. 3, in view of the Cor. of Prop. 11 of Chap. V, § 3, no. 10 and Prop. 12 of Chap. V, § 3, no. 10.

PROPOSITION 4. *Let* C′ *be a chamber of* $R^\vee$.

(i) *There exists a unique alcove* C *contained in* C′ *such that* $0 \in \overline{C}$.
(ii) *The union of the* $w(\overline{C})$ *for* $w \in W$ *is a neighbourhood of* 0 *in* E.
(iii) *Every wall of* C′ *is a wall of* C.

This follows from Prop. 11 of Chap. V, § 3, no. 10.

Assume now that R is irreducible. Let $(\alpha_i)_{i\in I}$ be a basis of R (§ 1, no. 5, Def. 2), and let $(\overline{\omega}_i)_{i\in I}$ be the dual basis. The $\overline{\omega}_i$ are the fundamental weights of $R^\vee$ for the chamber D′ of $R^\vee$ corresponding to the basis (α_i). Let

$$\tilde{\alpha} = \sum_{i\in I} n_i \alpha_i$$

be the highest root of R (§ 1, no. 8), and let J be the set of $i \in I$ such that $n_i = 1$.

PROPOSITION 5. *Let* C *be the alcove contained in* C′ *and containing* 0 *in its closure* (Prop. 4).

(i) C *is the set of* $x \in E$ *such that* $\langle \alpha_i, x \rangle > 0$ *for all* $i \in I$ *and* $\langle \tilde{\alpha}, x \rangle < 1$.

(ii) *The set* $\overline{C} \cap P(R\check{})$ *consists of* 0 *and the* $\overline{\omega}_i$ *for* $i \in J$.

Let D be the set of $x \in E$ such that $\langle \tilde{\alpha}, x \rangle < 1$ and set $C_1 = C' \cap D$. Since $0 \in \overline{C}$, we have $C \subseteq D$ and hence $C \subseteq C_1$. We are going to show that, for all $\alpha \in R$ and all $k \in \mathbf{Z}$, the sets C and C_1 are on the same side of the hyperplane $L_{\alpha,k}$. This will prove that $C_1 \subseteq C$ and so will establish assertion (i). If $k = 0$, the whole of the chamber C′ is on one side of $L_{\alpha,0}$, which establishes our assertion in this case. If $k \neq 0$, we may, by replacing α by $-\alpha$, assume that $k > 0$. Then $\langle \alpha, x \rangle < k$ on C, since $0 \in \overline{C}$. On the other hand, $\tilde{\alpha} - \alpha$ is positive on C′ (§ 1, no. 8, Prop. 25). Thus, for $y \in C_1$, we have $\langle \alpha, y \rangle \leqslant \langle \tilde{\alpha}, y \rangle < 1 \leqslant k$. Consequently, C and C_1 are on the same side of $L_{\alpha,k}$.

Now let $\overline{\omega} \in P(R\check{})$. Then $\overline{\omega} = \sum_i p_i \overline{\omega}_i$, with $p_i \in \mathbf{Z}$ (§ 1, no. 10), and $\overline{\omega} \in \overline{C'}$ if and only if the integers p_i are *positive*. If $\overline{\omega} \in \overline{C'}$, then $\overline{\omega} \in \overline{C}$ if and only if $\langle \tilde{\alpha}, \overline{\omega} \rangle = \sum_i n_i p_i$ is $\leqslant 1$, hence (ii).

COROLLARY. *The alcove* C *is an open simplex with vertices* 0 *and the* $\overline{\omega}_i / n_i$, $i \in I$.

This follows from (i).

3. NORMALISER OF W_a

In this no., we assume that the chosen scalar product on V is invariant not only under W but *under the whole of the group* A(R). We identify A(R) and A(R˘).

Let G be the normaliser of W_a in the group of displacements of the affine euclidean space E. If g is a displacement of E, and s is the orthogonal reflection with respect to a hyperplane L, the displacement gsg^{-1} is the orthogonal reflection with respect to the hyperplane $g(L)$. It follows that G is the set of displacements of E that permute the hyperplanes $L_{\alpha,k}$ (for $\alpha \in R$ and $k \in \mathbf{Z}$).

Now, the group of automorphisms of E is the semi-direct product of the orthogonal group U of V^* and the group T of translations. If $u \in U$ and $v \in V^*$, the hyperplane $L_{\alpha,k}$ is transformed by $g = u \circ t(v)$ into the hyperplane with equation

$$\langle {}^t u^{-1}(\alpha), x \rangle = k + \langle \alpha, v \rangle.$$

Consequently, $g \in G$ if and only if, on the one hand ${}^t u$ permutes the roots, in other words belongs to A(R), and on the other hand $\langle \alpha, v \rangle \in \mathbf{Z}$ for all $\alpha \in R$, that is $v \in P(R\check{})$. In other words, *the group* G *is the semi-direct product of* A(R) *by* P. Since $Q \subseteq P$ and $W \subseteq A(R)$, *the quotient group* G/W_a *is the semi-direct product of* A(R)/W *by* P(R˘)/Q(R˘); it is immediately checked that the corresponding action of A(R)/W on P(R˘)/Q(R˘) is the canonical action (§1, no. 9).

We denote by W'_a the subgroup of G formed by the semi-direct product of W by P. This is a normal subgroup of G, and G/W'_a is canonically isomorphic to A(R)/W; moreover, the canonical map from $P(R^\vee)$ to W'_a/W_a gives by passing to the quotient an isomorphism from $P(R^\vee)/Q(R^\vee)$ to W'_a/W_a.

Now let C be an alcove of E, and let G_C be the subgroup consisting of the elements $g \in G$ such that $g(C) = C$. Since W_a is simply-transitive on the alcoves, *the group* G *is the semi-direct product of* G_C *by* W_a. The corresponding isomorphism from G/W_a to G_C gives rise in particular to a canonical isomorphism from $P(R^\vee)/Q(R^\vee)$ to the group $\Gamma_C = G_C \cap W'_a$.

Assume that R is irreducible, and retain the notation of Prop. 5 of no. 2. Put $R_0 = R$, and let R_i $(i \in I)$ be the root system generated by the a_j, for $j \neq i$. For $i = 0$ (resp. $i \in I$), let w_i be the unique element of $W(R_i)$ (identified with a subgroup of W) which transforms the positive roots of R_i relative to the basis $(\alpha_j)_{j\neq i}$ into negative roots (§ 1, no. 6, Cor. 3 of Prop. 17).

PROPOSITION 6. *For all $i \in J$, the element $\gamma_i = t(\overline{\omega}_i)w_iw_0$ belongs to Γ_C and the map $i \mapsto \gamma_i$ is a bijection from J to $\Gamma_C - \{1\}$.*

We remark first of all that the root $w_i(\tilde{\alpha})$ is of the form

$$n_i\alpha_i + \sum_{j\neq i} b_{ij}\alpha_j,$$

and hence is *positive.*

We show that, if $i \in J$, then $\gamma_i \in \Gamma_C$. Indeed, let $a \in C$ and $b = \gamma_i(a)$. For $1 \leqslant j \leqslant l$ and $j \neq i$,

$$\begin{aligned}\langle b, \alpha_j\rangle &= \langle \overline{\omega}_i + w_iw_0(a), \alpha_j\rangle \\ &= \langle w_0(u), w_i(\alpha_j)\rangle > 0\end{aligned} \tag{2}$$

since $w_0(a) \in -C'$ and $w_i(\alpha_j)$ is negative. On the other hand,

$$\langle b, \alpha_i\rangle = 1 + \langle w_0(a), w_i(\alpha_i)\rangle \geqslant 1 + \langle w_0(a), \tilde{\alpha}\rangle > 0 \tag{3}$$

since $w_0(a) \in -C'$, $\tilde{\alpha} - w_i(\alpha_i)$ takes negative values on $-C'$, and $\langle w_0(a), \tilde{\alpha}\rangle > -1$. Finally,

$$\langle b, \tilde{\alpha}\rangle = n_i + \langle w_0(a), w_i(\tilde{\alpha})\rangle = 1 + \langle w_0(a), w_i(\tilde{\alpha})\rangle < 1 \tag{4}$$

since $w_0(a) \in -C'$ and $w_i(\tilde{\alpha})$ is a positive root. The relations (2), (3) and (4) then imply that $b \in C$, and hence that $\gamma_i \in \Gamma_C$. It is clear that the map $i \mapsto \gamma_i$ is *injective*, since $\gamma_i(0) = \overline{\omega}_i$. Finally, let $\gamma \in \Gamma_C$ with $\gamma \neq 1$, and put $\gamma = tw$ with $t \in P$ and $w \in W$. Then $t \neq 1$ since $\Gamma_C \cap W = \{1\}$. On the other hand, $t(0) = \gamma(0) \in \overline{C} \cap P(R^\vee)$ and Prop. 5 implies that there exists $i \in J$ such that $t(0) = \overline{\omega}_i$. Then $\gamma_i^{-1}\gamma(0) = 0$, hence $\gamma = \gamma_i$ since $\Gamma_C \cap W = \{1\}$. This completes the proof.

COROLLARY. *The $(\overline{\omega}_i)_{i\in J}$ form a system of representatives in* $P(R^\vee)$ *of the non-zero elements of* $P(R^\vee)/Q(R^\vee)$.

Indeed, if we identify Γ_c with $P(R^\vee)/Q(R^\vee)$, the element γ_i is identified with the class of $\overline{\omega}_i$ mod. $Q(R^\vee)$.

Remarks. 1) The map $\gamma \mapsto \gamma(0)$ is a bijection from Γ_C to $\overline{C} \cap P(R^\vee)$.

2) The group G is also the normaliser of W_a in the group of automorphisms of E provided only with its affine structure (cf. Exerc. 3).

4. APPLICATION: ORDER OF THE WEYL GROUP

Lemma 1. Let X *be a locally compact space countable at infinity,* G *a group acting continuously and properly on* X, μ *a measure on* X *invariant under* G, G′ *a subgroup of* G, U *and* U′ *two open subsets of* X *with finite non-zero measure. Assume that the* sU *for* $s \in G$ *(resp. the* s′U′ *for* $s' \in G'$*) are pairwise disjoint and that their union is of negligible complement. Then* G′ *is of finite index in* G *and* $(G : G') = \mu(U')/\mu(U)$.

Let $(s_\lambda)_{\lambda \in \Lambda}$ be a family of representatives of the right cosets of G′ in G. Let U_1 be the union of the $s_\lambda U$. Then the $s'U_1$, for $s' \in G'$, are pairwise disjoint and have union $M = \bigcup_{s \in G} sU$. Let $M' = \bigcup_{s' \in G'} s'U'$. The union of U′ (resp. U_1) and a suitable subset of $X - M'$ (resp. $X - M$) is a fundamental domain, evidently μ-measurable, for G′. By *Integration*, Chap. VII, § 2, no. 10, Cor. of Th. 4, $\mu(U') = \mu(U_1)$. This proves that $\operatorname{Card} \Lambda = (G : G')$ is finite, and that $\mu(U') = (\operatorname{Card} \Lambda)\mu(U)$.

PROPOSITION 7. *Assume that* R *is irreducible. Let* $B = \{\alpha_1, \ldots, \alpha_l\}$ *be a basis of* R, f *the connection index of* R (§ 1, no. 9) *and* $\tilde{\alpha} = n_1\alpha_1 + \cdots + n_l\alpha_l$ *the highest root of* R *(for the order defined by* B*). Then the order of* W *is equal to*

$$(l!)n_1 n_2 \ldots n_l f.$$

Let $(\overline{\omega}_1, \ldots, \overline{\omega}_l)$ be the basis of $P(R^\vee)$ dual to B. By the Cor. of Prop. 5, the open simplex C with vertices $0, n_1^{-1}\overline{\omega}_1, \ldots, n_l^{-1}\overline{\omega}_l$ is an alcove of E. Choose a Haar measure μ on the additive group V^*. Let A be the set of elements of V^* of the form $\xi_1\overline{\omega}_1 + \cdots + \xi_l\overline{\omega}_l$, with $0 < \xi_i < 1$ for $i = 1, \ldots, l$. By Cor. 2 of Prop. 15 of *Integration*, Chap. VII, § 1, no. 10,

$$\mu(A)/\mu(C) = (l!)n_1 n_2 \ldots n_l. \tag{5}$$

On the other hand, let A′ be the set of elements of V^* of the form

$$\xi_1\alpha_1^\vee + \cdots + \xi_l\alpha_l^\vee,$$

with $0 < \xi_i < 1$ for $i = 1, \ldots, l$. Since $(\alpha_1^\vee, \ldots, \alpha_l^\vee)$ is a basis of the **Z**-module $Q(R^\vee)$, we can apply Lemma 1 with $X = V^*$, $G = W_a$, $G' = Q$, $U = C$ and $U' = A'$. This gives

$$\mu(A')/\mu(C) = (W_a : Q) = \operatorname{Card} W. \tag{6}$$

Finally, Lemma 1 can be applied again, taking $X = V^*$, $G = P$, $G' = Q$, $U = A$ and $U' = A'$. This gives

$$\mu(A')/\mu(A) = (P : Q) = (P(R^\vee) : Q(R^\vee)) = f. \tag{7}$$

The proposition now follows by comparing formulas (5), (6) and (7).

5. ROOT SYSTEMS AND GROUPS GENERATED BY REFLECTIONS

PROPOSITION 8. *Let* F *be a real* Hilbert *space of finite dimension* l. *Let* $\mathfrak{H}$ *be the set of affine hyperplanes of* F *and* G *the group generated by the orthogonal reflections* s_H *with respect to the hyperplanes* $H \in \mathfrak{H}$. *Assume that the conditions of Chap.* V, § 3 *are satisfied (i.e. that* $g(H) \in \mathfrak{H}$ *for all* $H \in \mathfrak{H}$ *and* $g \in G$, *and that* G *acts properly on* F*). Assume also that* 0 *is a special point for* G *and that the group* T *of translations belonging to* G *is of rank* l. *Then there exists a unique reduced root system* R *in* $V = F^*$ *such that the canonical isomorphism from* F *to* V^* *transforms* G *to the affine Weyl group* W_a *of* R.

We remark first of all that the assumption on T implies that G is *essential*: otherwise, the affine space F would decompose into a product $F_0 \times F_1$, with $\dim F_1 < l$, the group G being identified with a group of displacements acting properly on F_1 (Chap. V, § 3, no. 8, Prop. 6), and T would not be of rank l.

Let $\mathfrak{H}_0$ be the set of $H \in \mathfrak{H}$ such that $0 \in H$. For $H \in \mathfrak{H}_0$, let $\mathfrak{H}_H$ be the set of elements of $\mathfrak{H}$ parallel to H. Since 0 is a special point, $\mathfrak{H}$ is the union of the $\mathfrak{H}_H$ for $H \in \mathfrak{H}_0$. Since T is of rank l, there exists a $v \in F$ such that the translation by the vector v belongs to T and $v \notin H$. The hyperplanes $H + kv$ for $k \in \mathbf{Z}$ are pairwise distinct and belong to $\mathfrak{H}_H$. Now let a be a unit vector of F orthogonal to H: then $H + (v|a)a \in \mathfrak{H}_H$ and since $\mathfrak{H}$ is locally finite (Chap. V, § 1, no. 1, Lemma 1), there is a smallest real number $\lambda > 0$ such that $H + \lambda a \in \mathfrak{H}$. We are going to show that $\mathfrak{H}_H$ is the set of hyperplanes $H + k\lambda a$ for $k \in \mathbf{Z}$. Indeed,

$$H' = H + \lambda a \in \mathfrak{H}_H$$

and the element $s_{H'} \circ s_H$ of G is the translation by the vector $2\lambda a$ (Chap. V, § 2, no. 4, Prop. 5). Consequently, $H + 2n\lambda a = (s_{H'}s_H)^n(H)$ and $H + (2n + 1)\lambda a = (s_{H'}s_H)^n(H')$ belongs to $\mathfrak{H}_H$. On the other hand, if $L \in \mathfrak{H}_H$, there exists $\xi \in \mathbf{R}$ such that $L = H + \xi\lambda a$ and there exists an integer n such that

$$\text{either } 2n < \xi \leqslant 2n + 1, \quad \text{or } 2n - 1 < \xi \leqslant 2n.$$

In the first case, $(s_H s_{H'})^n(L) = H + (\xi - 2n)\lambda a$ with

$$0 < (\xi - 2n)\lambda \leqslant \lambda$$

and the definition of λ implies that $\xi = 2n + 1$; in the second case,

$$s_{\rm H}(s_{\rm H}s_{\rm H'})^n({\rm L}) = {\rm H} + (2n-\xi)\lambda a \quad \text{with} \quad 0 \leqslant (2n-\xi)\lambda < \lambda$$

and the definition of λ implies that $\xi = 2n$.

It follows that if $\alpha_{\rm H}$ is the linear form on F such that

$$\mathrm{H}' = \{x \in \mathrm{F} \,|\, \langle \alpha_{\rm H}, x\rangle = 1\},$$

the set $\mathfrak{H}_{\rm H}$ *is the set of hyperplanes* $\mathrm{L}_{\alpha_{\rm H},k} = \{x \in \mathrm{F} \,|\, \langle\alpha_{\rm H}, x\rangle = k\}$ *for* $k \in \mathbf{Z}$, and $\alpha_{\rm H}$ and $-\alpha_{\rm H}$ are the only linear forms with this property.

Consequently, the proposition will be proved if we show that *the set* R *of elements of* V *of the form* $\pm\alpha_{\rm H}$ *is a reduced root system in* V.

a) We prove condition ($\mathrm{RS_I}$): it is clear that R is finite (since $\mathfrak{H}_0$ is finite) and does not contain 0. Moreover, R generates V. Indeed, if $x \in \mathrm{F}$ is orthogonal to R, then $x \in \mathrm{H}$ for all $\mathrm{H} \in \mathfrak{H}_0$ and the translation by the vector x commutes with every element of G. Since G is essential, this implies that $x = 0$.

b) We prove ($\mathrm{RS_{II}}$). For $v \in \mathrm{V}$ and $r \in \mathbf{R}$, put $\mathrm{L}_{v,r} = \{x \in \mathrm{F} \,|\, \langle v, x\rangle = r\}$ as above; if $\alpha \in \mathrm{R}$, put $\mathrm{H}_\alpha = \mathrm{L}_{\alpha,0}$, and let s_α be the transpose of s_{H_α}. There exists a unique element $\alpha\check{} \in \mathrm{F}$ orthogonal to H_α and such that $\langle\alpha\check{}, \alpha\rangle = 2$. Then $s_{\mathrm{H}_\alpha} = s_{\alpha\check{},\alpha}$ and $s_\alpha = s_{\alpha,\alpha\check{}}$. For $\beta \in \mathrm{R}$,

$$\mathrm{L}_{s_\alpha(\beta),1} = s_{\mathrm{H}_\alpha}(\mathrm{L}_{\beta,1}) \in \mathfrak{H}$$

and there exist $\gamma \in \mathrm{R}$ and $n \in \mathbf{N}^*$ such that $\mathrm{L}_{s_\alpha(\beta),1} = \mathrm{L}_{\gamma,n}$. Then

$$s_{\mathrm{H}_\alpha}(\mathrm{L}_{\gamma,1}) = \mathrm{L}_{\beta,1/n}$$

and so $1/n \in \mathbf{Z}$. Thus $n = 1$ and $s_\alpha(\beta) = \gamma \in \mathrm{R}$. This proves ($\mathrm{RS_{II}}$).

c) We prove ($\mathrm{RS_{III}}$). Let $\alpha \in \mathrm{R}$ and set $\mathrm{H}'_\alpha = \mathrm{L}_{\alpha,1}$. Then

$$\mathrm{H}'_\alpha = \mathrm{H}_\alpha + (1/2)\alpha\check{};$$

since the translation $t(\alpha\check{})$ by the vector $\alpha\check{}$ is the product $s_{\mathrm{H}'_\alpha} s_{\mathrm{H}_\alpha}$ (Chap. V, § 2, no. 4, Prop. 5), it belongs to T and $\alpha\check{} = t(\alpha\check{})(0)$ is a *special point* for G. Consequently, for all $\beta \in \mathrm{R}$, there exists a hyperplane $\mathrm{L}_{\beta,k}$ passing through $\alpha\check{}$, with k an integer, which shows that $\langle\beta, \alpha\check{}\rangle \in \mathbf{Z}$, and proves ($\mathrm{RS_{III}}$).

d) Finally, it is clear that R is *reduced*, for if $\mathrm{H}, \mathrm{H}' \in \mathfrak{H}_0$, $\mathrm{H} \neq \mathrm{H}'$, the linear forms $\alpha_{\rm H}$ and $\alpha_{\rm H'}$ are not proportional.

Remark. 1) The assumption that T is of rank l is satisfied in particular when G is *irreducible and infinite.* Indeed, the vector space generated by vectors corresponding to the translations in T is invariant under the canonical image of G in the linear group of F. It is different from $\{0\}$ if G is infinite and is thus equal to the whole of F if G is infinite and irreducible.

A finite group generated by reflections is not always the Weyl group of a root system. More precisely:

PROPOSITION 9. *Let* V *be a real vector space of finite dimension* l*, and let* G *be a finite subgroup of* **GL**(V)*, generated by reflections and essential. Give* V *a scalar product invariant under* G*. The following conditions are equivalent:*

(i) *There exists a discrete subgroup of* V *of rank* l *that is stable under* G.

(ii) *There exists a* **Q**-*structure on* V (*Algebra,* Chap. II, § 8, no. 1, Def. 1) *invariant under* G.

(iii) *There exists a root system in* V *whose Weyl group is* G.

(iv) *There exists a discrete group* G′ *of displacements of* V*, acting properly on* V*, and generated by reflections, such that* G′ *is the semi-direct product of* G *and a group of translations of rank* l.

(ii) $\Longrightarrow$ (i): let $V' \subseteq V$ be a **Q**-structure on V invariant under G. Let A be a finite subset of V′ generating the **Q**-vector space V′. Replacing A by $\bigcup_{s \in G} s(A)$, we can assume that A is stable under G. Let B be the subgroup of V generated by A. Then B is stable under G, of finite type and torsion-free, so has a basis over **Z** which is both a basis of V′ over **Q** and a basis of V over **R**.

(iii) $\Longrightarrow$ (ii): this follows from Prop. 1 of § 1, no. 1, for example.

(iv) $\Longrightarrow$ (iii): let G′ be a group satisfying condition (iv). The group of translations of G′ is of rank l, and 0 is a special point for G′ by Prop. 9 of Chap. V, § 3, no. 10. Prop. 6 shows that there exists a reduced root system R_0 in V^* such that G′ is identified with $W_a(R_0)$; the group G is then the Weyl group of the inverse root system of R_0.

(i) $\Longrightarrow$ (iv): assume that G leaves stable a discrete subgroup M of V, of rank l. For any reflection $s \in G$, $s(x) - x \in M$ for all $x \in M$, so the line D_s orthogonal to H_s meets M; let α_s, $-\alpha_s$ be the generators of the cyclic group $D_s \cap M$; the set A of the α_s and $-\alpha_s$ is stable under G, hence generates a subgroup M′ of M stable under G; the discrete group M′ is of rank l because G is essential. Let G′ be the group of affine transformations of V that is the semi-direct product of G and the group of translations whose vectors belong to M′. Let G'_1 be the subgroup of G′ generated by the reflections of G′. We shall show that $G'_1 = G'$, which will complete the proof. First, $G'_1 \supseteq G$ since G is generated by reflections. On the other hand, for any reflection s of G, let t_s be the translation with vector α_s. The transformation $s \circ t_s$ is a reflection, and $s \circ t_s \in G'$; thus t_s is a product of two reflections of G′; this being true for every reflection s of G, the translations whose vector belongs to M′ are all in G'_1.

DEFINITION 2. A *group* G *satisfying the equivalent conditions of Prop. 9 is called a crystallographic group.*

Remark. 2) Let G be a finite group generated by reflections and essential. Then G is crystallographic if and only if *every element of its Coxeter matrix is one of the integers* 1, 2, 3, 4, 6. Indeed, this condition is necessary by *Remark* 3) of § 1, no. 5. The fact that it is sufficient will follow from the classification of finite Coxeter groups given in § 4 (for a direct proof, see Chap. V, § 4, Exerc. 6).

§ 3. EXPONENTIAL INVARIANTS

In this section, the letter A denotes a commutative ring, with a unit element, and not reduced to 0.

1. GROUP ALGEBRA OF A FREE ABELIAN GROUP

Let P be a free **Z**-module of finite rank l. We denote by A[P] the group algebra of the additive group of P over A (*Algebra*, Chap. III, § 2, no. 6). For any $p \in \mathrm{P}$, denote by e^p the corresponding element of A[P]. Then $(e^p)_{p\in \mathrm{P}}$ is a *basis* of the A-module A[P], and, for any $p, p' \in \mathrm{P}$, we have

$$e^p e^{p'} = e^{p+p'}, \quad (e^p)^{-1} = e^{-p}, \quad e^0 = 1.$$

Lemma 1. Assume that A *is factorial (Commutative Algebra,* Chap. VII, § 3, no. 1, Def. 1*).*

(i) *The ring* A[P] *is factorial.*

(ii) *If* u, v *are non-proportional elements of* P, *the elements* $1 - e^u, 1 - e^v$ *of* A[P] *are relatively prime.*

Let $(p_1, p_2, \dots, p_l)$ be a basis of P, and $\mathrm{X}_1, \mathrm{X}_2, \dots, \mathrm{X}_l$ be indeterminates. The A-linear map from $\mathrm{A}[\mathrm{X}_1, \dots, \mathrm{X}_l, \mathrm{X}_1^{-1}, \dots, \mathrm{X}_l^{-1}]$ to A[P] that takes $\mathrm{X}_1^{n_1}\mathrm{X}_2^{n_2}\dots\mathrm{X}_l^{n_l}$ (where $n_1, n_2, \dots, n_l \in \mathbf{Z}$) to $e^{n_1p_1+\dots+n_lp_l}$ is an isomorphism of rings. Now $\mathrm{A}[\mathrm{X}_1, \dots, \mathrm{X}_l]$ is a factorial ring (*Commutative Algebra*, Chap. VII, § 3, no. 5), and $\mathrm{A}[\mathrm{X}_1, \dots, \mathrm{X}_l, \mathrm{X}_1^{-1}, \dots, \mathrm{X}_l^{-1}]$ is the ring of fractions of $\mathrm{A}[\mathrm{X}_1, \dots, \mathrm{X}_l]$, hence is also factorial.

Let P′ (resp. P″) be the set of elements of P of which some multiple belongs to $\mathbf{Z}u + \mathbf{Z}v$ (resp. $\mathbf{Z}u$). Then the groups P/P′ and P′/P″ are torsion-free, so there exists a complement of P″ in P′ and a complement of P′ in P. Consequently, there exists a basis $(z_1, z_2, \dots, z_l)$ of the **Z**-module P and rational integers j, m, n such that $u = jz_1, v = mz_1 + nz_2, j > 0, n > 0$. Putting $\mathrm{X}_i = e^{z_i}$ for $1 \leqslant i \leqslant l$, we then have $1 - e^u = 1 - \mathrm{X}_1^j, 1 - e^v = 1 - \mathrm{X}_1^m\mathrm{X}_2^n$. Let K be an algebraic closure of the field of fractions of A, so that A[P] can be identified with a subring of the ring $\mathrm{B} = \mathrm{K}[\mathrm{X}_1, \dots, \mathrm{X}_l, \mathrm{X}_1^{-1}, \dots, \mathrm{X}_l^{-1}]$. For any jth root of unity z, $1 - z\mathrm{X}_1$ is extremal in

$$\mathrm{K}[\mathrm{X}_1, \dots, \mathrm{X}_l];$$

moreover, the ideal generated by $1 - z\mathrm{X}_1$ contains no monomial in the X_i. We conclude that the ideal $(1 - z\mathrm{X}_1)\mathrm{B}$ of B is a prime ideal of height 1

(*Commutative Algebra*, Chap. VII, § 1, no. 6), hence that $1-zX_1$ is extremal in B. The extremal factors of $1-X_1^j$ in B are thus of the form $1-zX_1$. Now none of these factors divide $1-X_1^mX_2^n$ in B (for the homomorphism f from B to B such that $f(X_1)=z^{-1}, f(X_i)=X_i$ for $i \geqslant 2$, satisfies

$$f(1-zX_1)=0 \quad \text{and} \quad f(1-X_1^mX_2^n)=1-z^{-m}X_2^n \neq 0).$$

Thus, $1-X_1^j$ and $1-X_1^mX_2^n$ are relatively prime in B. Consequently, any common divisor of $1-X_1^j$ and $1-X_1^mX_2^n$ in A[P] is invertible in B and so, up to multiplication by an element of the form $X_1^{k_1}X_2^{k_2}\dots X_l^{k_l}$, is equal to an element a of A; in other words,a divides 1 in A, hence is invertible in A. Thus, finally, $1-X_1^j$ and $1-X_1^mX_2^n$ are relatively prime in A[P].

2. CASE OF THE GROUP OF WEIGHTS; MAXIMAL TERMS

We retain the notations of the preceding number and let R be a *reduced* root system in a real vector space V. In the remainder of this section, we take for P the group of *weights* of R (§ 1, no. 9). The group W = W(R) acts on P, hence also on the algebra A[P]; we have $w(e^p)=e^{w(p)}$ for $w \in W$ and $p \in P$.

Let C be a chamber of R (§ 1, no. 5) and let $B=(\alpha_i)_{1 \leqslant i \leqslant l}$ be the corresponding basis of R. We provide V (and hence also P) with the order structure defined by C. If $p, p' \in P$, $p \geqslant p'$ if and only if $p-p'$ is a linear combination of the α_i with positive coefficients.

DEFINITION 1. *Let* $x=\sum_{p \in P} x_pe^p$ *be an element of* A[P]. *The set* S *of* $p \in P$ *such that* $x_p \neq 0$ *is called the support of* x *and the set* X *of maximal elements of* S *is called the maximal support of* x. A *term* x_pe^p *with* $p \in X$ *is then called a maximal term of* x.

Lemma 2. Let $x \in A[P]$ *and let* $(x_pe^p)_{p\in X}$ *be the family of maximal terms of* x. *Let* $q \in P$ *and let* $y \in A[P]$ *be such that* e^q *is the unique maximal term of* y. *Then, the family of maximal terms of* xy *is* $(x_pe^{p+q})_{p \in X}$.

Put $x=\sum_p x_pe^p, y=\sum_r y_re^r$ and $xy=\sum_t z_te^t$. Then $r \leqslant q$ for all $r \in P$ such that $y_r \neq 0$ and $z_t=\sum_{p+r=t} x_py_r$.

If $t=p+q=p'+r$ with $p \in X$ and $x_{p'}y_r \neq 0$, then $r \leqslant q$, hence $p' \geqslant p$ and consequently $p'=p$. Thus $z_{p+q}=x_py_q=x_p \neq 0$. This shows that $X+q$ is contained in the support of the product xy.

On the other hand, if $t=p'+r$ with $x_{p'}y_r \neq 0$, there exists $p \in X$ such that $p' \leqslant p$ and we have $t \leqslant p+q$. The maximal support of xy is therefore contained in $X+q$. Since no two elements of $X+q$ are comparable, it follows that $X+q$ is exactly the maximal support of xy and we have seen above that $z_{p+q}=x_p$ for $p \in X$, which completes the proof of the lemma.

Remark. Since $x \neq 0$ means that the maximal support of x is non-empty, Lemma 2 shows that $x \neq 0$ implies $xy \neq 0$ whenever y admits a unique maximal term of the form e^q.

3. ANTI-INVARIANT ELEMENTS

We retain the notations of the preceding number. Denote by $\varepsilon(w)$ the determinant of the element $w \in \mathrm{W}$. Thus

$$\varepsilon(w) = (-1)^{l(w)},$$

the length $l(w)$ being taken relative to the family of reflections s_{α_i}.

DEFINITION 2. *An element* $x \in \mathrm{A[P]}$ *is said to be anti-invariant under* W *if*

$$w(x) = (-1)^{l(w)}.x$$

for all $w \in \mathrm{W}$.

The anti-invariant elements of A[P] form an A-submodule of A[P]. For any $x \in \mathrm{A[P]}$, put

$$\mathrm{J}(x) = \sum_{w \in \mathrm{W}} \varepsilon(w).w(x). \tag{1}$$

For $x \in \mathrm{A[P]}$ and $w \in \mathrm{W}$, we have

$$w(\mathrm{J}(x)) = \sum_{v \in \mathrm{W}} \varepsilon(v).wv(x) = \varepsilon(w) \sum_{v \in \mathrm{W}} \varepsilon(v).v(x) = \varepsilon(w).\mathrm{J}(x)$$

and $\mathrm{J}(x)$ is anti-invariant. On the other hand, let $q = \mathrm{Card(W)}$. For any anti-invariant element x of A[P], we have $\mathrm{J}(x) = q.x$. It follows that, if q is invertible in A, the map $q^{-1}\mathrm{J}$ is a *projection* from A[P] onto the submodule of anti-invariant elements.

Let $\overline{\omega}_1, \dots, \overline{\omega}_l$ be the fundamental weights corresponding to the chamber C. The elements of $\mathrm{P} \cap \overline{\mathrm{C}}$ (resp. $\mathrm{P} \cap \mathrm{C}$) are the weights of the form $n_1\overline{\omega}_1 + \cdots + n_l\overline{\omega}_l$ with $n_i \geqslant 0$ (resp. $n_i > 0$) for $1 \leqslant i \leqslant l$ (§ 1, no. 10). On the other hand,

$$\rho = \overline{\omega}_1 + \cdots + \overline{\omega}_l$$

is half the sum of the positive roots (*loc. cit.*) so the elements of $\mathrm{P} \cap \mathrm{C}$ are the weights of the form $\rho + p$ with $p \in \mathrm{P} \cap \overline{\mathrm{C}}$. Finally, if $p \in \mathrm{P} \cap \mathrm{C}$, then $w(p) < p$ for all $w \neq 1$ (§ 1, no. 6, Cor. to Prop. 18) and e^p is thus the unique maximal term of $\mathrm{J}(e^p)$.

PROPOSITION 1. *If* 2 *is not a zero divisor in* A, *the elements* $\mathrm{J}(e^p)$ *for* $p \in \mathrm{P} \cap \mathrm{C}$ *form a basis of the module of anti-invariant elements of* A[P].

The weights $w(p)$ for $w \in \mathrm{W}$ and $p \in \mathrm{P} \cap \mathrm{C}$ are pairwise distinct. It follows that the $\mathrm{J}(e^p)$ for $p \in \mathrm{P} \cap \mathrm{C}$ are linearly independent.

On the other hand, let $x = \sum_p x_p e^p$ be an anti-invariant element of A[P]. If p_0 belongs to a wall, it is invariant under a reflection $s \in \mathrm{W}$ and

$$x = \sum_p x_p e^p = -s(x) = -\sum_p x_p e^{s(p)}.$$

It follows that $2x_{p_0} = 0$, so $x_{p_0} = 0$. Since every element that does not belong to any wall can be written uniquely in the form $w(p)$ with $w \in \mathrm{W}$ and $p \in \mathrm{P} \cap \mathrm{C}$, we thus have

$$x = \sum_{p \in \mathrm{P} \cap \mathrm{C}} \sum_{w \in \mathrm{W}} x_{w(p)} e^{w(p)}. \tag{2}$$

Since $w(x) = \sum_p x_p e^{w(p)} = \varepsilon(w) \sum_p x_p e^p$, $x_{w(p)} = \varepsilon(w) x_p$ and we deduce from (2) that

$$x = \sum_{p \in \mathrm{P} \cap \mathrm{C}} x_p \mathrm{J}(e^p),$$

which completes the proof.

Consider now the element d of the algebra $\mathrm{A}[\frac{1}{2}\mathrm{P}]$ defined by

$$\begin{aligned} d &= \prod_{\alpha \in \mathrm{R}, \alpha > 0} (e^{\alpha/2} - e^{-\alpha/2}) \qquad (3) \\ &= e^{\rho} . \prod_{\alpha \in \mathrm{R}, \alpha > 0} (1 - e^{-\alpha}) \\ &= e^{-\rho} . \prod_{\alpha \in \mathrm{R}, \alpha > 0} (e^{\alpha} - 1). \end{aligned}$$

Since $\rho \in \mathrm{P}$, $d \in \mathrm{A}[\mathrm{P}]$.

PROPOSITION 2. (i) *The element d defined by (3) is an anti-invariant element of* A[P]*; its unique maximal term* (no. 2, Def. 1) *is* e^{ρ} *and* $d = \mathrm{J}(e^{\rho})$.

(ii) *For any* $p \in \mathrm{P}$*, the element* $\mathrm{J}(e^p)$ *is divisible uniquely by d and the quotient* $\mathrm{J}(e^p)/d$ *is an element of* A[P] *invariant under* W.

(iii) *If* 2 *is not a zero divisor in* A*, multiplication by d is a bijection from the set of elements of* A[P] *invariant under* W *to the set of anti-invariant elements of* A[P].

We know that, for $1 \leqslant i \leqslant l$, the reflection $s_i = s_{\alpha_i}$ leaves stable the set of positive roots other than α_i and that $s_i(\alpha_i) = -\alpha_i$ (§ 1, no. 6, Cor. 1 of Prop. 17). Hence,

$$\begin{aligned} s_i(d) &= (e^{-\alpha_i/2} - e^{\alpha_i/2}) . \prod_{\alpha \in \mathrm{R}, \alpha > 0, \alpha \neq \alpha_i} (e^{\alpha/2} - e^{-\alpha/2}) \\ &= -d = \varepsilon(s_i).d. \end{aligned}$$

Since the s_i generate W, this proves the first assertion in (i). The second assertion in (i) follows immediately from (3) and Lemma 2, noting that 1 is the unique maximal term of $1 - e^{-\alpha}$ for $\alpha \in \mathrm{R}$, $\alpha > 0$.

Assume now that $\mathrm{A} = \mathbf{Z}$. By Prop. 1,

$$d = \prod_{p \in \mathrm{P} \cap \mathrm{C}} c_p \mathrm{J}(e^p) \text{ with } c_p \in \mathbf{Z}. \tag{4}$$

On the other hand, it is clear that

$$d = e^\rho + \sum_{q<\rho} c'_q e^q. \tag{5}$$

If $p \in \mathrm{P} \cap \mathrm{C}$ with $p \neq \rho$, then $p > \rho$ and the coefficient of e^p in d is zero by (5). Thus, $c_p = 0$. Moreover, comparison of the coefficients of e^ρ in (4) and (5) shows that $c_\rho = 1$ and hence that $d = \mathrm{J}(e^\rho)$.

We continue to assume that $\mathrm{A} = \mathbf{Z}$. Let $p \in \mathrm{P}$, $\alpha \in \mathrm{R}$ and M be a system of representatives of the right cosets of W with respect to the subgroup $\{1, s_\alpha\}$. Then,

$$\mathrm{J}(e^p) = \sum_{w \in \mathrm{M}} \varepsilon(w) e^{w(p)} + \sum_{w \in \mathrm{M}} \varepsilon(s_\alpha w) e^{s_\alpha w(p)}.$$

Now $s_\alpha w(p) = w(p) - \langle \alpha^\vee, w(p) \rangle \alpha = w(p) + n_w \alpha$, with $n_w \in \mathbf{Z}$. Thus,

$$\mathrm{J}(e^p) = \sum_{w \in \mathrm{M}} \varepsilon(w) e^{w(p)} (1 - e^{n_w \alpha}).$$

If $n_w \geqslant 0$, it is clear that $1 - e^{n_w \alpha}$ is divisible by $1 - e^\alpha$ and this is also true when $n_w < 0$ since $1 - e^{n_w \alpha} = -e^{n_w \alpha}(1 - e^{-n_w \alpha})$. Hence, $\mathrm{J}(e^p)$ is divisible by $1 - e^\alpha$ in $\mathbf{Z}[\mathrm{P}]$.

By Lemma 1, $\mathbf{Z}[\mathrm{P}]$ is factorial and the elements $1 - e^\alpha$ for $\alpha \in \mathrm{R}$ and $\alpha > 0$ are mutually prime. It follows that $\mathrm{J}(e^p)$ is divisible in $\mathbf{Z}[\mathrm{P}]$ by the product $\prod_{\alpha > 0} (1 - e^\alpha)$, and hence also by $d = e^{-\rho} \prod_{\alpha > 0} (1 - e^\alpha)$.

Returning to the general case, by extension of scalars from $\mathbf{Z}$ to A, we deduce from the above that $d = \mathrm{J}(e^\rho)$ and that every element $\mathrm{J}(e^p)$ is divisible by d. Since e^ρ is the unique maximal term of d, the *Remark* of no. 2 shows that there exists a unique element $y \in \mathrm{A}[\mathrm{P}]$ such that $\mathrm{J}(e^p) = dy$ and it follows immediately that y is invariant under W, and hence that d and $\mathrm{J}(e^p)$ are anti-invariant. This proves (i) and (ii).

Finally, if 2 is not a zero divisor in A, the *Remark* of no. 2 and Prop. 1 imply (iii).

Remarks. 1) If 2 is not a zero divisor in A, it is easy to check that d is the unique anti-invariant element of $\mathrm{A}[\mathrm{P}]$ with e^ρ as its maximal term.

2) Lemma 2 of no. 2 shows that the unique maximal term of the quotient $\mathrm{J}(e^p)/d$ (for $p \in \mathrm{P} \cap \mathrm{C}$) is $e^{p-\rho}$.

4. INVARIANT ELEMENTS

Let $A[P]^W$ be the subalgebra of A[P] consisting of the elements invariant under W. For $p \in P$, denote by W.p the orbit of p under W, and let $S(e^p) = \sum_{q \in W.p} e^q$ be the sum of the W-transforms of e^p; this is a W-invariant element. If $p \in P \cap \overline{C}$, $w(p) \leqslant p$ for all $w \in W$ (§ 1, no. 6, Prop. 18) and e^p is the unique maximal term of $S(e^p)$.

Let $x = \sum_p x_p e^p \in A[P]^W$; then $x_{w(p)} = x_p$ for all $p \in P$ and all $w \in W$. On the other hand, every orbit of W in P meets $P \cap \overline{C}$ in exactly one point (§ 1, no. 5, Th. 2). Hence,

$$x = \sum_{P \cap \overline{C}} x_p S(e^p). \tag{6}$$

We deduce:

Lemma 3. The $S(e^p)$ *for* $p \in P \cap \overline{C}$ *form a basis of the A-module* $A[P]^W$.

More generally:

PROPOSITION 3. *For any* $p \in P \cap \overline{C}$, *let* x_p *be an element of* $A[P]^W$ *with unique maximal term* e^p. *Then the family* $(x_p)_{p \in P \cap \overline{C}}$ *is a basis of the A-module* $A[P]^W$.

We first prove a lemma.

Lemma 4. Let I *be an ordered set satisfying the following condition:*

(MIN) *Every non-empty subset of* I *contains a minimal element.*

Let E *be an A-module,* $(e_i)_{i \in I}$ *a basis of* E *and* $(x_i)_{i \in I}$ *a family of elements of* E *such that*

$$x_i = e_i + \sum_{j<i} a_{ij} e_j,$$

for all $i \in I$ *(with* $a_{ij} \in A$, *the support of the family* (a_{ij}) *being finite for all* i*). Then,* $(x_i)_{i \in I}$ *is a basis of* E.

For any subset J of I, let E_J be the submodule of E with basis $(e_i)_{i \in J}$. Let $\mathfrak{S}$ be the set of subsets J of I with the following properties:

(*a*) If $i' \leqslant i$ and $i \in J$, then $i' \in J$;

(*b*) $(x_i)_{i \in J}$ is a basis of E_J.

It is immediate that $\mathfrak{S}$, ordered by inclusion, is inductive and non-empty. It therefore has a maximal element J. If $J \neq I$, let i_0 be a minimal element of $I - J$ and put $J' = J \cup \{i_0\}$. Every element $i \in I$ such that $i < i_0$ then belongs to J: it follows that J′ satisfies (*a*). On the other hand, J′ also satisfies (*b*): indeed,

$$e_{i_0} = x_{i_0} - \sum_{j<i_0} a_{i_0 j} e_j,$$

from which (*b*) follows. Hence $J' \in \mathfrak{S}$, a contradiction. Thus, $J = I$ and the lemma is proved.

We now prove Prop. 3. We apply Lemma 4 with $I = P \cap \overline{C}$. Let $q \in I$, and let I_q be the set of $p \in I$ such that $p \leqslant q$. If $p \in I_q$, the relations

$$q - p \geqslant 0, \quad p \in \overline{C}, \quad q \in \overline{C}$$

imply that

$$(q - p|p) \geqslant 0 \quad \text{and} \quad (q - p|q) \geqslant 0,$$

and hence that

$$(p|p) \leqslant (p|q) \leqslant (q|q).$$

The set I_q is thus *bounded.* Since I is discrete, it follows that I_q is *finite*, and it is clear that I satisfies the condition (MIN). On the other hand, for all $p \in I$,

$$x_p = e^p + \sum_{q<p} c_{pq} e^q$$

so by (6),

$$x_p = S(e^p) + \sum_{q<p, q\in I} c_{pq} S(e^q).$$

The proposition now follows from Lemmas 3 and 4.

THEOREM 1. *Let $\overline{\omega}_1, \dots, \overline{\omega}_l$ be the fundamental weights corresponding to the chamber C, and, for $1 \leqslant i \leqslant l$, let x_i be an element of $A[P]^W$ with $e^{\overline{\omega}_i}$ as its unique maximal term. Let*

$$\varphi : A[X_1, \dots, X_l] \to A[P]^W$$

be the homomorphism from the polynomial algebra $A[X_1, \dots, X_l]$ to $A[P]^W$ that takes X_i to x_i. Then, the map φ is an isomorphism.

Lemma 2 implies that the image under φ of the monomial $X_1^{n_1} \dots X_l^{n_l}$ is an element with unique maximal term $e^{n_1\overline{\omega}_1 + \dots + n_l\overline{\omega}_l}$. Since every element of $P \cap \overline{C}$ can be written uniquely in the form $n_1\overline{\omega}_1 + \dots + n_l\overline{\omega}_l$, Prop. 3 shows that the images under φ of the monomials $X_1^{n_1} \dots X_l^{n_l}$ are a basis of $A[P]^W$, hence the theorem.

Examples. 1) We can take $x_i = S(e^{\overline{\omega}_i})$.

2) By *Remark* 2 of no. 3, we can take $x_i = J(e^{\rho + \overline{\omega}_i})/d$ (with the notation in no. 3).

§ 4. CLASSIFICATION OF ROOT SYSTEMS

1. FINITE COXETER GROUPS

In this section, we are going to determine, up to isomorphism, all root systems, and consequently all crystallographic groups (§ 2, no. 5). More generally, we shall start by determining all finite groups generated by reflections in a finite-dimensional real vector space: this is equivalent (Chap. V, § 4, no. 8) to determining all finite Coxeter groups, or (Chap. V, § 4, no. 8, Th. 2) to determining all Coxeter matrices of finite order such that the associated bilinear form is positive and non-degenerate.

Let $\mathrm{M} = (m_{ij})_{i,j\in \mathrm{I}}$ be a Coxeter matrix of finite order l. Put

$$q_{ij} = -\cos(\pi/m_{ij}).$$

Recall that $q_{ii} = 1$ and that $q_{ij} = q_{ji}$ is zero or $\leqslant -1/2$ for $i \neq j$. Put $\mathrm{E} = \mathbf{R}^{\mathrm{I}}$ and let $(e_i)_{i\in\mathrm{I}}$ be the canonical basis of E. Denote by $(x|y)$ the bilinear form on E associated to M (Chap. V, § 4, no. 1) and q the quadratic form $x \mapsto (x|x)$ on E. For $x = \sum_{i\in\mathrm{I}} \xi_i x_i$,

$$\| x \|^2 = q(x) = \sum_{i,j\in\mathrm{I}} q_{ij}\xi_i\xi_j.$$

Denote by (X, f) the *Coxeter graph* of M (Chap. IV, § 1, no. 9). If a is an edge of X, $f(a)$ is called the *order* of a.

In the remainder of this number, the Coxeter group W(M) defined by M (Chap. V, § 4, no. 3) is assumed to be *finite*, so that q is positive and non-degenerate and X is a *forest* (Chap. V, § 4, no. 8, Prop. 8). We also assume that X is *connected* (in other words that the Coxeter group W(M) is *irreducible*), so that X is a *tree.*

From the condition that q is positive and non-degenerate, we shall obtain conditions on the m_{ij} that will enable us to list all the possibilities for the corresponding Coxeter graphs; it will only remain to show that these possibilities are actually realised, in other words that the corresponding groups W(M) are finite.

Lemma 1. For all i, $\sum_{j\neq i} q_{ij}^2 < 1$.

Let J be the set of $j \in \mathrm{I}$ such that $q_{ij} \neq 0$, in other words such that $\{i, j\}$ is an edge of X. If $j, j' \in \mathrm{J}$ and $j \neq j'$, $\{j, j'\}$ is not an edge (otherwise i, j, j' would form a circuit), so $(e_j|e_{j'}) = 0$. Let $\mathrm{F} = \sum_{j\in\mathrm{J}} \mathbf{R}e_j$. Then $(e_j)_{j\in\mathrm{J}}$ is an orthonormal basis of F. The distance d from e_i to F is given by $d^2 = 1 - \sum_{j\in\mathrm{J}} (e_i|e_j)^2 = 1 - \sum_{j\in\mathrm{J}} q_{ij}^2 = 1 - \sum_{j\neq i} q_{ij}^2$, hence the lemma.

Lemma 2. Any vertex of X *belongs to at most 3 edges.*

Indeed, if i is linked to h other vertices, the relations $q_{ij}^2 \geqslant \frac{1}{4}$ for these other vertices implies that $\frac{h}{4} < 1$ by Lemma 1, so $h \leqslant 3$.

Lemma 3. If i *belongs to 3 edges, these edges are of order 3.*

If not, we would have, in view of the relation $\cos\frac{\pi}{4} = \frac{\sqrt{2}}{2}$,

$$\sum_{j \neq i} q_{ij}^2 \geqslant \frac{1}{4} + \frac{1}{4} + (\frac{\sqrt{2}}{2})^2 = 1$$

which is impossible (Lemma 1).

Lemma 4. If there exists an edge of order $\geqslant 6$, *then* $l = 2$.

Indeed, let $\{i, j\}$ be such an edge. If $l > 2$, one of the edges i, j (say i) would be linked to a third vertex j', since X is connected. In view of the relation $\cos\frac{\pi}{6} = \frac{\sqrt{3}}{2}$ we would have

$$\sum_{k \neq i} q_{ik}^2 \geqslant \frac{1}{4} + (\frac{\sqrt{3}}{2})^2 = 1$$

which is impossible (Lemma 1).

Lemma 5. A *vertex cannot belong to two distinct edges of order* $\geqslant 4$.

Let i be such a vertex. We would have $\sum_{j \neq i} q_{ij}^2 \geqslant (\frac{\sqrt{2}}{2})^2 + (\frac{\sqrt{2}}{2})^2 = 1$, which is impossible (Lemma 1).

Let $\{i, j\}$ be an edge of X. We are going to define a new Coxeter graph, which will be obtained from the graph of M *by identifying* i *and* j. The set I' of its vertices is the quotient of I obtained by identifying i and j. Put $p = \{i, j\}$, which is an element of I', and identify the elements of I distinct from i and j with their canonical images in I'. Let k, k' be two distinct elements of I'. Then, $\{k, k'\}$ is an edge of the new graph in the following cases:

1) k and k' are distinct from p and $\{k, k'\}$ is an edge of X; in this case, the order of this edge is defined to be $m_{kk'}$;

2) $k = p$, and one of the sets $\{i, k'\}, \{j, k'\}$ is an edge of X; the order of $\{p, k'\}$ is defined to be $m_{ik'}$ if $\{i, k'\}$ is an edge of X, and $m_{jk'}$ if $\{j, k'\}$ is an edge of X (these two possibilities are mutually exclusive because X is a tree).

Let $\mathrm{M}' = (m'_{ij})_{i,j \in \mathrm{I}'}$ be the new Coxeter matrix thus defined, and put $q'_{ij} = -\cos\frac{\pi}{m'_{ij}}$. Then, for $k \neq p$, $q'_{pk} = q_{ik} + q_{jk}$. Thus, if $(\xi_i) \in \mathbf{R}^{\mathrm{I}'}$,

$$\sum_{k,k' \in \mathrm{I}'} q'_{kk'}\xi_k\xi_{k'} = \sum_{k,k' \in \mathrm{I}} q_{kk'}\xi_k\xi_{k'} + \xi_p^2 - \xi_i^2 - \xi_j^2 - 2q_{ij}\xi_i\xi_j \qquad (1)$$

$$= \sum_{k,k' \in \mathrm{I}} q_{kk'}\xi_k\xi_{k'} - (1 + 2q_{ij})\xi_p^2.$$

Lemma 6. If $\{i, j\}$ *is of order 3,* W(M′) *is a finite Coxeter group.*

Indeed, $q_{ij} = -\frac{1}{2}$, so (1) becomes

$$\sum_{k,k' \in \mathrm{I}'} q'_{kk'} \xi_k \xi_{k'} = \sum_{k,k' \in \mathrm{I}} q_{kk'} \xi_k \xi_{k'}$$

and $(\xi_k)_{k \in \mathrm{I}'} \mapsto \sum_{k,k' \in \mathrm{I}'} q'_{kk'} \xi_k \xi_{k'}$ is a positive non-degenerate quadratic form. It now suffices to apply Th. 2 of Chap. V, § 4, no. 8.

Lemma 7. We have one of the following:

a) X *has a unique ramification point* (Chap. IV, Appendix, no. 1), *and all the edges of* X *are of order 3.*

b) X *is a chain and has at most one edge of order* $\geqslant 4$.

We argue by induction on l.

a) Assume that X has a ramification point i. Then i belongs to 3 edges of order 3, $\{i, k_1\}, \{i, k_2\}, \{i, k_3\}$ (Lemmas 2 and 3). If $l = 4$ the lemma is proved. If not, then k_1, say, belongs to an edge distinct from those just mentioned since X is connected. Identify i and k_1 in the Coxeter graph of M. This gives a new graph to which the induction hypothesis can be applied, in view of Lemma 6. Now the image p of i is a ramification point of the new graph X′. Thus X′ has no other ramification point and all its edges are of order 3. Thus all the edges of X are of order 3, and i and k_1 are its only possible ramification points. But if k_1 were a ramification point of X, p would belong to at least 4 edges in X′, contrary to Lemma 2.

b) Assume that X has no ramification point. Then X is a chain (Chap. IV, Appendix, no. 3, Prop. 3). Let $\{i, j\}$ be an edge of order $\geqslant 4$. If $l = 2$, the lemma is trivial. If not, then i, say, belongs to an edge $\{i, k\}$ with $k \neq j$ (since X is connected). This edge is of order 3 (Lemma 5). Identify i and k in the Coxeter graph of M. By Lemma 6, the induction hypothesis can be applied. Let p be the image of i in the new graph X′. In X′, $\{p, j\}$ is an edge of order $\geqslant 4$, so X′ has no other edge of order $\geqslant 4$, and hence $\{i, j\}$ is the only edge of order $\geqslant 4$ in X.

Lemma 8. Let $i_1, i_2, \ldots, i_p$ *be vertices of* X *such that* $\{i_1, i_2\}, \{i_2, i_3\}, \ldots$ $\ldots, \{i_{p-1}, i_p\}$ *are edges of order 3. Then* $q(\sum_{r=1}^{p} r e_{i_r}) = \frac{1}{2} p(p+1)$.

We have $(e_{i_r}|e_{i_r}) = 1, (e_{i_r}|e_{i_{r+1}}) = -\frac{1}{2}, (e_{i_r}|e_{i_s}) = 0$ if $s > r+1$. Thus

$$q(\sum_{r=1}^{p} r e_{i_r}) = \sum_{r=1}^{p} r^2 - 2 \sum_{r=1}^{p-1} \frac{1}{2} r(r+1) = p^2 - \sum_{r=1}^{p-1} r.$$

By *Theory of Sets*, Chap. III, § 5, no. 8, Cor. to Prop. 14, this is equal to

$$p^2 - \frac{1}{2} p(p-1) = \frac{1}{2} p(p+1).$$

Lemma 9. Assume that X *is a chain with vertices* $1, 2, \dots, l$ *and edges* $\{1,2\}, \{2,3\}, \dots, \{l-1, l\}$.

(i) *If one of the edges* $\{2,3\}, \{3,4\}, \dots, \{l-2, l-1\}$ *is of order* $\geqslant 4$, *this edge is of order 4 and the graph is the following:*

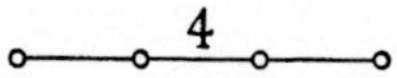

(ii) *If the edge* $\{1,2\}$ *is of order 5, the graph is one of the following:*

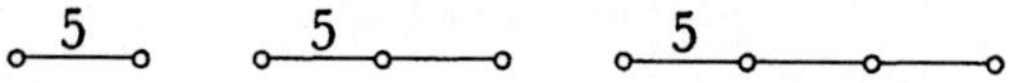

We can assume that $l > 2$ (Lemma 4). Assume that $\{i, i+1\}$ is of order $\geqslant 4$, with $1 \leqslant i \leqslant l-1$. Put

$$x = e_1 + 2e_2 + \cdots + ie_i, \; y = e_i + 2e_{l-1} + \cdots + (l-i)e_{i+1}, \text{ and } j = l-i.$$

By Lemma 8, $\| x \|^2 = \frac{1}{2}i(i+1), \| y \|^2 = \frac{1}{2}j(j+1)$. On the other hand, $(x|y) = ij(e_i|e_{i+1}) = -ij\cos\frac{\pi}{m}$ with $m = 4$ or 5 (Lemma 4). Now

$$(x|y)^2 < \| x \|^2 \| y \|^2,$$

which gives

$$\frac{1}{4}ij(i+1)(j+1) > i^2 j^2 \cos^2\frac{\pi}{m}$$

so

$$(i+1)(j+1) > 4ij\cos^2\frac{\pi}{m} \geqslant 2ij.$$

This gives, first of all, $ij - i - j - 1 < 0$, or $(i-1)(j-1) < 2$. If

$$1 < i < l-1,$$

then $1 < j < l-1$, so $i = j = 2$, and so [1]

$$9 > 16\cos^2\frac{\pi}{m}, \quad \text{thus} \quad \cos^2\frac{\pi}{m} < \cos^2\frac{\pi}{5}$$

and hence $m = 4$. This proves (i). If $i = 1$ and $m = 5$, then $2j + 2 > 4j\frac{3+\sqrt{5}}{8}$, or $j\frac{\sqrt{5}-1}{2} < 2$, $j < \sqrt{5}+1 < 4$, and so $l = j+1 \leqslant 4$. This proves (ii).

---

[1] The 5th roots of 1 distinct from 1 are the solutions of $z^4 + z^3 + z^2 + z + 1 = 0$. Putting $x = \frac{1}{2}(z + \frac{1}{z})$, this equation becomes $(2x)^2 - 2 + 2x + 1 = 0$, or $4x^2 + 2x - 1 = 0$, so $x = \frac{-1\pm\sqrt{5}}{4}$. Hence,

$$2\cos^2\frac{\pi}{5} - 1 = \cos\frac{2\pi}{5} = \frac{\sqrt{5}-1}{4}, \; \cos^2\frac{\pi}{5} = \frac{3+\sqrt{5}}{8} > \frac{5}{8} > \frac{9}{16}, \; \cos\frac{\pi}{5} = \frac{1+\sqrt{5}}{4}.$$

Lemma 10. If X *has a ramification point* i, *the full subgraph* $\mathrm{X}-\{i\}$ *is the union of three chains, and if* $p-1$, $q-1$, $r-1$ *are the lengths of these chains, the triple* $\{p,q,r\}$ *is equal, up to a permutation, to one of the triples* $\{1,2,2\}$, $\{1,2,3\}$, $\{1,2,4\}$, $\{1,1,m\}$ *(for some* $m \geqslant 1$*).*

The vertex i belongs to 3 edges (Lemma 2), and there is no other ramification point (Lemma 7), so the full subgraph $\mathrm{X}-\{i\}$ is the sum of 3 chains X_1, X_2, X_3 each of which has a terminal vertex linked to i in X. Let $\{i_1,i_2\}$, $\{i_2,i_3\},\ldots,\{i_{p-1},i_p\}$ be the edges of X_1, $\{j_1,j_2\}$, $\{j_2,j_3\},\ldots,\{j_{q-1},j_q\}$ those of X_2, and $\{k_1,k_2\}$, $\{k_2,k_3\},\ldots,\{k_{r-1},k_r\}$ those of X_3, with i_1, j_1, k_1 linked to i in X. We can assume that $p \geqslant q \geqslant r \geqslant 1$. Put

$$\begin{aligned} x &= e_{i_p} + 2e_{i_{p-1}} + \cdots + pe_{i_1} \\ y &= e_{j_q} + 2e_{j_{q-1}} + \cdots + qe_{j_1} \\ z &= e_{k_r} + 2e_{k_{r-1}} + \cdots + re_{k_1}. \end{aligned}$$

Since all the edges of X are of order 3 (Lemma 7), Lemma 8 gives $\| x \|^2 = \frac{1}{2}p(p+1)$, $\| y \|^2 = \frac{1}{2}q(q+1)$, $\| z \|^2 = \frac{1}{2}r(r+1)$. On the other hand, e_i is orthogonal to $e_{i_2}, e_{i_3}, \ldots, e_{i_p}$, so $(e_i|x) = p(e_i|e_{i_1}) = -\frac{1}{2}p$; similarly $(e_i|y) = -\frac{1}{2}q$, $(e_i|z) = -\frac{1}{2}r$. The unit vectors $\| x \|^{-1} x$, $\| y \|^{-1} y$, $\| z \|^{-1} z$ are mutually orthogonal, and e_i does not belong to the subspace F that they generate; the square of the distance from e_i to F is

$$\begin{aligned} 1 - (e_i|\frac{x}{\| x \|})^2 - (e_i|\frac{y}{\| y \|})^2 - (e_i|\frac{z}{\| z \|})^2 & \\ &= 1 - \frac{1}{2}\frac{p}{p+1} - \frac{1}{2}\frac{q}{q+1} - \frac{1}{2}\frac{r}{r+1} \\ &= 1 - \frac{1}{2} + \frac{1}{2}\frac{1}{p+1} - \frac{1}{2} + \frac{1}{2}\frac{1}{q+1} - \frac{1}{2} + \frac{1}{2}\frac{1}{r+1}. \end{aligned}$$

Since this quantity is > 0, we have

$$(p+1)^{-1} + (q+1)^{-1} + (r+1)^{-1} > 1. \tag{4}$$

Hence $3(r+1)^{-1} > 1$, so $r < 2$ and finally $r = 1$. Then (4) gives

$$(p+1)^{-1} + (q+1)^{-1} > \frac{1}{2} \tag{5}$$

hence $2(q+1)^{-1} > \frac{1}{2}$, so $q \leqslant 2$. Finally, if $q = 2$, (5) gives

$$(p+1)^{-1} > \frac{1}{6}, \quad \text{hence } p \leqslant 4.$$

THEOREM 1. *The graph of any irreducible finite Coxeter system* (W, S) *is isomorphic to one of the following:*

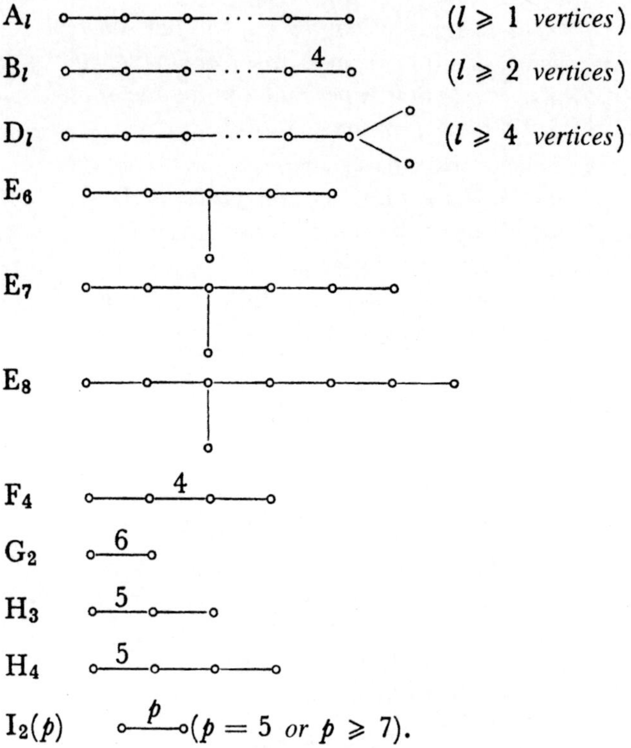

No two of these graphs are isomorphic.

Indeed, let $W = (m_{ij})$ be the Coxeter matrix of (W, S), and let $l =$ Card(S). If one of the m_{ij} is $\geqslant 6$, then $l = 2$ (Lemma 4) and the Coxeter graph of (W, S) is of type G_2 or $I_2(p)$ with $p \geqslant 7$. Assume now that all the $m_{ij} \leqslant 5$.

a) If the m_{ij} are not all equal to 3, the graph X of (W, S) is a chain and exactly one of the m_{ij} is equal to 4 or 5 (Lemma 7). If one of the m_{ij} is equal to 5, Lemma 9 shows that we have one of the types H_3, H_4 or $I_2(5)$. If one of the m_{ij} is equal to 4, Lemma 9 shows that we have one of the types B_l or F_4.

b) Assume now that all the m_{ij} are equal to 3. If X is a chain, the Coxeter graph is of type A_l. If not, Lemma 10 shows that it is of type E_6, E_7, E_8 or D_l.

The fact that no two of the Coxeter graphs listed are isomorphic is clear.

Conversely:

THEOREM 2. *The Coxeter groups defined by the Coxeter graphs* $A_l, B_l, \ldots,$ $I_2(p)$ *of Th. 1 are finite.*

This is clear for $I_2(p)$, the corresponding group being the dihedral group of order $2p$ (Chap. IV, § 1, no. 9). For H_4 the corresponding quadratic form is

$$\begin{aligned}
&\xi_1^2 + \xi_2^2 + \xi_3^2 + \xi_4^2 - \xi_1\xi_2 - \xi_2\xi_3 - 2(\cos\frac{\pi}{5})\xi_3\xi_4 \\
&= \xi_1^2 + \xi_2^2 + \xi_3^2 + \xi_4^2 - \xi_1\xi_2 - \xi_2\xi_3 - \frac{1+\sqrt{5}}{2}\xi_3\xi_4 \\
&= (\xi_2 - \frac{\xi_1+\xi_3}{2})^2 + (\xi_4 - \frac{1+\sqrt{5}}{4}\xi_3)^2 + \frac{3}{4}(\xi_1 - \frac{1}{3}\xi_3)^2 + \frac{7-3\sqrt{5}}{24}\xi_3^2.
\end{aligned}$$

Since $7 - 3\sqrt{5}$ is > 0, this form is positive non-degenerate, and the corresponding Coxeter group is finite. The same holds for that corresponding to H_3, since it is isomorphic to a subgroup of the preceding (Chap. IV, § 1, no. 8).

For the types A_l, $B_l, \dots, G_2$, we shall construct, in Nos. 5 to 13, root systems having the corresponding groups as Weyl groups. We shall see that these groups are not only finite, but *crystallographic* (§ 2, no. 5).

2. DYNKIN GRAPHS

By abuse of language, we shall call a *normed graph* a pair (Γ, f) having the following properties:

1) Γ is a graph (called the *underlying* graph of (Γ, f)).

2) If E denotes the set of pairs (i, j) such that $\{i, j\}$ is an edge of Γ, f is a map from E to $\mathbf{R}$ such that $f(i, j)f(j, i) = 1$ for all $(i, j) \in E$.

There is an obvious notion of isomorphism of normed graphs.

Let R be a reduced root system in a real vector space V. We are going to associate to it a normed graph (X, f), called the *Dynkin graph* of R. The vertices of X will be the elements of the set I of orbits of W(R) in the union of the sets $\{B\} \times B$ (where B is the set of bases of R). If $N = (n_{ij})_{i,j\in I}$ (resp. $M = (m_{ij})_{i,j\in I}$) is the canonical Cartan matrix (resp. the Coxeter matrix) of R (§ 1, no. 5, *Remark* 7), two vertices i and j of X are linked if and only if $n_{ij} \neq 0$ and we then put

$$f(i, j) = \frac{n_{ij}}{n_{ji}}.$$

Since $n_{ij} = 0$ implies $n_{ji} = 0$, this defines a normed graph (X, f).

Let $(x|y)$ be a scalar product on V, invariant under W(R), and let $B = (\alpha_i)_{i\in I}$ be a basis of R, indexed canonically. Formulas (7) and (9) of § 1, no. 1 show that vertices i and j of the graph X are linked if and only if

$$(\alpha_i|\alpha_j) \neq 0$$

and that

$$f(i, j) = \frac{(\alpha_i|\alpha_i)}{(\alpha_j|\alpha_j)}.$$

In view of the results of § 1, Nos. 3 and 5, the only possibilities are the following, up to interchanging i and j:

1) i and j are not linked; $n_{ij} = n_{ji} = 0$; $m_{ij} = 2$;
2) $f(i,j) = f(j,i) = 1$; $n_{ij} = n_{ji} = -1$; $m_{ij} = 3$;
3) $f(i,j) = 2$, $f(j,i) = 1/2$; $n_{ij} = -2$, $n_{ji} = -1$; $m_{ij} = 4$;
4) $f(i,j) = 3$, $f(j,i) = 1/3$; $n_{ij} = -3$, $n_{ji} = -1$; $m_{ij} = 6$.

We see from this that the Dynkin graph R determines the Cartan matrix and the Coxeter matrix of R, and hence determines R up to isomorphism. More precisely, the Cor. of Prop. 15 of § 1, no. 5 implies the following result:

PROPOSITION 1. *Let* R_1 *and* R_2 *be two reduced root systems in vector spaces* V_1 *and* V_2. *Let* $B_1 = (\alpha_i)_{i \in I_1}$ *and* $B_2 = (\alpha_i)_{i \in I_2}$ *be bases of* R_1 *and* R_2, *indexed canonically. Let* λ *be an isomorphism from the Dynkin graph of* R_1 *to the Dynkin graph of* R_2. *Then, there exists a unique isomorphism from* V_1 *to* V_2 *transforming* R_1 *into* R_2 *and* α_i *into* $\alpha_{\lambda(i)}$ *for all* $i \in I_1$.

It is clear that an automorphism of R defines an automorphism of the Dynkin graph of R, and hence a homomorphism φ from the group A(R) to the group of automorphisms of the Dynkin graph of R.

COROLLARY. *The homomorphism* φ *defines by passage to the quotient an isomorphism from the group* A(R)/W(R) *to the group of automorphisms of the Dynkin graph of* R.

Clearly, $\varphi(g) = \mathrm{Id}$ for all $g \in W(R)$. On the other hand, Prop. 1 shows that there exists an isomorphism ψ from the group of isomorphisms of the Dynkin graph of R to the subgroup E of elements of A(R) leaving fixed a given basis B of R, such that $\varphi \circ \psi = \mathrm{Id}$. Since A(R) is the semi-direct product of E and W(R) (§ 1, no. 5, Prop. 16), the corollary follows.

In practice, the Dynkin graph (X, f) is represented by a diagram composed of nodes and bonds in the following way. The nodes correspond to the vertices of X; two nodes corresponding to two distinct vertices i and j are joined by 0, 1, 2 or 3 bonds in cases 1), 2), 3) and 4) above (up to interchanging i and j). Moreover, in cases 3) and 4), that is when $f(i,j) > 1$, or when the roots α_1 and α_j are not orthogonal and not of the same length, an inequality sign $>$ is placed on the double or triple bond joining the nodes corresponding to i and j oriented towards the node corresponding to j (that is, the shortest root):

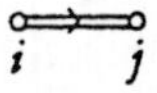 (for $f(i,j) = 2$), 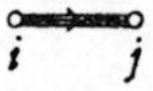 (for $f(i,j) = 3$).

It is clear that the Dynkin graph (X, f) can be recovered from this diagram.

We remark that the diagram associated to the Coxeter graph of W(R) can be obtained from that associated to the Dynkin graph of R by keeping the nodes and the single bonds and replacing the double (resp. triple) bonds by a bond surmounted by the number 4 (resp. 6). Conversely, given the Coxeter graph of W(R), the diagram associated to the Dynkin graph of R can be recovered using the inverse of this procedure, except for the inequality signs on the double or triple bonds. Th. 1 thus gives immediately the list of possible Dynkin graphs. More precisely:

THEOREM 3. *If* R *is an irreducible reduced root system, its Dynkin graph is isomorphic to one of the graphs represented by the following diagrams:*

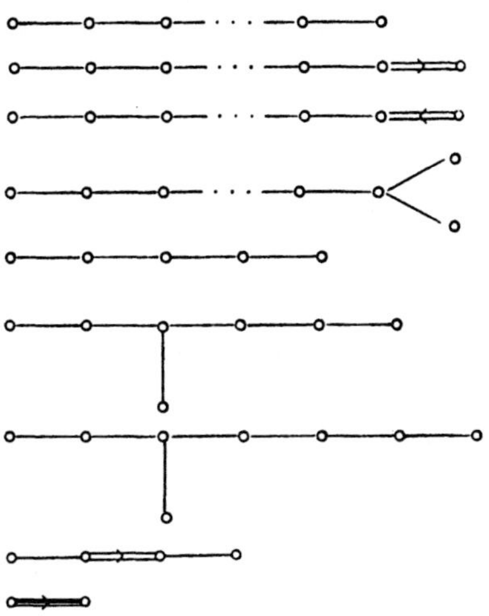

A_l ($l \geqslant 1$ *vertices*)
B_l ($l \geqslant 2$ *vertices*)
C_l ($l \geqslant 3$ *vertices*)
D_l ($l \geqslant 4$ *vertices*)
E_6
E_7
E_8
F_4
G_2

No two of these graphs are isomorphic and there are irreducible reduced root systems having each of them as their Dynkin graph (up to isomorphism).

The first assertion follows immediately from Th. 1, in view of the preceding remarks, the fact that the Coxeter groups of the graphs H_3, H_4 and $I_2(p)$ (for $p = 5$ and $p \geqslant 7$) are not crystallographic, and the fact that the two possible inequalities for the double (resp. triple) bond of the Dynkin graph associated to the Coxeter graph F_4 (resp. G_2) give isomorphic Dynkin graphs. The second assertion is clear and the third will follow from the explicit construction of an irreducible reduced root system for each type, a construction that will be carried out in Nos. 5 to 13.

Remarks. 1) The graph A_1 reduces to a single node; we denote it also by B_1 or C_1. The graph B_2 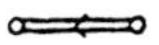 is also denoted by C_2. The graph A_3 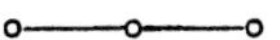 is also denoted by D_3. Finally, D_2 denotes the graph consisting of two unconnected nodes. (These conventions are derived from the properties of the corresponding root systems, cf. nos. 5 to 8.)

2) If (X, f) is the Dynkin graph of a reduced root system R, the Dynkin graph of the inverse system can be identified with (X, f^{-1}). In other words, the diagram associated to the Dynkin graph of $R^\vee$ can be obtained from that associated to the Dynkin graph of R by reversing the inequality signs. If R is irreducible, we see that R is isomorphic to $R^\vee$ unless R is of type B_l or C_l, in which case $R^\vee$ is of type C_l or B_l.

3. AFFINE WEYL GROUP AND COMPLETED DYNKIN GRAPH

Let R be an irreducible reduced root system and let (X, f) be its Dynkin graph. We are going to define another normed graph $(\tilde{X}, \tilde{f})$ that we shall call the *completed Dynkin graph* of R. The set $\tilde{I}$ of vertices of $\tilde{X}$ consists of the set I of vertices of X and a vertex denoted by 0, not belonging to I. To define $\tilde{f}$, choose a basis $B = (\alpha_i)_{i \in I}$ of R and a scalar product $(x|y)$ invariant under W(R). Let α_0 be *the negative of the highest root* for the order defined by B. Two distinct vertices $i, j \in \tilde{I}$ are linked if and only if $(\alpha_i|\alpha_j) \neq 0$ and we then put

$$\tilde{f}(i,j) = \frac{(\alpha_i|\alpha_i)}{(\alpha_j|\alpha_j)}.$$

It is immediate that the graph $\tilde{X}$ and the map $\tilde{f}$ thus defined do not depend on the choice of B or the scalar product.

If the rank l of R is equal to 1, then $I = \{i\}$ and $\alpha_0 = -\alpha_1$; hence $\tilde{f}(0,i) = 1$. If $l \geqslant 2$, α_0 is not proportional to any of the α_i and $(\alpha_0|\alpha_i)$ is $\leqslant 0$ (§ 1, no. 8, Prop. 25). For any pair (i,j) of distinct elements of $\tilde{I}$, the only possibilities are those denoted by 1), 2), 3), 4) in the preceding number (putting, for example, $n_{0i} = n(\alpha_0, \alpha_i)$ and m_{0i} = order of $s_{\alpha_0} s_{\alpha_i}$ for all $i \in I$).

In the case $l \geqslant 2$, the completed Dynkin graph is represented by a diagram with the same conventions as in the preceding number, sometimes indicating by dotted lines the bonds joining the vertex 0 to the other vertices. We remark that the inequality sign $>$ on such a bond, if it exists, is always directed towards the vertex distinct from 0, since α_0 is a longest root (§ 1, no. 8, Prop. 25). The graph (X, f) is the subgraph obtained from $(\tilde{X}, \tilde{f})$ by deleting the vertex 0.

The action of A(R) on (X, f) extends to an action on $(\tilde{X}, \tilde{f})$, leaving 0 fixed, and W(R) acts trivially on $(\tilde{X}, \tilde{f})$.

We retain the notations of § 2. Prop. 5 of § 2, no. 2, together with Th. 1 of Chap. V, § 3, no. 2, shows that the Coxeter graph Σ of the affine Weyl group $W_a(R)$ can be obtained from $(\tilde{X}, \tilde{f})$ by the same rules by which the Coxeter graph of W(R) is obtained from (X, f). On the other hand, let G be the normaliser of $W_a(R)$ (§ 2, no. 3). To any $g \in G$ corresponds an automorphism $\varphi(g)$ of Σ and $\varphi(g) = \mathrm{Id}$ if $g \in W_a(R)$. Conversely, given an automorphism λ of Σ there is, by Prop. 11 of Chap. V, § 4, no. 9, a unique element $g = \psi(\lambda)$ preserving a given alcove C and such that $\varphi(g) = \lambda$. Since G is the semi-direct product of the subgroup G_C of elements preserving C and $W_a(R)$ (§ 2, no. 3), we deduce that φ defines by passage to the quotient an *isomorphism from* G/W_a *(or from* G_C*) to* $\mathrm{Aut}(\Sigma)$. It is immediate that the composite of this isomorphism with the canonical map from A(R)/W(R) to G/W_a coincides with the homomorphism from A(R)/W(R) to $\mathrm{Aut}(\Sigma)$ induced by the homomorphism from A(R)/W(R) to $\mathrm{Aut}(\tilde{X}, \tilde{f})$ defined above. By § 2, no. 3, the group $\mathrm{Aut}(\Sigma)$ is isomorphic to the semi-direct product of

A(R)/W(R) by P(R˘)/Q(R˘), and P(R˘)/Q(R˘) is isomorphic to the group $\Gamma_C = G_C \cap W'_a$ (with the notation of § 2, no. 3); the element of $\mathrm{Aut}(\Sigma)$ corresponding to the element γ_i of Γ_C transforms the vertex 0 to the vertex i of Σ.

Remark. It can be shown that the canonical map

$$\mathrm{Aut}(\tilde{X}, \tilde{f}) \to \mathrm{Aut}(\Sigma)$$

is an isomorphism.

THEOREM 4. *Let* (W, S) *be an irreducible Coxeter system with* S *finite. The associated quadratic form* (Chap. V, § 4, no. 1) *is positive and degenerate if and only if the Coxeter graph of* (W, S) *is isomorphic to one of the following:*

$\tilde{A}_1$ 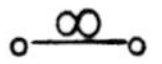

$\tilde{A}_l$ $(l \geqslant 2)$ 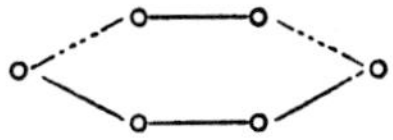 *(circuit with* $l + 1$ *vertices)*

$\tilde{B}_2$ 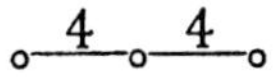

$\tilde{B}_l$ $(l \geqslant 3)$ 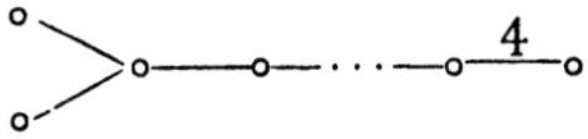

($l + 1$ *vertices*)

$\tilde{C}_l$ $(l \geqslant 3)$ 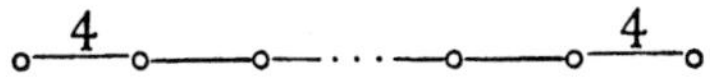

($l + 1$ *vertices*)

$\tilde{D}_l$ $(l \geqslant 4)$ 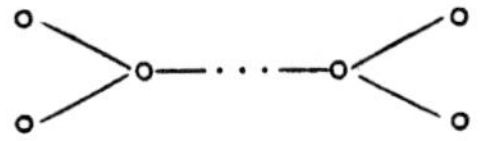 ($l + 1$ *vertices*)

$\tilde{E}_6$ 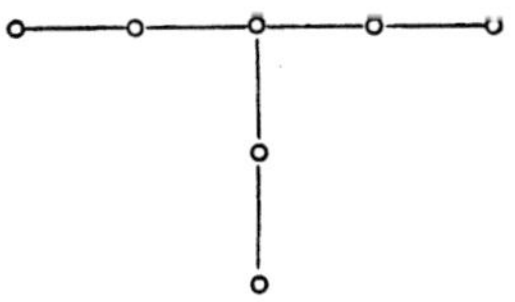

$\tilde{E}_7$ 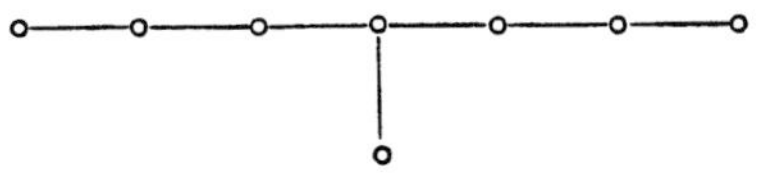

$\tilde{E}_8$ 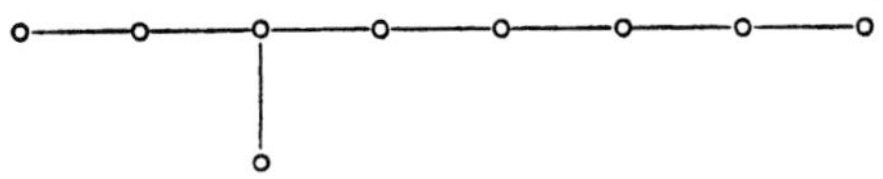

$\tilde{F}_4$ 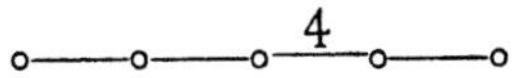

$\tilde{G}_2$ 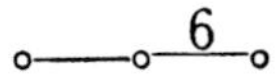

No two of these Coxeter graphs are isomorphic.

By Chap. V, § 4, no. 9 and Prop. 8 of § 2, no. 5, the Coxeter systems whose quadratic form is positive and degenerate are those which correspond to the affine Weyl groups of irreducible reduced root systems. The theorem therefore follows from the determination of the completed Dynkin graphs made in nos. 5 to 13 below.

4. PRELIMINARIES TO THE CONSTRUCTION OF ROOT SYSTEMS

Let V be a real vector space of dimension $l \geqslant 1$ equipped with a scalar product $(x|y)$, L a discrete subgroup of V, Λ a finite set of numbers > 0, and R the set of $\alpha \in$ L such that $(\alpha|\alpha) \in \Lambda$. Assume that R generates V and that, for any pair (α, β) of points of R, the number $2\frac{(\alpha|\beta)}{(\alpha|\alpha)}$ is an integer. Then, R *is a root system in* V. Indeed, R clearly satisfies $(\mathrm{RS_I})$. Let $\alpha \in$ R; let s_α be the orthogonal reflection $x \mapsto x - 2\frac{(x|\alpha)}{(\alpha|\alpha)}\alpha$; then, if $\beta \in$ R, we have $2\frac{(\beta|\alpha)}{(\alpha|\alpha)} \in \mathbf{Z}$, so $s_\alpha(\beta) \in$ L, and moreover $\| s_\alpha(\beta) \| = \| \beta \|$, so $s_\alpha(\beta) \in$ R; thus, R satisfies $(\mathrm{RS_{II}})$ and $(\mathrm{RS_{III}})$, and is reduced if Λ does not contain two numbers of the form λ and 4λ.

Now let V be a subspace of $\mathrm{E} = \mathbf{R}^n$. Let $(\varepsilon_1, \ldots, \varepsilon_n)$ be the canonical basis of E; we equip E with the scalar product for which this basis is orthonormal and identify E^* with E (resp. V^* with V) by means of this scalar product. We define subgroups $\mathrm{L_0}, \mathrm{L_1}, \mathrm{L_2}, \mathrm{L_3}$ of E as follows:

1) $\mathrm{L_0}$ is the $\mathbf{Z}$-module with basis (ε_i). We have $(\alpha|\beta) \in \mathbf{Z}$ for all $\alpha, \beta \in \mathrm{L_0}$. The vectors $\alpha \in \mathrm{L_0}$ for which $(\alpha|\alpha) = 1$ are the $\pm\varepsilon_i$ $(1 \leqslant i \leqslant n)$; those for which $(\alpha|\alpha) = 2$ are the $\pm\varepsilon_i \pm \varepsilon_j$ for $i < j$ (the two signs $\pm$, in $\pm\varepsilon_i \pm \varepsilon_j$, are chosen independently of each other; we adopt an analogous convention throughout the remainder of this section).

2) $\mathrm{L_1}$ is the $\mathbf{Z}$-submodule of $\mathrm{L_0}$ consisting of the $x = \sum_{i=1}^{n} \xi_i\varepsilon_i \in \mathrm{L_0}$ such that $\sum_{i=1}^{n} \xi_i$ is even; since ξ_i and ξ_i^2 have the same parity, this is equivalent to requiring that $(x|x)$ is even. Let L'_1 be the submodule of $\mathrm{L_1}$ generated by the $\varepsilon_i \pm \varepsilon_j$; we have $\sum_{i=1}^{n} \xi_i\varepsilon_i \equiv (\sum_{i=1}^{n} \xi_i)\varepsilon_n \pmod{\mathrm{L}'_1}$, and since $2\varepsilon_n = (\varepsilon_1 + \varepsilon_n) - (\varepsilon_1 - \varepsilon_n) \in \mathrm{L}'_1$, it follows that $\mathrm{L}'_1 = \mathrm{L_1}$. Since $\mathrm{L_0}$ is generated by $\mathrm{L_1}$ and ε_1, $\mathrm{L_0}/\mathrm{L_1}$ is isomorphic to $\mathbf{Z}/2\mathbf{Z}$.

3) $\mathrm{L_2} = \mathrm{L_0} + \mathbf{Z}(\frac{1}{2}\sum_{i=1}^{n} \varepsilon_i)$. It is clear that an element $x = \sum_{i=1}^{n} \xi_i\varepsilon_i$ of V is in $\mathrm{L_2}$ if and only if

$$2\xi_i \in \mathbf{Z}, \quad \xi_i - \xi_j \in \mathbf{Z} \text{ for all } i \text{ and } j. \tag{6}$$

Since $(\varepsilon_k|\frac{1}{2}\sum_{i=1}^{n} \varepsilon_i) = \frac{1}{2}$ for all k, and since $\| \frac{1}{2}\sum_{i=1}^{n} \varepsilon_i \|^2 = \frac{n}{4}$, we have $(\alpha|\beta) \in \frac{1}{2}\mathbf{Z}$ for $\alpha, \beta \in \mathrm{L_2}$ if n is even. The group $\mathrm{L_2}/\mathrm{L_0}$ is isomorphic to $\mathbf{Z}/2\mathbf{Z}$.

4) $L_3 = L_1 + \mathbf{Z}(\frac{1}{2}\sum_{i=1}^{n}\varepsilon_i)$. If n is a multiple of 4, L_3 is the set of $\sum_{i=1}^{n}\xi_i\varepsilon_i$ satisfying (6) and the condition $\sum_{i=1}^{n}\xi_i \in 2\mathbf{Z}$; in this case, $(\alpha|\beta) \in \mathbf{Z}$ for all $\alpha, \beta \in L_3$.

It is immediate that the subgroup of E associated to L_0 (resp. L_1, L_2) is L_0 (resp. L_2, L_1). The subgroup of E associated to L_3 is the set of

$$x = \sum_{i=1}^{n}\xi_i\varepsilon_i \in L_2$$

such that $(x|\frac{1}{2}\sum_{i=1}^{n}\varepsilon_i) \in \mathbf{Z}$, that is, such that $\sum_{i=1}^{n}\xi_i \in 2\mathbf{Z}$; if $n \equiv 0 \pmod{4}$, this associated subgroup is therefore L_3.

The abelian group L_2/L_1 is of order 4, and hence is isomorphic to $\mathbf{Z}/4\mathbf{Z}$ or $\mathbf{Z}/2\mathbf{Z} \times \mathbf{Z}/2\mathbf{Z}$ (*Algebra*, Chap. VII, § 4, no. 6, Th. 3). If n is odd,

$$p(\frac{1}{2}\sum_{i=1}^{n}\varepsilon_i) \in L_1 \Leftrightarrow p \equiv 0 \ (\text{mod. } 4)$$

so L_2/L_1 is cyclic of order 4. If n is even,

$$p(\frac{1}{2}\sum_{i=1}^{n}\varepsilon_i) \in L_1 \Leftrightarrow p \equiv 0 \ (\text{mod. } 2)$$

so L_2/L_1, which contains two distinct elements of order 2, is isomorphic to $\mathbf{Z}/2\mathbf{Z} \times \mathbf{Z}/2\mathbf{Z}$.

We shall use this notation throughout the next nine nos. and in the plates. For each type of Dynkin graph in Th. 3, we shall describe explicitly:

(I) A root system R and the number of roots.

(II) A basis B of R, and the corresponding positive roots. The basis B will be indexed by the integers $1, \dots, l$.

(III) The Coxeter number h (§ 1, no. 11).

(IV) The highest root $\tilde{\alpha}$ (for the order defined by B) and the completed Dynkin graph (no. 3). We shall indicate next to each vertex the corresponding root of B.

(V) The inverse system $R^\vee$, the canonical bilinear form and the constant $\gamma(R)$ (§ 1, no. 12).

(VI) The fundamental weights relative to B (§ 1, no. 10).

(VII) The sum of the positive roots.

(VIII) The groups $P(R), Q(R), P(R)/Q(R)$ and the connection index (§ 1, no. 9).

(IX) The exponents of W(R) (Chap. V, § 6, no. 2, Def. 2). In the cases A_l, B_l, C_l and D_l we determine the symmetric invariants.

(X) The order of W(R) (and in some cases its structure).

(XI) The group A(R)/W(R), its action on the Dynkin graph, and the element w_0 of W(R) that transforms B to $-$B.

(XII) The action of P(R˘)/Q(R˘) on the completed Dynkin graph and the action of A(R)/W(R) on P(R˘)/Q(R˘).

For each Dynkin graph in Th. 3, these data will be collected in Plates I to IX, and ordered in a uniform way as above. We also give:

(XIII) The Cartan matrix, from which the Dynkin graph is derived as described in no. 2.

5. SYSTEMS OF TYPE B_l ($l \geqslant 2$)

(I) We consider the group L_0 in $V = \mathbf{R}^l$ (no. 4). Let R be the set of $\alpha \in L_0$ such that $(\alpha|\alpha) = 1$ or $(\alpha|\alpha) = 2$, in other words the set of vectors $\pm\varepsilon_i$ $(1 \leqslant i \leqslant l)$ and $\pm\varepsilon_i \pm \varepsilon_j$ $(1 \leqslant i < j \leqslant l)$. It is clear that R generates V and that $2(\alpha|\beta)/(\alpha|\alpha) \in \mathbf{Z}$ for all $\alpha, \beta \in$ R. Thus R is a reduced root system in V (no. 4). The number of roots is $n = 2l + 4\frac{l(l-1)}{2} = 2l^2$.

(II) Put

$$\alpha_1 = \varepsilon_1 - \varepsilon_2,\ \alpha_2 = \varepsilon_2 - \varepsilon_3, \ldots, \alpha_{l-1} = \varepsilon_{l-1} - \varepsilon_l,\ \alpha_l = \varepsilon_l.$$

Then

$$\begin{aligned} \varepsilon_i &= \alpha_i + \alpha_{i+1} + \cdots + \alpha_l \quad (1 \leqslant i \leqslant l) \\ \varepsilon_i + \varepsilon_j &= (\alpha_i + \alpha_{i+1} + \cdots + \alpha_l) + (\alpha_j + \alpha_{j+1} + \cdots + \alpha_l) \ (1 \leqslant i < j \leqslant l) \\ \varepsilon_i - \varepsilon_j &= \alpha_i + \alpha_{i+1} + \cdots + \alpha_{j-1} \quad (1 \leqslant i < j \leqslant l). \end{aligned}$$

Thus $(\alpha_1, \alpha_2, \ldots, \alpha_l)$ is a basis of R (§ 1, no. 7, Cor. 3 of Prop. 20). Moreover, $\| \alpha_i \|^2 = 2$ for $i < l$, $\| \alpha_l \|^2 = 1$, $(\alpha_i|\alpha_{i+1}) = -1$ for $1 \leqslant i \leqslant l-1$, $(\alpha_i|\alpha_j) = 0$ for $j > i+1$; the Dynkin graph of R is thus of type B_l, which shows that R is irreducible. The positive roots are the ε_i and the $\varepsilon_i \pm \varepsilon_j$ $(i < j)$.

(III) By Th. 1 (ii) of Chap. V, § 6, no. 2,

$$h = n/l = 2l.$$

(IV) Let $\tilde{\alpha} = \varepsilon_1 + \varepsilon_2 = \alpha_1 + 2\alpha_2 + 2\alpha_3 + \cdots + 2\alpha_l$, which is a root. The sum of its coordinates relative to the basis (α_i) is $2l - 1 = h - 1$. In view of Prop. 31 of § 1, no. 11, $\tilde{\alpha}$ is the highest root of R. We have $(\tilde{\alpha}|\alpha_i) = 0$ for $i \neq 2$ and $(\tilde{\alpha}|\alpha_2) = 1$. Since α_2 is of length 1 (resp. $\sqrt{2}$) when $l = 2$ (resp. $l \geqslant 3$), the completed Dynkin graph of R is as follows:

for $l = 2$

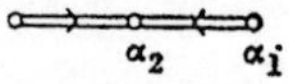

for $l \geqslant 3$

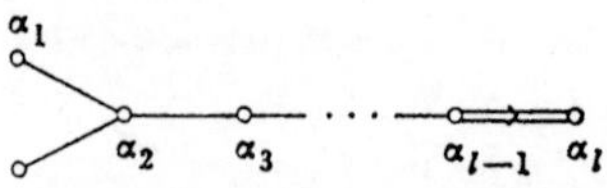

(V) The formula $\alpha^{\check{}} = \frac{2\alpha}{(\alpha|\alpha)}$ gives for $R^{\check{}}$ the set of vectors $\pm 2\varepsilon_i$ $(1 \leqslant i \leqslant l)$, $\pm\varepsilon_i \pm \varepsilon_j$ $(1 \leqslant i < j \leqslant l)$. The Dynkin graph of $R^{\check{}}$ is obtained from that of R by the procedure explained in no. 2, and we see that $R^{\check{}}$ is of type C_l.

There are $4l-2$ roots not orthogonal to $\beta = \varepsilon_1$, namely $\pm\varepsilon_1$ and $\pm\varepsilon_1 \pm \varepsilon_j$ for $2 \leqslant j \leqslant l$; for each such root α, $n(\alpha, \beta) = \pm 2$. Formula (17) of § 1, no. 12 shows that, for Φ_R, the square of the length of β is $(4l-2)^{-1}$; hence $\Phi_R(x, y) = (x|y)/(4l-2)$. Apply formula (18) of § 1, no. 12 with $x = y = \beta$. This gives

$$2 + \frac{1}{4}(4l-4) = \gamma(R)\frac{1}{4l-2}$$

and so $\gamma(R) = (l+1)(4l-2)$.

(VI) The fundamental weights ω_i $(1 \leqslant i \leqslant l)$ such that $(\omega_i|\alpha_j) = \delta_{ij}$ are easily calculated, and we find that

$$\begin{aligned}\omega_i &= \varepsilon_1 + \varepsilon_2 + \cdots + \varepsilon_i \\ &= \alpha_1 + 2\alpha_2 + \cdots + (i-1)\alpha_{i-1} + i(\alpha_1 + \alpha_{i+1} + \cdots + \alpha_l) \quad (i < l) \\ \omega_l &= \frac{1}{2}(\varepsilon_1 + \varepsilon_2 + \cdots + \varepsilon_l) = \frac{1}{2}(\alpha_1 + 2\alpha_2 + \cdots + l\alpha_l).\end{aligned}$$

(VII) The sum of the positive roots is

$$\begin{aligned}2\rho &= (2l-1)\varepsilon_1 + (2l-3)\varepsilon_2 + \cdots + 3\varepsilon_{l-1} + \varepsilon_l \\ &= (2l-1)\alpha_1 + 2(2l-2)\alpha_2 + \cdots + i(2l-i)\alpha_i + \cdots + l^2\alpha_l.\end{aligned}$$

(VIII) We have $Q(R) = L_0$ (no. 4), and P(R) is generated by Q(R) and ω_l, hence is equal to L_2 (no. 4). Hence, P(R)/Q(R) is isomorphic to $\mathbf{Z}/2\mathbf{Z}$, and the connection index is equal to 2.

(IX) and (X) In $\mathbf{R}^l$, the orthogonal reflection $s_{\varepsilon_i - \varepsilon_j}$ $(i \neq j)$ interchanges ε_i and ε_j and leaves ε_k invariant when the index k is distinct from i and j. The $s_{\varepsilon_i-\varepsilon_j}$ generate a group G_1 isomorphic to the symmetric group $\mathfrak{S}_l$. The orthogonal reflection s_{ε_i} transforms ε_i to $-\varepsilon_i$ and leaves invariant the ε_k when the index k is distinct from i. The s_{ε_i} generate a group G_2 isomorphic to $(\mathbf{Z}/2\mathbf{Z})^l$. The Weyl group W(R) is generated by G_1 and G_2, and G_2 is normal in W(R), so W(R) is isomorphic to the semi-direct product of $\mathfrak{S}_l$ by $(\mathbf{Z}/2\mathbf{Z})^l$. Its order is therefore $2^l.l!$.

The symmetric algebra $\mathbf{S}(\mathbf{R}^l)$ can be identified canonically with the algebra of polynomial functions $P(\xi_1, \ldots, \xi_l)$ on $\mathbf{R}^l$. For such a polynomial to be invariant under W(R), it is first of all necessary that

$$P(\xi_1, \xi_2, \ldots, \xi_l) = P(\pm\xi_1, \pm\xi_2, \ldots, \pm\xi_l)$$

for all choices of the signs on the right-hand side, so that

$$P(\xi_1, \ldots, \xi_l) = Q(\xi_1^2, \ldots, \xi_l^2)$$

where Q is a polynomial, and further that Q is a symmetric polynomial; and these conditions are sufficient. Consequently (*Algebra*, Chap. V, App. I), $\mathbf{S}(\mathbf{R}^l)^{\mathrm{W(R)}}$ is the algebra generated by the l polynomial functions

$$t_i = \sum_{\tau \in \mathfrak{S}_l} \xi^2_{\tau(1)}\xi^2_{\tau(2)} \cdots \xi^2_{\tau(l)} \quad (1 \leqslant i \leqslant l).$$

Moreover, the transcendence degree over $\mathbf{R}$ of the field of fractions of $\mathbf{S}(\mathbf{R}^l)^{\mathrm{W(R)}}$ is l, so the t_i are algebraically independent. Since the t_i have degree $2, 4, \ldots, 2l$, we conclude that the exponents of W(R) (Chap. V, § 6, no. 3, Prop. 3) are:

$$1, 3, 5, \ldots, 2l-1.$$

(XI) The only automorphism of the Dynkin graph is the identity element. Thus, $\mathrm{A(R)} = \mathrm{W(R)}$ and $-1 \in \mathrm{W(R)}$. Since -1 transforms B to $-$B, we conclude that $w_0 = -1$.

(XII) The group $\mathrm{P(R^\vee)/Q(R^\vee)}$ is dual to $\mathrm{P(R)/Q(R)}$, and hence is isomorphic to $\mathbf{Z}/2\mathbf{Z}$. Its non-trivial element permutes the vertices corresponding to α_0 and α_1 and leaves the others fixed.

6. SYSTEMS OF TYPE C_l $(l \geqslant 2)$

(I) The existence of root systems of type C_l has been proved in no. 5, since we have seen that the inverse system of a system of type B_l is of type C_l. A root system of type C_l is thus obtained by taking in $\mathbf{R}^l$ the vectors $\pm 2\varepsilon_i$ $(1 \leqslant i \leqslant l)$, and $\pm\varepsilon_i \pm \varepsilon_j$ $(1 \leqslant i < j \leqslant l)$. The number of roots is $2l^2$.

(II) A basis of R can be obtained by taking the image under the map $\alpha \mapsto \frac{2\alpha}{(\alpha|\alpha)}$ of the basis of the system considered in no. 5. We obtain:

$$\alpha_1 = \varepsilon_1 - \varepsilon_2,\ \alpha_2 = \varepsilon_2 - \varepsilon_3, \ldots,\ \alpha_{l-1} = \varepsilon_{l-1} - \varepsilon_l,\ \alpha_l = 2\varepsilon_l.$$

The positive roots are the $2\varepsilon_i$ and the $\varepsilon_i \pm \varepsilon_j$ $(i < j)$.

(III) The Coxeter number is the same as for the inverse system: $h = 2l$.

(IV) Let $\tilde{\alpha} = 2\varepsilon_1 = 2\alpha_1 + 2\alpha_2 + \cdots + 2\alpha_{l-1} + \alpha_l$, which is a root. The sum of its coordinates relative to (α_i) is $2l - 1 = h - 1$. Hence, $\tilde{\alpha}$ is the highest root. We have $(\tilde{\alpha}|\alpha_i) = 0$ for $i \neq l$, $(\tilde{\alpha}|\alpha_l) = 2$. Thus, the completed Dynkin graph is

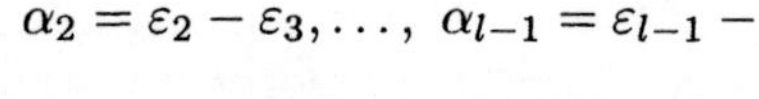

(V) We have already determined $\mathrm{R}^\vee$, which is of type B_l. By formula (19) of § 1, no. 12 and by no. 5 (V), the square of the length of $2\varepsilon_i$ for Φ_{R} is

$$((l+1)(4l-2))^{-1}((4l-2)^{-1})^{-1} = (l+1)^{-1};$$

thus, $\Phi_{\mathrm{R}}(x, y) = (x|y)/4(l+1)$.

We have $\gamma(\mathrm{R}) = \gamma(\mathrm{R}^\vee) = (l+1)(4l-2)$.

(VI) The fundamental weights are easily found:

$$\begin{aligned}\omega_i &= \varepsilon_1 + \varepsilon_2 + \cdots + \varepsilon_i \\ &= \alpha_1 + 2\alpha_2 + \cdots + (i-1)\alpha_{i-1} + i(\alpha_i + \alpha_{i+1} + \cdots + \frac{1}{2}\alpha_l) \quad (i \leqslant l).\end{aligned}$$

(VII) The sum of the positive roots is

$$\begin{aligned}2\rho &= 2l\varepsilon_1 + (2l-2)\varepsilon_2 + \cdots + 4\varepsilon_{l-1} + 2\varepsilon_l \\ &= 2l\alpha_1 + 2(2l-1)\alpha_3 + \cdots + i(2l-i+1)\alpha_i + \cdots \\ &\qquad \cdots + (l-1)(l+2)\alpha_{l-1} + \frac{1}{2}l(l+1)\alpha_l.\end{aligned}$$

(VIII) By no. 4 and no. 5 (VIII), $\mathrm{Q(R)} = \mathrm{L}_1$, $\mathrm{P(R)} = \mathrm{L}_0$; $\mathrm{P(R)/Q(R)}$ is isomorphic to $\mathbf{Z}/2\mathbf{Z}$, and the connection index is 2.

(IX) and (X) These data depend only on W(R), and so are the same as for type B_l.

(XI) The same argument as in no. 5 shows that $\mathrm{A(R)} = \mathrm{W(R)}$ and $w_0 = -1$.

(XII) The single non-identity element of $\mathrm{P(R^\vee)/Q(R^\vee)}$ defines the unique non-trivial automorphism of the completed Dynkin graph: it interchanges the vertices corresponding to α_j and α_{l-j} for $0 \leqslant j \leqslant l$.

7. SYSTEMS OF TYPE A_l ($l \geqslant 1$)

(I) and (II) Let V be the hyperplane in $\mathrm{E} = \mathbf{R}^{l+1}$ with equation $\sum_{i=1}^{l+1} \xi_i = 0$. Replacing l by $l+1$ in no. 5, we obtain a system R′ of type B_{l+1} in E with basis

$$\alpha_1 = \varepsilon_1 - \varepsilon_2,\ \alpha_2 = \varepsilon_2 - \varepsilon_3, \ldots, \alpha_l = \varepsilon_l - \varepsilon_{l+1},\ \alpha_{l+1} = \varepsilon_{l+1}.$$

Since $\alpha_1, \ldots, \alpha_l$ generate V, $\mathrm{R} = \mathrm{R}' \cap \mathrm{V}$ is a root system in V with basis $(\alpha_1, \ldots, \alpha_l)$ (§ 1, no. 7, Cor. 4 of Prop. 20). By the calculation of the scalar products in no. 5, it is immediate that R is of type A_l. The elements of R are the $\varepsilon_i - \varepsilon_j$ ($i \neq j, 1 \leqslant i \leqslant l+1, 1 \leqslant j \leqslant l+1$). There are $n = l(l+1)$ roots. The positive roots are the $\varepsilon_i - \varepsilon_j$ where $i < j$.

(III) We have $h = n/l = l+1$.

(IV) Let $\tilde{\alpha} = \varepsilon_1 - \varepsilon_{l+1} = \alpha_1 + \alpha_2 + \cdots + \alpha_l$, which is a root. The sum of its coordinates relative to (α_i) is $l = h-1$. Hence $\tilde{\alpha}$ is the highest root.

For $l = 1$, $\tilde{\alpha} = \alpha_1$ so $(\tilde{\alpha}|\alpha_1) = 2$; the Coxeter graph of the group $\mathrm{W}_a(\mathrm{R})$ is

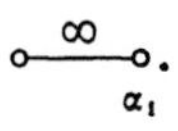

For $l \geqslant 2$, $(\tilde{\alpha}|\alpha_i) = 0$ for $0 < i < l$ and $(\tilde{\alpha}|\alpha_1) = (\tilde{\alpha}|\alpha_l) = 1$. Hence the completed Dynkin graph is:

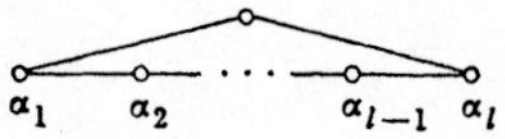

(V) Identifying V with its dual using the scalar product, we have $\alpha^\vee = \frac{2\alpha}{(\alpha|\alpha)} = \alpha$ for all $\alpha \in \mathrm{R}$, so $\mathrm{R}^\vee = \mathrm{R}$.

For the form Φ_R, the length of the roots is $h^{-1/2} = (l+1)^{-1/2}$ (§ 1, no. 12); so $\Phi_r(x,y) = (x|y)/2(l+1)$.

We have $\gamma(\mathrm{R}) = (l+1)^2$ (§ 1, no. 12, formula (20)).

(VI) Let $(\omega_i)_{1 \leqslant i \leqslant l}$ be the family of fundamental weights. Put

$$\omega_i = \sum_{j=1}^{l+1} \xi_{ij}\varepsilon_j, \qquad \text{with } \xi_{ij} \in \mathbf{R}.$$

The conditions $(\omega_i|\alpha_j) = \delta_{ij}$ and $\omega_i \in \mathrm{V}$ give

$$\xi_{ii} - \xi_{i,i+1} = 1, \quad \xi_{ij} - \xi_{i,j+1} = 0 \text{ for } j \neq i, \quad \sum_{j=1}^{l+1} \xi_{ij} = 0,$$

which easily lead to

$$\begin{aligned}\omega_i &= \varepsilon_1 + \cdots + \varepsilon_i - \frac{i}{l+1}(\varepsilon_1 + \cdots + \varepsilon_{l+1}) \\ &= \frac{1}{l+1}((l-i+1)(\alpha_1 + 2\alpha_2 + \cdots + (i-1)\alpha_{i-1}) \\ &\qquad + i((l-i+1)\alpha_i + (l-i)\alpha_{i+1} + \cdots + \alpha_l)).\end{aligned}$$

(VII) The sum of the positive roots is

$$\begin{aligned}2\rho &= l\varepsilon_1 + (l-2)\varepsilon_2 + (l-4)\varepsilon_3 + \cdots - (l-2)\varepsilon_l - l\varepsilon_{l+1} \\ &= l\alpha_1 + 2(l-1)\alpha_2 + \cdots + i(l-i+1)\alpha_i + \cdots + l\alpha_l.\end{aligned}$$

(VIII) Introduce in $\mathrm{E} = \mathbf{R}^{l+1}$ the subgroup L_0 of no. 4. Let p be the orthogonal projection of E onto V. By § 1, no. 10, Prop. 28, we have

$$\mathrm{Q}(\mathrm{R}) = \mathrm{Q}(\mathrm{R}') \cap \mathrm{V} = \mathrm{L}_0 \cap \mathrm{V}, \quad \text{and} \quad \mathrm{P}(\mathrm{R}) = p(\mathrm{P}(\mathrm{R}'));$$

in view of the fact that the last fundamental weight of R' is orthogonal to V, we have $\mathrm{P}(\mathrm{R}) = p(\mathrm{Q}(\mathrm{R}')) = p(\mathrm{L}_0)$. Thus, P(R) is the group generated by the $\varepsilon_i - \varepsilon_j$ and by $p(\varepsilon_1) = \varepsilon_1 - (l+1)^{-1}\sum_{i=1}^{l+1}\varepsilon_i$, so

$$\mathrm{P}(\mathrm{R}) = \mathrm{Q}(\mathrm{R}) + \mathbf{Z}(\varepsilon_1 - (l+1)^{-1}\sum_{i=1}^{l+1}\varepsilon_i).$$

Now $l+1$ is the smallest integer $m > 0$ such that $mp(\varepsilon_1) \in \mathrm{Q(R)}$. Thus $\mathrm{P(R)/Q(R)}$ is isomorphic to $\mathbf{Z}/(l+1)\mathbf{Z}$ and the connection index is $l+1$.

(IX) and (X) For any automorphism g of V, let $\varphi(g)$ be the automorphism of E that extends g and leaves $\varepsilon_1+\varepsilon_2+\cdots+\varepsilon_l$ invariant. If g is the orthogonal reflection $s_{\varepsilon_i-\varepsilon_j}|\mathrm{V}$, $\varphi(g)$ is equal to $s_{\varepsilon_i-\varepsilon_j}$, which interchanges ε_i and ε_j and leaves fixed the ε_k with k distinct from i and j. Let

$$\mathrm{X} = \{\varepsilon_1, \varepsilon_2, \dots, \varepsilon_{l+1}\}.$$

Then $g \mapsto \varphi(g)|\mathrm{X}$ is an isomorphism from W(R) to the symmetric group of X. Thus, W(R) is isomorphic to the symmetric group $\mathfrak{S}_{l+1}$, and so is of order $(l+1)!$.

The symmetric algebra $\mathbf{S}(\mathrm{E})$ can be identified canonically with the algebra of polynomial functions $\mathrm{P}(\xi_1, \xi_2, \dots, \xi_{l+1})$ on E. Let $\mathrm{G} = \varphi(\mathrm{W(R)})$. By the preceding paragraph, the set $\mathbf{S}(\mathrm{E})^{\mathrm{G}}$ of elements of $\mathbf{S}(\mathrm{E})$ invariant under G is the set of symmetric polynomials (*Algebra*, Chap. V, App. I), and consequently (*ibid.*) is the algebra generated by the functions

$$s'_i = \sum_{\tau \in \mathfrak{S}_{l+1}} \xi_{\tau(1)}\xi_{\tau(2)}\cdots\xi_{\tau(i)} \qquad (1 \leqslant i \leqslant l+1).$$

The algebra $\mathbf{S}(\mathrm{V})$ can be identified with the restrictions to V of the polynomial functions on E. If $\mathrm{P} \in \mathbf{S}(\mathrm{E})^{\mathrm{G}}$, the restriction of P to V is clearly invariant under W(R). Conversely, if $\mathrm{Q} \in \mathbf{S}(\mathrm{V})^{\mathrm{W(R)}}$, there exists $\mathrm{P} \in \mathbf{S}(\mathrm{E})$ extending Q; replacing P by $((l+1)!)^{-1} \sum_{g \in \mathrm{G}} g(\mathrm{P})$, which has the same restriction as P to V, we can assume that $\mathrm{P} \in \mathbf{S}(\mathrm{E})^{\mathrm{G}}$. Thus, $\mathbf{S}(\mathrm{V})^{\mathrm{W(R)}}$ is generated by the $s_i = s'_i|\mathrm{V}$. Now $s_1 = 0$. Moreover, the transcendence degree over $\mathbf{R}$ of the field of fractions of $\mathbf{S}(\mathrm{V})^{\mathrm{W(R)}}$ is l, so the s_i $(2 \leqslant i \leqslant l+1)$ are algebraically independent. Since the s_i are of degrees $2, 3, \dots, l+1$, the exponents of W(R) are

$$1, 2, 3, \dots, l.$$

(XI) For $l = 1$, $\mathrm{A(R)} = \mathrm{W(R)} = \mathbf{Z}/2\mathbf{Z}$ and $w_0 = -1$.

For $l \geqslant 2$, let $\varepsilon \in \mathrm{A(R)}$ be the automorphism that transforms α_i to α_{l+1-i}. It is clear that the automorphism induced by ε is the unique non-trivial automorphism of the Dynkin graph. The group A(R)/W(R) is isomorphic to $\mathbf{Z}/2\mathbf{Z}$. Since -1 is an element of A(R) which does not belong to W(R) by (IX) and (X), we see that A(R) is isomorphic to $\mathrm{W(R)} \times \mathbf{Z}/2\mathbf{Z}$. We have $w_0 = -\varepsilon$.

(XII) The group $\mathrm{P(R^\vee)/Q(R^\vee)}$ is cyclic of order $l+1$ and acts on the completed Dynkin graph by circular permutations. If $l \geqslant 2$, the unique non-identity element of A(R)/W(R) acts on $\mathrm{P(R^\vee)/Q(R^\vee)}$ by the automorphism $x \mapsto -x$.

8. SYSTEMS OF TYPE D_l ($l \geqslant 3$)

(I) Consider in $V = \mathbf{R}^l$ the group L_0 (no. 4). The set R of $\alpha \in L_0$ such that $(\alpha|\alpha) = 2$ consists of the vectors $\pm\varepsilon_i \pm \varepsilon_j$ $(1 \leqslant i < j \leqslant l)$. It is clear that R generates V and that $2(\alpha|\beta)/(\alpha|\alpha) \in \mathbf{Z}$ for all $\alpha, \beta \in R$. Thus R is a reduced root system in V (no. 4). The number of roots is $n = 2l(l-1)$.

(II) Put

$$\alpha_1 = \varepsilon_1 - \varepsilon_2,\ \alpha_2 = \varepsilon_2 - \varepsilon_3, \ldots, \alpha_{l-1} = \varepsilon_{l-1} - \varepsilon_l,\ \alpha_l = \varepsilon_{l-1} + \varepsilon_l.$$

The following formulas are immediate:

$$\begin{aligned}
\varepsilon_i - \varepsilon_j &= \alpha_i + \alpha_{i+1} + \cdots + \alpha_{j-1} \quad (i<j)\\
\varepsilon_i + \varepsilon_j &= \alpha_i + \alpha_{i+1} + \cdots + \alpha_{j-1} + 2\alpha_j + 2\alpha_{j+1} + \cdots\\
&\qquad \cdots + 2\alpha_{l-2} + \alpha_{l-1} + \alpha_l \quad (i<j\leqslant l-2)\\
\varepsilon_i + \varepsilon_{l-1} &= \alpha_i + \alpha_{i+1} + \cdots + \alpha_l \quad (i<l-1)\\
\varepsilon_i + \varepsilon_l &= \alpha_i + \alpha_{i+1} + \cdots + \alpha_{l-2} + \alpha_l \quad (i<l-1)\\
\varepsilon_{l-1} + \varepsilon_l &= \alpha_l,
\end{aligned}$$

so $(\alpha_1, \ldots, \alpha_l)$ is a basis if R (§ 1, no. 2, Cor. 3 of Prop. 20). Further, $\| \alpha_i \|^2 = 2$ for all i, $(\alpha_i|\alpha_j) = 0$ for $i+1<j$ except for $i = l-2, j = l$ in which case $(\alpha_{l-2}|\alpha_l) = -1$, $(\alpha_i|\alpha_{i+1}) = -1$ for $i \leqslant l-2$, and finally $(\alpha_{l-1}|\alpha_l) = -1$; the Dynkin graph of R is thus of type D_l. The positive roots are the $\varepsilon_i \pm \varepsilon_j$ for $i<j$.

(III) We have $h = n/l = 2(l-1)$.

(IV) Let $\tilde{\alpha} = \varepsilon_1 + \varepsilon_2 = \alpha_1 + 2\alpha_2 + \cdots + 2\alpha_{l-2} + \alpha_{l-1} + \alpha_l$, which is a root. The sum of its coordinates relative to (α_i) is

$$2l - 3 = h - 1.$$

Hence $\tilde{\alpha}$ is the highest root.

If $l = 3$, we have

$$(\tilde{\alpha}|\alpha_1) = 0, \quad (\tilde{\alpha}|\alpha_2) = (\tilde{\alpha}|\alpha_3) = 1.$$

If $l \geqslant 4$, we have $(\tilde{\alpha}|\alpha_i) = 0$ for $i \neq 2$ and $(\tilde{\alpha}|\alpha_2) = 1$. Hence the completed Dynkin graph is:

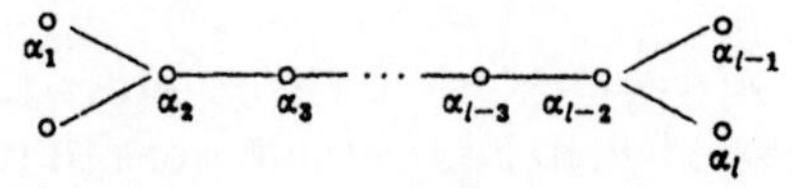

(V) Since $(\alpha|\alpha) = 2$ for all $\alpha \in R$, we have $R^\vee = R$.
The length of the roots for Φ_R is $h^{-1/2} = (2l-2)^{-1/2}$. Hence

$$\Phi_R(x,y) = (x|y)/(4l-4) \quad \text{and} \quad \gamma(R) = 4(l-1)^2.$$

(VI) A calculation analogous to that in no. 7 gives the fundamental weights:

$$\begin{aligned}\omega_i &= \varepsilon_1 + \varepsilon_2 + \cdots + \varepsilon_i \\ &= \alpha_1 + 2\alpha_2 + \cdots + (i-1)\alpha_{i-1} + i(\alpha_i + \alpha_{i+1} + \cdots + \alpha_{l-2}) \\ &\qquad + \frac{1}{2}i(\alpha_{l-1} + \alpha_l)\end{aligned}$$

for $i < l-1$,

$$\begin{aligned}\omega_{l-1} &= \frac{1}{2}(\varepsilon_1 + \varepsilon_2 + \cdots + \varepsilon_{l-2} + \varepsilon_{l-1} - \varepsilon_l) \\ &= \frac{1}{2}(\alpha_1 + 2\alpha_2 + \cdots + (l-2)\alpha_{l-2} + \frac{1}{2}l\alpha_{l-1} + \frac{1}{2}(l-2)\alpha_l), \\ \omega_l &= \frac{1}{2}(\varepsilon_1 + \varepsilon_2 + \cdots + \varepsilon_{l-2} + \varepsilon_{l-1} + \varepsilon_l) \\ &= \frac{1}{2}(\alpha_1 + 2\alpha_2 + \cdots + (l-2)\alpha_{l-2} + \frac{1}{2}(l-2)\alpha_{l-1} + \frac{1}{2}l\alpha_l).\end{aligned}$$

(VII) The sum of the positive roots is

$$\begin{aligned}2\rho &= 2(l-1)\varepsilon_1 + 2(l-2)\varepsilon_2 + \cdots + 2\varepsilon_{l-1} \\ &= \sum_{i=1}^{l-2} 2(il - \frac{i(i+1)}{2})\alpha_i + \frac{l(l-1)}{2}(\alpha_{l-1} + \alpha_l).\end{aligned}$$

(VIII) The $\pm\varepsilon_i \pm \varepsilon_j$ generate L_1 (no. 4), so $\mathrm{Q(R)} = \mathrm{L}_1$. Hence $\mathrm{Q(R^\vee)} = \mathrm{L}_1$ and consequently $\mathrm{P(R)} = \mathrm{L}_2$ (no. 4). By no. 4, $\mathrm{P(R)/Q(R)}$ is isomorphic to $\mathbf{Z}/4\mathbf{Z}$ for l odd, and to $\mathbf{Z}/2\mathbf{Z} \times \mathbf{Z}/2\mathbf{Z}$ for l even. In the first case, $\mathrm{P(R)/Q(R)}$ is generated by the canonical image of ω_l (and also by that of ω_{l-1}). In the second case, $\mathrm{P(R)/Q(R)}$ is generated by the canonical images of ω_{l-1} and ω_l. In both cases the connection index is 4.

(IX) and (X) In $\mathbf{R}^l$, the orthogonal reflection $s_{\varepsilon_i - \varepsilon_j}$ $(i \neq j)$ interchanges ε_i and ε_j and leaves invariant the ε_k with k distinct from i and j. The $s_{\varepsilon_i - \varepsilon_j}$ generate a group G_1 isomorphic to the symmetric group $\mathfrak{S}_l$. On the other hand, $s_{ij} = s_{\varepsilon_i - \varepsilon_j} s_{\varepsilon_i + \varepsilon_j}$ transforms ε_i to $-\varepsilon_i$, ε_j to $-\varepsilon_j$ and leaves invariant the ε_k with k distinct from i and j. The s_{ij} generate a group G_2, the set of automorphisms u of the vector space $\mathbf{R}^l$ such that $u(\varepsilon_i) = (-1)^{\nu_i}\varepsilon_i$ with $\prod_{i=1}^{l}(-1)^{\nu_i} = 1$. The group G_2 is isomorphic to $(\mathbf{Z}/2\mathbf{Z})^{l-1}$, and G_2 is normal in $\mathrm{W(R)}$, so $\mathrm{W(R)}$ is isomorphic to the semi-direct product of $\mathfrak{S}_l$ by $(\mathbf{Z}/2\mathbf{Z})^{l-1}$. Consequently, its order is $2^{l-1}.l!$.

The polynomial functions t_i of no. 5 are invariant under $\mathrm{W(R)}$, and so is $t = \xi_1\xi_2\ldots\xi_l$; moreover, $t_l = t^2$. Let $\mathrm{P}(\xi_1, \ldots, \xi_l)$ be a polynomial invariant under $\mathrm{W(R)}$. Let $\xi_1^{\nu_1}\xi_2^{\nu_2}\ldots\xi_l^{\nu_l}$ be a monomial featuring in P such that ν_i is odd; then ν_j is odd for all j because the monomial $(-1)^{\nu_i+\nu_j}\xi_1^{\nu_1}\xi_2^{\nu_2}\ldots\xi_l^{\nu_l}$ features in $s_{ij}(\mathrm{P})$, so $\nu_i + \nu_j \equiv 0 \pmod{2}$ and $\nu_j \equiv 1 \pmod{2}$. Thus

$P = P_1 + tP_2$, where all the monomials featuring in P_1 and P_2 have only even exponents. Since P is invariant under the permutations of the ξ_i, P_1 and P_2 have the same property, and so can be written as polynomials in $t_1, t_2, \ldots, t_l$. This proves that the algebra $\mathbf{S}(\mathbf{R}^l)^{W(R)}$ is generated by $t_1, t_2, \ldots, t_{l-1}, t$. Moreover, the transcendence degree of the field of fractions of $\mathbf{S}(\mathbf{R}^l)^{W(R)}$ is l, so $t_1, t_2, \ldots, t_{l-1}, t$ are algebraically independent. We conclude that the sequence of exponents, suitably ordered, is:

$$1, 3, 5, \ldots, 2l-5, 2l-3, l-1.$$

Note that $l-1$ appears twice if l is even, and once if l is odd.

(XI) The automorphisms of the Dynkin graph are those of the underlying graph. Thus:

1) If $l = 3$, A(R)/W(R) is isomorphic to $\mathbf{Z}/2\mathbf{Z}$.

2) If $l = 4$, every permutation of the terminal vertices defines an automorphism of the graph, so A(R)/W(R) is isomorphic to $\mathfrak{S}_3$.

3) If $l \geqslant 5$, the chains starting at the ramification point have length 1, 1, and $l-3 \geqslant 2$. The only automorphism of the graph distinct from the identity thus corresponds to the automorphism $\varepsilon \in A(R)$ which interchanges α_{l-1} and α_l and leaves fixed the α_i for $1 \leqslant i \leqslant l-2$. Thus A(R)/W(R) is isomorphic to $\mathbf{Z}/2\mathbf{Z}$; moreover, A(R) is the semi-direct product of the group $G_1 \cong \mathfrak{S}_l$ defined in (IX) by the group G_3 consisting of the automorphisms u of $\mathbf{R}^l$ such that $u(\varepsilon_i) = \pm\varepsilon_i$ for all i.

If l is even, $-1 \in W(R)$, so $w_0 = -1$. If l is odd, $-1 \notin W(R)$, so $A(R) = W(R) \times \{1, -1\}$ and $w_0 = -\varepsilon$.

(XII) For l even, $P(R^\vee)/Q(R^\vee)$ has three elements of order 2, namely ω_1, ω_{l-1} and ω_l. Since ω_l (resp. ω_{l-1}) interchanges the vertices corresponding to α_0 and α_l (resp. α_{l-1}), it interchanges those corresponding to α_1 and α_{l-1} (resp. α_l) and also those corresponding to α_j and α_{l-j} for

$$2 \leqslant j \leqslant l-2.$$

We have $\omega_1 = \omega_l\omega_{l-1}$.

For l odd, $P(R^\vee)/Q(R^\vee)$ has two elements of order 4, namely ω_{l-1} and ω_l, and one element of order 2, equal to ω_1. Indeed, ω_1 interchanges the vertices corresponding to α_0 and α_1, so it leaves fixed the vertices corresponding to α_j for $2 \leqslant j \leqslant l-2$ and is necessarily of order 2. Consequently ω_l is of order 4 and transforms the vertex corresponding to α_0 (resp. α_l, resp. α_1, resp. α_{l-1}) to that corresponding to α_l (resp. α_1, resp. α_{l-1}, resp. α_0), and interchanges the vertices corresponding to α_j and α_{l-j} for $2 \leqslant j \leqslant l-2$. We have $\omega_1 = \omega_l^2$ and $\omega_{l-1} = \omega_l^3$.

For $l \neq 4$, the non-identity element of A(R)/W(R) interchanges the vertices corresponding to α_{l-1} and α_l, and consequently interchanges the elements ω_{l-1} and ω_l of $P(R^\vee)/Q(R^\vee)$. For l odd, the automorphism of $P(R^\vee)/Q(R^\vee)$ thus obtained is the map $x \mapsto -x$.

For $l = 4$, A(R)/W(R) can be identified with the group of permutations of $\{1, 3, 4\}$ and acts by permutations of the indices on $\{\omega_1, \omega_3, \omega_4\}$.

9. SYSTEM OF TYPE F_4

(I) Consider the group L_2 (no. 4) in $\mathbf{R}^4$. Let R be the set of $\alpha \in L_2$ such that $(\alpha|\alpha) = 1$ or $(\alpha|\alpha) = 2$; it contains the vectors

$$\pm\varepsilon_i, \quad \pm\varepsilon_i \pm \varepsilon_j \ (i < j), \quad \frac{1}{2}(\pm\varepsilon_1 \pm \varepsilon_2 \pm \varepsilon_3 \pm \varepsilon_4).$$

Conversely, if $\alpha \in R$, the coordinates of α can only take the values $0, \pm\frac{1}{2}, \pm 1$ (since $(\frac{3}{2})^2 > 2$); either these coordinates are all integers, giving the vectors $\pm\varepsilon_i, \pm\varepsilon_i \pm \varepsilon_j$, or they are all equal to $\pm\frac{1}{2}$, giving the vectors $\frac{1}{2}(\pm\varepsilon_1 \pm \varepsilon_2 \pm \varepsilon_3 \pm \varepsilon_4)$.

We show that, for $\alpha, \beta \in R$, we have $2(\alpha|\beta)/(\alpha|\alpha) \in \mathbf{Z}$. If $\alpha = \pm\varepsilon_i$ or $\alpha = \frac{1}{2}(\pm\varepsilon_1 \pm \varepsilon_2 \pm \varepsilon_3 \pm \varepsilon_4)$, then $(\alpha|\alpha) = 1$ and we have seen in no. 4 that $(\alpha|\beta) \in \frac{1}{2}\mathbf{Z}$ since $\alpha, \beta \in L_2$. If $\alpha = \pm\varepsilon_i \pm \varepsilon_j$, then $(\alpha|\alpha) = 2$ and we have seen in no. 4 that $(\alpha|\beta) \in \mathbf{Z}$ since $\alpha \in L_1$ and $\beta \in L_2$. Hence, R is a reduced root system in $\mathbf{R}^4$ (no. 4). The number of roots is $n = 8 + \binom{4}{2}4 + 2^4 = 48$.

(II) Give $\mathbf{R}^4$ the lexicographic order defined by the basis $(\varepsilon_1, \varepsilon_2, \varepsilon_3, \varepsilon_4)$ (§ 1, no. 7). In particular, we have $\varepsilon_1 > \varepsilon_2 > \varepsilon_3 > \varepsilon_4$. The positive roots are

$$\varepsilon_i, \quad \varepsilon_i \pm \varepsilon_j \ (i < j), \quad \frac{1}{2}(\varepsilon_1 \pm \varepsilon_2 \pm \varepsilon_3 \pm \varepsilon_4).$$

The smallest root is $\alpha_3 = \varepsilon_4$. Among the roots belonging to $\mathbf{R}\varepsilon_3 + \mathbf{R}\varepsilon_4$ but not to $\mathbf{R}\varepsilon_4$, the smallest is $\alpha_2 = \varepsilon_3 - \varepsilon_4$. Among the positive roots belonging to $\mathbf{R}\varepsilon_2 + \mathbf{R}\varepsilon_3 + \mathbf{R}\varepsilon_4$ but not to $\mathbf{R}\varepsilon_3 + \mathbf{R}\varepsilon_4$, the smallest is $\alpha_1 = \varepsilon_2 - \varepsilon_3$. Among the positive roots not belonging to $\mathbf{R}\varepsilon_2 + \mathbf{R}\varepsilon_3 + \mathbf{R}\varepsilon_4$, the smallest is $\alpha_4 = \frac{1}{2}(\varepsilon_1 - \varepsilon_2 - \varepsilon_3 - \varepsilon_4)$. None of the α_i is a sum of 2 positive roots. Hence, $(\alpha_1, \alpha_2, \alpha_3, \alpha_4)$ is a basis of R (§ 1, no. 6, Cor. 1 to Prop. 19). We have $\| \alpha_1 \|^2 = \| \alpha_2 \|^2 = 2$, $\| \alpha_3 \|^2 = \| \alpha_4 \|^2 = 1$, $(\alpha_1|\alpha_2) = (\alpha_2|\alpha_3) = -1$, $(\alpha_3|\alpha_4) = -\frac{1}{2}$, $(\alpha_1|\alpha_3) = (\alpha_1|\alpha_4) = (\alpha_2|\alpha_4) = 0$. We see that the Dynkin graph of R is of type F_4, and hence is irreducible.

(III) We have $h = \frac{n}{l} = 12$.

(IV) Let $\tilde{\alpha} = \varepsilon_1 + \varepsilon_2 = 2\alpha_1 + 3\alpha_2 + 4\alpha_3 + 2\alpha_4$. The sum of the coordinates of $\tilde{\alpha}$ with respect to (α_i) is $11 = h - 1$, so $\tilde{\alpha}$ is the highest root. We have $(\tilde{\alpha}|\alpha_1) = 1, (\tilde{\alpha}|\alpha_2) = (\tilde{\alpha}|\alpha_3) = (\tilde{\alpha}|\alpha_4) = 0$.

The completed Dynkin graph is

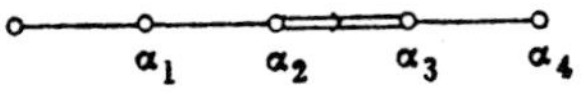

(V) The formula $\alpha^{\vee} = \frac{2\alpha}{(\alpha|\alpha)}$ gives for $R^{\vee}$ the set of vectors $\pm 2\varepsilon_i$, $\pm\varepsilon_i \pm \varepsilon_j$, $\pm\varepsilon_1 \pm \varepsilon_2 \pm \varepsilon_3 \pm \varepsilon_4$. The Dynkin graph of $R^{\vee}$ is obtained from that of R by the procedure explained in no. 2, and we see that $R^{\vee}$ is of type F_4.

The roots not orthogonal to $\beta = \varepsilon_1$ are $\pm\varepsilon_1, \pm\varepsilon_1 \pm \varepsilon_j$ ($j \geqslant 2$), and $\frac{1}{2}(\pm\varepsilon_1 \pm \varepsilon_2 \pm \varepsilon_3 \pm \varepsilon_4)$; the number $n(\alpha|\beta) = 2(\alpha|\beta)$ is equal to ± 2 for the first 14 of these roots and to ± 1 for the last 16; thus, for Φ_{R}, the square of the length of β is $4(14.4 + 16.1)^{-1} = \frac{1}{18}$; hence

$$\Phi_{\mathrm{R}}(x, y) = \frac{(x|y)}{18}.$$

We now apply formula (18) of § 1, no. 12, with $x = y = \beta$; this gives

$$2 + 12.\frac{1}{4} + 16.\frac{1/4}{1} = \gamma(\mathrm{R}).\frac{1}{18}$$

so

$$\gamma(\mathrm{R}) = 2.3^4.$$

(VI) Calculating the fundamental weights gives

$$\begin{aligned}
\omega_1 &= \varepsilon_1 + \varepsilon_2 = 2\alpha_1 + 3\alpha_2 + 4\alpha_3 + 2\alpha_4 = \tilde{\alpha} \\
\omega_2 &= 2\varepsilon_1 + \varepsilon_2 + \varepsilon_3 = 3\alpha_1 + 6\alpha_2 + 8\alpha_3 + 4\alpha_4 \\
\omega_3 &= \frac{1}{2}(3\varepsilon_1 + \varepsilon_2 + \varepsilon_3 + \varepsilon_4) = 2\alpha_1 + 4\alpha_2 + 6\alpha_3 + 3\alpha_4 \\
\omega_4 &= \varepsilon_1 = \alpha_1 + 2\alpha_2 + 3\alpha_3 + 2\alpha_4.
\end{aligned}$$

(VII) The sum of the positive roots is

$$2\rho = 11\varepsilon_1 + 5\varepsilon_2 + 3\varepsilon_3 + \varepsilon_4 = 16\alpha_1 + 30\alpha_2 + 42\alpha_3 + 22\alpha_4.$$

(VIII) We have $\mathrm{Q(R)} = \mathrm{L}_2$ (no. 4), and $\mathrm{P(R)} = \mathrm{Q(R)}$ by (VI). Hence, the connection index is 1.

(IX) The family of exponents has 4 terms, and since $h = 12$, it must contain the integers $1, 5, 7, 11$, coprime to 12 (§ 1, no. 11, Prop. 30); consequently, these are all the exponents of W(R).

(X) and (XI) The only automorphism of the Dynkin graph is the identity, so $\mathrm{A(R)} = \mathrm{W(R)}$ and $w_0 = -1$. Let R' be the set of longest elements of R, that is, the $\pm\varepsilon_i \pm \varepsilon_j$: R' is the root system of type D_4 constructed in no. 8. Clearly, every element of A(R) is an element of $\mathrm{A(R')}$. Conversely, an element of $\mathrm{A(R')}$ leaves L_1 stable (since it is generated by R'), hence also its associated L_2, and hence also R. So $\mathrm{W(R)} = \mathrm{A(R)} = \mathrm{A(R')}$. By no. 8, W(R) is the semi-direct product of $\mathfrak{S}_3$ by $\mathrm{W(R')}$, $\mathrm{W(R')}$ itself being the semi-direct product of $\mathfrak{S}_4$ by $(\mathbf{Z}/2\mathbf{Z})^3$. The order of W(R) is $3!4!2^3 = 2^7.3^2$.

10. SYSTEM OF TYPE E_8

(I) Consider the group L_3 (no. 4) in $\mathbf{R}^8$. Let R be the set of $\alpha \in L_3$ such that $(\alpha|\alpha) = 2$; it contains the vectors

$$\pm\varepsilon_i \pm \varepsilon_j \ (i < j), \ \frac{1}{2}\sum_{i=1}^{8}(-1)^{\nu(i)}\varepsilon_i \quad (\sum_{i=1}^{8}\nu(i) \text{ even}).$$

Conversely, if an element $\alpha \in L_3$ is such that $(\alpha|\alpha) = 2$, its coordinates must be among the values $0, \pm\frac{1}{2}, \pm 1$; by no. 4, either these coordinates are all integers, giving the vectors $\pm\varepsilon_i \pm \varepsilon_j$, or they are all equal to $\pm\frac{1}{2}$ with an integer sum, giving the vectors

$$\frac{1}{2}\sum_{i=1}^{8}(-1)^{\nu(i)}\varepsilon_i$$

with $\sum_{i=1}^{8}\nu(i)$ even.

We have seen (no. 4) that $(\alpha|\beta) \in \mathbf{Z}$ for all $\alpha, \beta \in L_3$. Hence, R is a reduced root system. The number of roots is $n = \binom{8}{2}.4 + 2^7 = 240$.

(II) Let ρ be the vector $(0, 1, 2, 3, 4, 5, 6, 23)$ of L_3. No element of R is orthogonal to ρ (this is clear for the $\pm\varepsilon_i \pm \varepsilon_j$; if $\frac{1}{2}\sum_{i=1}^{8}(-1)^{\nu(i)}\varepsilon_i$ were orthogonal to ρ, we would have $\sum_{i=1}^{6} i(-1)^{\nu(i+1)} + 23(-1)^{\nu(8)} = 0$, which is impossible since $\sum_{i=1}^{6} i < 23$). Hence (§ 1, no. 7, Cor. 2 of Prop. 20) the $\alpha \in R$ such that $(\alpha|\rho) > 0$ are the positive roots relative to a certain chamber. These roots are the $\pm\varepsilon_i + \varepsilon_j$ $(i < j)$, and the

$$\frac{1}{2}(\varepsilon_8 + \sum_{i=1}^{7}(-1)^{\nu(i)}\varepsilon_i)$$

with $\sum_{i=1}^{7}\nu(i)$ even. We have $(\alpha|\rho) \in \mathbf{Z}$ for all $\alpha \in R$ (no. 4), and $(\alpha|\rho)$ is equal to 1 for the following roots:

$$\alpha_1 = \frac{1}{2}(\varepsilon_1 + \varepsilon_8) - \frac{1}{2}(\varepsilon_2 + \varepsilon_3 + \varepsilon_4 + \varepsilon_5 + \varepsilon_6 + \varepsilon_7),$$
$$\alpha_3 = \varepsilon_1 + \varepsilon_2, \ \alpha_3 = \varepsilon_2 - \varepsilon_1, \ \alpha_4 = \varepsilon_3 - \varepsilon_2, \ \alpha_5 = \varepsilon_4 - \varepsilon_3,$$
$$\alpha_6 = \varepsilon_5 - \varepsilon_4, \ \alpha_7 = \varepsilon_6 - \varepsilon_5, \ \alpha_8 = \varepsilon_7 - \varepsilon_6,$$

and these eight vectors form a basis of $\mathbf{R}^8$. By § 1, no. 6, Cor. 1 of Prop. 19, $(\alpha_1, \alpha_2, \ldots, \alpha_8)$ is a basis of R for which the positive roots are those which have been defined above. We have

$$(\alpha_4|\alpha_5) = (\alpha_5|\alpha_6) = (\alpha_6|\alpha_7) = (\alpha_7|\alpha_8) = (\alpha_4|\alpha_2) = (\alpha_4|\alpha_3) = (\alpha_3|\alpha_1) = -1,$$

and $(\alpha_i|\alpha_j) = 0$ for all other pairs of indices. Hence, the Dynkin graph of R is of type E_8, and R is irreducible.

(III) We have $h = \frac{n}{8} = 30$.

(IV) Let

$$\tilde{\alpha} = \varepsilon_7 + \varepsilon_8 = 2\alpha_1 + 3\alpha_2 + 4\alpha_3 + 6\alpha_4 + 5\alpha_5 + 4\alpha_6 + 3\alpha_7 + 2\alpha_8,$$

which is a root. The sum of its coordinates with respect to (α_i) is $29 = h-1$, so $\tilde{\alpha}$ is the highest root. It is orthogonal to all the α_i except α_8, and $(\tilde{\alpha}|\alpha_8) = 1$. Hence, the completed Dynkin graph is:

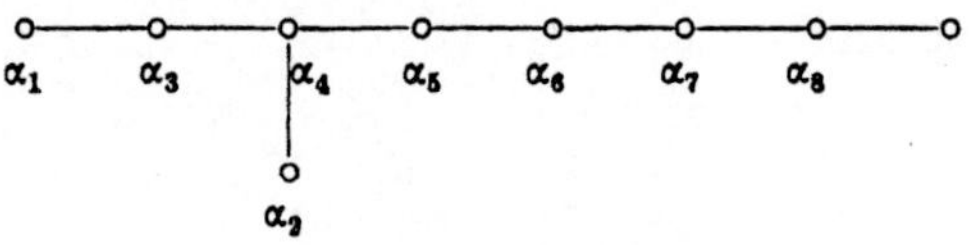

(V) Since $(\alpha|\alpha) = 2$ for all $\alpha \in R$, we have $R^\vee = R$.

For Φ_R, the squared length of the roots is $\frac{1}{30}$ (§ 1, no. 12). Hence, $\Phi_R(x, y) = (x|y)/60$ and $\gamma(R) = 900$ (§ 1, no. 12, formula (20)).

(VI) Calculating the fundamental weights gives

$$\begin{aligned}
\omega_1 &= 2\varepsilon_8 = 4\alpha_1 + 5\alpha_2 + 7\alpha_3 + 10\alpha_4 + 8\alpha_5 + 6\alpha_6 + 4\alpha_7 + 2\alpha_8 \\
\omega_2 &= \frac{1}{2}(\varepsilon_1 + \varepsilon_2 + \varepsilon_3 + \varepsilon_4 + \varepsilon_5 + \varepsilon_6 + \varepsilon_7 + 5\varepsilon_8) \\
&= 5\alpha_1 + 8\alpha_2 + 10\alpha_3 + 15\alpha_4 + 12\alpha_5 + 9\alpha_6 + 6\alpha_7 + 3\alpha_8 \\
\omega_3 &= \frac{1}{2}(-\varepsilon_1 + \varepsilon_2 + \varepsilon_3 + \varepsilon_4 + \varepsilon_5 + \varepsilon_6 + \varepsilon_7 + 7\varepsilon_8) \\
&= 7\alpha_1 + 10\alpha_2 + 14\alpha_3 + 20\alpha_4 + 16\alpha_5 + 12\alpha_6 + 8\alpha_7 + 4\alpha_8 \\
\omega_4 &= \varepsilon_3 + \varepsilon_4 + \varepsilon_5 + \varepsilon_6 + \varepsilon_7 + 5\varepsilon_8 \\
&= 10\alpha_1 + 15\alpha_2 + 20\alpha_3 + 30\alpha_4 + 24\alpha_5 + 18\alpha_6 + 12\alpha_7 + 6\alpha_8 \\
\omega_5 &= \varepsilon_4 + \varepsilon_5 + \varepsilon_6 + \varepsilon_7 + 4\varepsilon_8 \\
&= 8\alpha_1 + 12\alpha_2 + 16\alpha_3 + 24\alpha_4 + 20\alpha_5 + 15\alpha_6 + 10\alpha_7 + 5\alpha_8 \\
\omega_6 &= \varepsilon_5 + \varepsilon_6 + \varepsilon_7 + 3\varepsilon_8 \\
&= 6\alpha_1 + 9\alpha_2 + 12\alpha_3 + 18\alpha_4 + 15\alpha_5 + 12\alpha_6 + 8\alpha_7 + 4\alpha_8 \\
\omega_7 &= \varepsilon_6 + \varepsilon_7 + 2\varepsilon_8 \\
&= 4\alpha_1 + 6\alpha_2 + 8\alpha_3 + 12\alpha_4 + 10\alpha_5 + 8\alpha_6 + 6\alpha_7 + 3\alpha_8 \\
\omega_8 &= \varepsilon_7 + \varepsilon_8 \\
&= 5\alpha_1 + 8\alpha_2 + 10\alpha_3 + 15\alpha_4 + 12\alpha_5 + 9\alpha_6 + 6\alpha_7 + 3\alpha_8 = \tilde{\alpha}.
\end{aligned}$$

(VII) Half the sum of the positive roots is the sum of the fundamental weights (§ 1, no. 10, Prop. 29); this gives

$$\begin{aligned}
\rho &= \varepsilon_2 + 2\varepsilon_3 + 3\varepsilon_4 + 4\varepsilon_5 + 5\varepsilon_6 + 6\varepsilon_7 + 23\varepsilon_8 \\
&= 46\alpha_1 + 68\alpha_2 + 91\alpha_3 + 135\alpha_4 + 110\alpha_5 + 84\alpha_6 + 57\alpha_7 + 29\alpha_8.
\end{aligned}$$

(VIII) The group Q(R) is generated by the $\varepsilon_i \pm \varepsilon_j$ and $\frac{1}{2}\sum_{i=1}^{8} \varepsilon_i$, and is equal to L_3 (no. 4). Hence P(R), which is associated to $Q(R^\vee) = Q(R) = L_3$, is L_3 (no. 4). The connection index is 1.

(IX) The family of exponents has 8 terms, and since $h = 30$, the integers $1, 7, 11, 13, 17, 19, 23, 29$, coprime to 30, must feature in this family; consequently, these are the exponents of W(R).

(X) From (IX) and Chap. V, § 6, no. 2, Cor. 1 of Prop. 3, it follows that the order of W(R) is

$$2.8.12.14.18.20.24.30 = 2^{14}.3^5.5^2.7.$$

(XI) The only automorphism of the Dynkin graph is the identity since the three chains issuing from the ramification point have distinct lengths. Hence, $A(R) = W(R)$ and $w_0 = -1$.

11. SYSTEM OF TYPE E_7

(I) and (II) Let $E = \mathbf{R}^8$, and let R_8 be the root system in E constructed in no. 10. Let V be the hyperplane in E generated by the roots $\alpha_1, \dots, \alpha_7$ of R_8; it is orthogonal to the eighth fundamental weight $\omega = \varepsilon_7 + \varepsilon_8$ of R_8.

Let $R = R_8 \cap V$. Then R is a reduced root system with basis $(\alpha_1, \dots, \alpha_7)$, cf. § 1, no. 7, Cor. 4 of Prop. 20; hence, this system is of type E_7. Its elements are:

$$\pm\varepsilon_i \pm \varepsilon_j \ (1 \leqslant i \leqslant j \leqslant 6), \quad \pm(\varepsilon_7 - \varepsilon_8),$$

$$\pm\frac{1}{2}(\varepsilon_7 - \varepsilon_8 + \sum_{i=1}^{8}(-1)^{\nu(i)}\varepsilon_i) \quad \text{with } \sum_{i=1}^{8}\nu(i) \text{ odd.}$$

The number of roots is $n = 2 + \binom{6}{2}.4 + 2^6 = 126$. The positive roots are

$$\pm\varepsilon_i + \varepsilon_j \ (1 \leqslant i < j \leqslant 6), \quad -\varepsilon_7 + \varepsilon_8,$$

$$\frac{1}{2}(-\varepsilon_7 + \varepsilon_8 + \sum_{i=1}^{6}(-1)^{\nu(i)}\varepsilon_i) \quad \text{with } \sum_{i=1}^{6}\nu(i) \text{ odd.}$$

(III) We have $h = \frac{n}{l} = 18$.

(IV) Let $\tilde{\alpha} = \varepsilon_8 - \varepsilon_7 = 2\alpha_1 + 2\alpha_2 + 3\alpha_3 + 4\alpha_4 + 3\alpha_5 + 2\alpha_6 + \alpha_7$, which is a root. The sum of its coordinates with respect to (α_i) is $17 = h - 1$. It is therefore the highest root. It is orthogonal to α_i for $2 \leqslant i \leqslant 7$, and $(\tilde{\alpha}|\alpha_1) = 1$. The completed Dynkin graph is

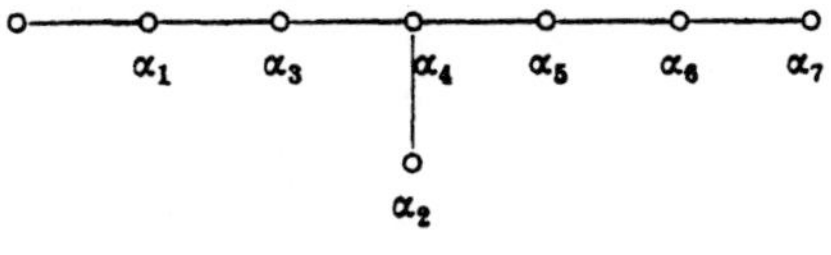

(V) Since $(\alpha|\alpha) = 2$ for all $\alpha \in \mathrm{R}$, we have $\mathrm{R}^{\vee} = \mathrm{R}$.
For Φ_{R}, the squared length of the roots is $\frac{1}{18}$, so

$$\Phi_{\mathrm{R}}(x, y) = (x|y)/36, \quad \text{and} \quad \gamma(\mathrm{R}) = 2^2.3^4$$

(§ 1, no. 12, formula (20)).

(VI) Calculating the fundamental weights gives

$$\begin{aligned}
\omega_1 &= \varepsilon_8 - \varepsilon_7 = 2\alpha_1 + 2\alpha_2 + 3\alpha_3 + 4\alpha_4 + 3\alpha_5 + 2\alpha_6 + \alpha_7 \\
\omega_2 &= \frac{1}{2}(\varepsilon_1 + \varepsilon_2 + \varepsilon_3 + \varepsilon_4 + \varepsilon_5 + \varepsilon_6 - 2\varepsilon_7 + 2\varepsilon_8) \\
&= \frac{1}{2}(4\alpha_1 + 7\alpha_2 + 8\alpha_3 + 12\alpha_4 + 9\alpha_5 + 8\alpha_6 + 3\alpha_7) \\
\omega_3 &= \frac{1}{2}(-\varepsilon_1 + \varepsilon_2 + \varepsilon_3 + \varepsilon_4 + \varepsilon_5 + \varepsilon_6 - 3\varepsilon_7 + 3\varepsilon_8) \\
&= 3\alpha_1 + 4\alpha_2 + 6\alpha_3 + 8\alpha_4 + 6\alpha_5 + 4\alpha_6 + 2\alpha_7 \\
\omega_4 &= \varepsilon_3 + \varepsilon_4 + \varepsilon_5 + \varepsilon_6 + 2(\varepsilon_8 - \varepsilon_7) \\
&= 4\alpha_1 + 6\alpha_2 + 8\alpha_3 + 12\alpha_4 + 9\alpha_5 + 6\alpha_6 + 3\alpha_7 \\
\omega_5 &= \varepsilon_4 + \varepsilon_5 + \varepsilon_6 + \frac{3}{2}(\varepsilon_8 - \varepsilon_7) \\
&= \frac{1}{2}(6\alpha_1 + 9\alpha_2 + 12\alpha_3 + 18\alpha_4 + 15\alpha_5 + 10\alpha_6 + 5\alpha_7) \\
\omega_6 &= \varepsilon_5 + \varepsilon_6 - \varepsilon_7 + \varepsilon_8 \\
&= 2\alpha_1 + 3\alpha_2 + 4\alpha_3 + 6\alpha_4 + 5\alpha_5 + 4\alpha_6 + 2\alpha_7 \\
\omega_7 &= \varepsilon_6 + \frac{1}{2}(\varepsilon_8 - \varepsilon_7) \\
&= \frac{1}{2}(2\alpha_1 + 3\alpha_2 + 4\alpha_3 + 6\alpha_4 + 5\alpha_5 + 4\alpha_6 + 3\alpha_7).
\end{aligned}$$

(VII) The sum 2ρ of the positive roots is $2\sum_{i=1}^{7}\omega_i$ (§ 1, no. 10, Prop. 29), so

$$\begin{aligned}
2\rho &= 2\varepsilon_2 + 4\varepsilon_3 + 6\varepsilon_4 + 8\varepsilon_5 + 10\varepsilon_6 - 17\varepsilon_7 + 17\varepsilon_8 \\
&= 34\alpha_1 + 49\alpha_2 + 66\alpha_3 + 96\alpha_4 + 75\alpha_5 + 52\alpha_6 + 27\alpha_7.
\end{aligned}$$

(VIII) By no. 10 (VIII) and § 1, no. 10, Prop. 28, we have

$$\mathrm{Q}(\mathrm{R}) = \mathrm{Q}(\mathrm{R}_8) \cap \mathrm{V} = \mathrm{L}_3 \cap \mathrm{V} \quad \text{and} \quad \mathrm{P}(\mathrm{R}) = p(\mathrm{P}(\mathrm{R}_8)) = p(\mathrm{L}_3),$$

where p denotes the orthogonal projection of E onto V. The group Q(R) has basis $(\alpha_1, \ldots, \alpha_7)$; the group P(R) is generated by Q(R) and

$$p(\alpha_8) = \alpha_8 - \frac{1}{2}\omega.$$

We have $\omega \in \mathrm{P}(\mathrm{R}_8)$, $\frac{1}{2}\omega \notin \mathrm{P}(\mathrm{R}_8)$, so $2p(\alpha_8) \in \mathrm{Q}(\mathrm{R})$ and $p(\alpha_8) \notin \mathrm{Q}(\mathrm{R})$. Thus, P(R)/Q(R) is isomorphic to $\mathbf{Z}/2\mathbf{Z}$ and is generated by, for example, the image of ω_7.

The connection index is 2.

(IX) The sequence of exponents of W(R) has 7 terms. The numbers $1, 5, 7, 11, 13, 17$, coprime to $h = 18$, feature in this sequence. The last exponent m must be such that $m + m = 18$ (Chap. V, § 6, no. 2, formula (2)). Hence, the sequence of exponents is

$$1, 5, 7, 9, 11, 13, 17.$$

(X) From (IX) and Chap. V, § 6, no. 2, Cor. 1 of Prop. 3, it follows that the order of W(R) is

$$2.6.8.10.12.14.18 = 2^{10}.3^4.5.7.$$

(XI) The only automorphism of the Dynkin graph is the identity, so $\mathrm{A}(\mathrm{R}) = \mathrm{W}(\mathrm{R})$ and $w_0 = -1$.

(XII) $\mathrm{P}(\mathrm{R}^\vee)/\mathrm{Q}(\mathrm{R}^\vee)$ has only one non-identity element. It interchanges the vertices corresponding to α_0 and α_7, α_1 and α_6, α_3 and α_5, and leaves α_2 and α_4 fixed.

12. SYSTEM OF TYPE E_6

(I) and (II) Let $\mathrm{E} = \mathbf{R}^8$, and let R_8 be the root system in E constructed in no. 10. Let V be the vector subspace of E generated by the roots $\alpha_1, \dots, \alpha_6$ of R_8; this is the orthogonal complement of the plane generated by the last two fundamental weights $\omega = \varepsilon_7 + \varepsilon_8$ and $\pi = \varepsilon_6 + \varepsilon_7 + 2\varepsilon_8$ of R_8.

Let $\mathrm{R} = \mathrm{R}_8 \cap \mathrm{V}$. This is a reduced root system with basis $(\alpha_1, \dots, \alpha_6)$, and hence of type E_6. Its elements are:

$$\pm\varepsilon_i \pm \varepsilon_j \quad (1 \leqslant i < j \leqslant 5),$$

$$\pm\frac{1}{2}(\varepsilon_8 - \varepsilon_7 - \varepsilon_6 + \sum_{i=1}^{5}(-1)^{\nu(i)}\varepsilon_i) \text{ with } \sum_{i=1}^{5}\nu(i) \text{ even.}$$

The number of roots is $n = \binom{5}{2}.4 + 2^5 = 72$. The positive roots are

$$\pm\varepsilon_i + \varepsilon_j \quad (1 \leqslant i < j \leqslant 5),$$

$$\frac{1}{2}(\varepsilon_8 - \varepsilon_7 - \varepsilon_6 + \sum_{i=1}^{5}(-1)^{\nu(i)}\varepsilon_i) \text{ with } \sum_{i=1}^{5}\nu(i) \text{ even.}$$

(III) We have $h = \frac{n}{6} = 12$.

(IV) Let

$$\begin{aligned}\tilde{\alpha} &= \frac{1}{2}(\varepsilon_1 + \varepsilon_2 + \varepsilon_3 + \varepsilon_4 + \varepsilon_5 - \varepsilon_6 - \varepsilon_7 + \varepsilon_8)\\ &= \alpha_1 + 2\alpha_2 + 2\alpha_3 + 3\alpha_4 + 2\alpha_5 + \alpha_6,\end{aligned}$$

which is a root. The sum of its coordinates with respect to (α_i) is $11 = h-1$, so $\tilde{\alpha}$ is the highest root. It is orthogonal to $\alpha_1, \alpha_3, \alpha_4, \alpha_5, \alpha_6$, and $(\tilde{\alpha}|\alpha_2) = 1$. The completed Dynkin graph is

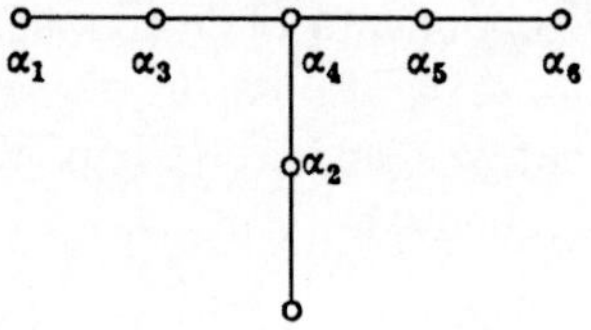

(V) Since $(\alpha|\alpha) = 2$ for all $\alpha \in \mathrm{R}$, we have $\mathrm{R}^\vee = \mathrm{R}$.
For Φ_{R}, the squared length of the roots is $\frac{1}{12}$, so

$$\Phi_{\mathrm{R}}(x, y) = (x|y)/24, \quad \text{and} \quad \gamma(\mathrm{R}) = 144.$$

(VI) Calculating the fundamental weights gives:

$$\omega_1 = \frac{2}{3}(\varepsilon_8 - \varepsilon_7 - \varepsilon_6) = \frac{1}{3}(4\alpha_1 + 3\alpha_2 + 5\alpha_3 + 6\alpha_4 + 4\alpha_5 + 2\alpha_6)$$
$$\omega_2 = \frac{1}{2}(\varepsilon_1 + \varepsilon_2 + \varepsilon_3 + \varepsilon_4 + \varepsilon_5 - \varepsilon_6 - \varepsilon_7 + \varepsilon_8)$$
$$= \alpha_1 + 2\alpha_2 + 2\alpha_3 + 3\alpha_4 + 2\alpha_5 + \alpha_6 = \tilde{\alpha}$$
$$\omega_3 = \frac{5}{6}(\varepsilon_8 - \varepsilon_7 - \varepsilon_6) + \frac{1}{2}(-\varepsilon_1 + \varepsilon_2 + \varepsilon_3 + \varepsilon_4 + \varepsilon_5)$$
$$= \frac{1}{3}(5\alpha_1 + 6\alpha_2 + 10\alpha_3 + 12\alpha_4 + 8\alpha_5 + 4\alpha_6)$$
$$\omega_4 = \varepsilon_3 + \varepsilon_4 + \varepsilon_5 - \varepsilon_6 - \varepsilon_7 + \varepsilon_8$$
$$= 2\alpha_1 + 3\alpha_2 + 4\alpha_3 + 6\alpha_4 + 4\alpha_5 + 2\alpha_6$$
$$\omega_5 = \frac{2}{3}(\varepsilon_8 - \varepsilon_7 - \varepsilon_6) + \varepsilon_4 + \varepsilon_5$$
$$= \frac{1}{3}(4\alpha_1 + 6\alpha_2 + 8\alpha_3 + 12\alpha_4 + 10\alpha_5 + 5\alpha_6)$$
$$\omega_6 = \frac{1}{3}(\varepsilon_8 - \varepsilon_7 - \varepsilon_6) + \varepsilon_5$$
$$= \frac{1}{3}(2\alpha_1 + 3\alpha_2 + 4\alpha_3 + 6\alpha_4 + 5\alpha_5 + 4\alpha_6).$$

(VII) Half the sum of the positive roots is $\sum_{i=1}^{6} \omega_i$, so

$$\rho = \varepsilon_2 + 2\varepsilon_3 + 3\varepsilon_4 + 4\varepsilon_5 + 4(\varepsilon_8 - \varepsilon_7 - \varepsilon_6)$$
$$= 8\alpha_1 + 11\alpha_2 + 15\alpha_3 + 21\alpha_4 + 15\alpha_5 + 8\alpha_6.$$

(VIII) By no. 10 (VIII) and § 1, no. 10, Prop. 28,

$$\mathrm{Q(R)} = \mathrm{Q(R_8)} \cap \mathrm{V} = \mathrm{L}_3 \cap \mathrm{V} \quad \text{and} \quad \mathrm{P(R)} = p(\mathrm{P(R_8)}) = p(\mathrm{L}_3),$$

where p denotes the orthogonal projection of E onto V. We have

$$p(\alpha_7) = \alpha_7 - \frac{2}{3}\pi + \omega, \quad p(\alpha_8) = \alpha_8 + \pi - 2\omega.$$

The group Q(R) has basis $(\alpha_1, \dots, \alpha_6)$. The group P(R) is generated by Q(R) and $p(\alpha_7)$, since $p(\alpha_8) \in \mathrm{P}(\mathrm{R}_8) \cap \mathrm{V} = \mathrm{Q}(\mathrm{R}_8) \cap \mathrm{V} = \mathrm{Q}(\mathrm{R})$. We have $3p(\alpha_7) \in \mathrm{Q}(\mathrm{R})$ and $p(\alpha_7) \notin \mathrm{Q}(\mathrm{R})$. Hence, the group P(R)/Q(R) is isomorphic to $\mathbf{Z}/3\mathbf{Z}$; it is generated, for example, by the image of ω_6.

The connection index is 3.

(IX) and (X) By § 2, no. 4, Prop. 7, the order of the Weyl group is $6!1.2.2.3.2.1.3 = 2^7.3^4.5$. The sequence of exponents has 6 terms between 1 and 11, and contains the integers $1, 5, 7, 11$ which are coprime to 12. The other exponents m, m' are integers such that

$$m + m' = 12,$$
$$(m+1)(m'+1)(1+1)(5+1)(7+1)(11+1) = 2^7.3^4.5,$$

in view of Chap. V, § 6, no. 2, formula (2) and Cor. 1 of Prop. 3. The second relation gives $(m+1)(m'+1) = 45$, and since $m + m' + 2 = 14$, we obtain $m = 4, m' = 8$. Hence, the sequence of exponents is

$$1, 4, 5, 7, 8, 11.$$

(XI) and (XII) Since the roots all have the same length, the automorphisms of the Dynkin graph are those of the underlying graph. Apart from the identity, there is only the automorphism ε which transforms $\alpha_1, \alpha_3, \alpha_4, \alpha_5, \alpha_6, \alpha_2$ into $\alpha_6, \alpha_5, \alpha_4, \alpha_3, \alpha_1, \alpha_2$, respectively. Hence, A(R)/W(R) is isomorphic to $\mathbf{Z}/2\mathbf{Z}$; since $-1 \in \mathrm{W}(\mathrm{R})$ (Chap. V, §6, no. 2, Cor. 3 of Prop. 3), A(R) is isomorphic to $\mathrm{W}(\mathrm{R}) \times \{1, -1\}$ and w_0 can be identified with $-\varepsilon$. It follows that the non-identity element of A(R)/W(R) defines the automorphism $x \mapsto -x$ of $\mathrm{P}(\mathrm{R}^\vee)/\mathrm{Q}(\mathrm{R}^\vee)$.

Moreover, $\mathrm{P}(\mathrm{R}^\vee)/\mathrm{Q}(\mathrm{R}^\vee)$ has two non-identity elements of order 3. They define the two automorphisms of order 3 of the completed Dynkin graph.

13. SYSTEM OF TYPE G_2

(I) Let E be the hyperplane in $\mathbf{R}^3$ with equation

$$\xi_1 + \xi_2 + \xi_3 = 0.$$

Let R be the set of $\alpha \in \mathrm{L}_0 \cap \mathrm{V}$ such that $(\alpha|\alpha) = 2$ or $(\alpha|\alpha) = 6$. The elements of R are

$$\pm(\varepsilon_1 - \varepsilon_2), \ \pm(\varepsilon_1 - \varepsilon_3), \ \pm(\varepsilon_2 - \varepsilon_3), \ \pm(2\varepsilon_1 - \varepsilon_2 - \varepsilon_3),$$
$$\pm(2\varepsilon_2 - \varepsilon_1 - \varepsilon_3), \ \pm(2\varepsilon_3 - \varepsilon_1 - \varepsilon_2).$$

Then, R generates V, and $\frac{2(\alpha|\beta)}{(\beta|\beta)} \in \mathbf{Z}$ for all $\alpha, \beta \in \mathrm{R}$: this is clear if $\beta = \pm(\varepsilon_i - \varepsilon_j)$ with $i \neq j$; if $\beta = 2\varepsilon_1 - \varepsilon_2 - \varepsilon_3$ for example, we have $(\alpha|\beta) \in 3\mathbf{Z}$, and again our assertion holds. Hence, R is a reduced root system in V. The number of roots is $n = 12$.

(II) Put $\alpha_1 = \varepsilon_1 - \varepsilon_2, \alpha_2 = -2\varepsilon_1 + \varepsilon_2 + \varepsilon_3$. Then the roots are

$$\pm\alpha_1, \quad \pm(\alpha_1 + \alpha_2), \quad \pm(2\alpha_1 + \alpha_2), \quad \pm\alpha_2,$$
$$\pm(3\alpha_1 + \alpha_2), \quad \pm(3\alpha_1 + 2\alpha_2).$$

Hence, (α_1, α_2) is a basis of R. We have $\| \alpha_1 \|^2 = 2, \| \alpha_2 \|^2 = 6, (\alpha_1|\alpha_2) = -3$, so R is a system of type G_2. The positive roots are $\alpha_1, \alpha_1 + \alpha_2, 2\alpha_1 + \alpha_2$, $3\alpha_1 + \alpha_2$, $3\alpha_1 + 2\alpha_2$.

(III) We have $h = \frac{n}{2} = 6$.

(IV) The highest root is $\tilde{\alpha} = 3\alpha_1 + 2\alpha_2 = -\varepsilon_1 - \varepsilon_2 + 2\varepsilon_3$. We have $(\tilde{\alpha}|\alpha_1) = 0, (\tilde{\alpha}|\alpha_2) = 3$. The completed Dynkin graph is

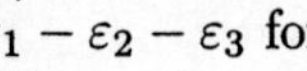

(V) The inverse system is the following set of vectors:

$$\pm\alpha_1, \quad \pm(\alpha_1 + \alpha_2), \quad \pm(2\alpha_1 + \alpha_2), \quad \pm\frac{1}{3}\alpha_2,$$
$$\pm\frac{1}{3}(3\alpha_1 + \alpha_2), \quad \pm\frac{1}{3}(3\alpha_1 + 2\alpha_2).$$

There are 10 roots not orthogonal to α_1; we have $n(\beta, \alpha_1) = \pm 1$ for 4 of these roots, $n(\beta, \alpha_1) = \pm 3$ for 4 others, and $n(\beta, \alpha_1) = \pm 2$ for $\beta = \pm\alpha_1$. Hence, the squared length of α_1 for Φ_{R} is $4(4.1 + 4.9 + 2.4)^{-1} = \frac{1}{12}$. Hence, $\Phi_{\mathrm{R}}(x, y) = (x|y)/24$. We now apply formula (18) of § 1, no. 12, with $x = y = \alpha_1$; this gives

$$2 + 4.\frac{1}{4} + 4.\frac{1}{4} = \gamma(\mathrm{R}).\frac{1}{12}$$

so $\gamma(\mathrm{R}) = 48$.

(VI) and (VII) Half the sum of the positive roots is

$$\rho = 5\alpha_1 + 3\alpha_2.$$

The fundamental weights ω_1 and ω_2 are orthogonal to α_2 and α_1, hence proportional to $2\alpha_1 + \alpha_2$ and $3\alpha_1 + 2\alpha_2$. We have

$$\omega_1 + \omega_2 = \rho = 5\alpha_1 + 3\alpha_2 = (2\alpha_1 + \alpha_2) + (3\alpha_1 + 2\alpha_2).$$

Hence,

$$\omega_1 = 2\alpha_1 + \alpha_2, \quad \omega_2 = 3\alpha_1 + 2\alpha_2 = \tilde{\alpha}.$$

(VIII) Q(R) is generated by $\varepsilon_1 - \varepsilon_2$ and $\varepsilon_1 - \varepsilon_3$, for example. By (VI) and (VII), P(R) = Q(R). The connection index is 1.

(IX) The family of exponents has 2 terms; since 1 and $h - 1 = 5$ are exponents, they are the only ones.

(X) We have $(\widehat{\alpha_1, \alpha_2}) = \frac{5\pi}{6}$, so W(R) is isomorphic to the dihedral group of order 12.

(XI) The only automorphism of the Dynkin diagram is the identity, so A(R) = W(R) and $w_0 = -1$.

14. IRREDUCIBLE NON-REDUCED ROOT SYSTEMS

The irreducible, non-reduced root systems can be obtained from the irreducible, reduced systems by using Props. 13 and 14 of § 1, no. 4. For each integer $l \geqslant 1$, there exists, up to isomorphism, a unique irreducible, non-reduced root system of rank l: let R be a root system of type B_l, A the set of shortest roots of R; take the union of R and 2A. With the notation of no. 5, we obtain the $2l(l+1)$ vectors

$$\pm\varepsilon_i, \quad \pm 2\varepsilon_i, \quad \varepsilon_i \pm \varepsilon_j \quad (i < j).$$

EXERCISES

§1.

All the root systems considered below are relative to *real* vector spaces. We denote by $(x|y)$ a scalar product invariant under the Weyl group (cf. no. 3).

1) Let R be a root system, $R = R_1 \cup R_2$ a partition of R. Assume that, if x, y are two elements of R_i and if $x + y$ (resp. $x - y$) is a root, then $x + y \in R_i$ (resp. $x - y \in R_i$), where $i = 1, 2$. Then, R is the direct sum of R_1 and R_2. (By using the Cor. of Th. 1, no. 3, show that if $x \in R_1$ and $y \in R_2$ then $(x|y) = 0$.)

2) Let R be a root system, α and β two roots. If t is a scalar such that $\beta + t\alpha \in$ R, then $2t \in \mathbf{Z}$. (For $n(\beta + t\alpha, \alpha) = n(\beta, \alpha) + 2t$.) If α is indivisible, then $t \in \mathbf{Z}$. (If not, show, by using Prop. 9, that there exists a root γ orthogonal to α such that $\gamma + \frac{1}{2}\alpha \in$ R; then $(\gamma + \frac{1}{2}\alpha|\alpha) > 0$, so $\frac{1}{2}\alpha \in$ R.)

3) Let R be an irreducible non-reduced root system in V. There exists a non-degenerate symmetric bilinear form Φ on V such that, if we identify V with V^* using Φ, we have $R = R^\vee$. (Use Prop. 13.)

4) Let Γ be a free $\mathbf{Z}$-module of finite rank l, Γ^* the dual $\mathbf{Z}$-module, I a finite set of indices, $(x_i, x_i^*)_{i \in I}$ a family of elements of $\Gamma \times \Gamma^*$ such that $\langle x_i, x_i^* \rangle = 2$ for all $i \in I$, $s_i = s_{x_i, x_i^*}$. Let V be the real vector space $\Gamma \otimes_{\mathbf{Z}} \mathbf{R}$, whose dual V^* can be identified with $\Gamma^* \otimes_{\mathbf{Z}} \mathbf{R}$. We also denote by s_i the reflection $s_i \otimes 1$ in V. Let R (resp. R′) be the set of x_i (resp. x_i^*). Let E (resp. E′) be the subspace of V (resp. V^*) generated by R (resp. R′). Assume that $s_i(R) = R$ for all i. Then, R is a root system in E, E′ is canonically identified with the dual of E and x_i^* with $x_i{}^\vee$ for all i. If F (resp. F′ is the subspace of V (resp. V^*) consisting of the points invariant under all the s_i (resp. ${}^t s_i$), then $\Gamma \cap F$ (resp. $\Gamma^* \cap F'$) generates F (resp. F′). If we put $\Gamma_1 = (\Gamma \cap E) \oplus (\Gamma \cap F)$ (resp. $\Gamma_1^* = (\Gamma^* \cap E') \oplus (\Gamma^* \cap F')$), then Γ / Γ_1 and Γ^* / Γ_1^* are isomorphic finite groups.

5) Let R be an irreducible root system. For any $\beta \in$ R,

$$16\gamma(\mathrm{R}) = (\sum_{\alpha\in\mathrm{R}} n(\alpha,\beta)^2)(\sum_{\alpha\in\mathrm{R}} n(\beta,\alpha)^2)$$

and consequently $\gamma(\mathrm{R}) = \gamma(\lambda\mathrm{R})$ for any non-zero scalar λ. (Use formulas (17) and (19) of no. 12.)

6) *a*) Let A be an abelian group of finite type, and T a finite subset of A not containing 0. There exists a subgroup H of A of finite index such that $\mathrm{H} \cap \mathrm{T} = \varnothing$. (Let $t \in \mathrm{T}$. By using the structure of abelian groups of finite type, construct a subgroup of A of finite index that does not contain t. Now proceed by induction on Card(T).)

b) Let R be a root system and P a closed symmetric subset of R. There exists a subgroup H of Q(R) of finite index such that $\mathrm{P} = \mathrm{H} \cap \mathrm{R}$. (Pass to the quotient by the subgroup of Q(R) generated by P, and use *a*) and Prop. 23.)

7) The connection index of a root system is equal to the determinant of its Cartan matrix. (Use formula (14) of no. 10. Show on the other hand that, in a real vector space with a scalar product, if $(\varepsilon_1, \dots, \varepsilon_n), (\varepsilon'_1, \dots, \varepsilon'_n)$ are two bases such that $(\varepsilon_i|\varepsilon'_j) = \delta_{ij}$, then $\det_{(\varepsilon_1,\dots,\varepsilon_n)}(\varepsilon'_1, \dots, \varepsilon'_n) > 0$.)

8) Let R be a reduced root system, C a chamber, 2σ the sum of the positive elements of $\mathrm{R}^\vee$, $\mathrm{P}'(\mathrm{R})$ the set of $x \in \mathrm{P}(\mathrm{R})$ such that $\langle x, \sigma\rangle \in \mathbf{Z}$. Then, $\mathrm{Q}(\mathrm{R}) \subseteq \mathrm{P}'(\mathrm{R}) \subseteq \mathrm{P}(\mathrm{R})$, and $\mathrm{P}(\mathrm{R})/\mathrm{P}'(\mathrm{R})$ is of order 1 or 2. Let $(\beta_1, \dots, \beta_l)$ be the basis of $\mathrm{R}^\vee$ corresponding to C, and put $2\sigma = n_1\beta_1 + \cdots + n_l\beta_l$ where the n_i are integers > 0. Then, $\mathrm{P}(\mathrm{R}) = \mathrm{P}'(\mathrm{R})$ if and only if all the n_i are even.

¶ 9) Let R be a root system, C a chamber. Put $\mathrm{B}(\mathrm{C}) = \{\alpha_1, \dots, \alpha_l\}$,

$$\mathrm{R}_+(\mathrm{C}) = \{\alpha_1, \dots, \alpha_l, \alpha_{l+1}, \dots, \alpha_s\}$$

(the α_i being pairwise distinct), and $\alpha = \alpha_1 + \cdots + \alpha_s$.

a) For $i = 1, 2, \dots, s$, put $\varepsilon_i = \pm 1$. Let $\alpha^* = \varepsilon_1\alpha_1 + \cdots + \varepsilon_s\alpha_s$. If $(\alpha^*|\alpha_i) > 0$ for $i = 1, \dots, l$, then $\alpha^* = \alpha$ and $\varepsilon_i = 1$ for all i. (Let γ (resp. δ) be the sum of the α_i for which $\varepsilon_i = 1$ (resp. -1). Then, $(\gamma|\alpha_i) - (\delta|\alpha_i) > 0, (\gamma|\alpha_i) + (\delta|\alpha_i) = (\alpha_i|\alpha_i)$, so

$$2(\gamma|\alpha_i) > (\alpha_i|\alpha_i);$$

since $2(\gamma|\alpha_i)/(\alpha_i|\alpha_i) \in \mathbf{Z}$, $(\gamma|\alpha_i) \geqslant (\alpha_i|\alpha_i) = (\alpha|\alpha_i)$, so $\gamma - \alpha \in \overline{\mathrm{C}}$, $\gamma \geqslant \alpha$, $\gamma = \alpha$ and $\delta = 0$.)

b) For $i = 1, 2, \dots, s$, let $\varepsilon_i = \pm 1$. The set of $\varepsilon_i\alpha_i$ is the set of roots > 0 relative to a chamber if and only if $\alpha^* = \sum_i \varepsilon_i\alpha_i$ belongs to a chamber. (To show that the condition is sufficient, let $\mu_i = \pm 1$ be such that $(\alpha^*|\mu_i\alpha_i) > 0$. There exists an element $w \in \mathrm{W}(\mathrm{R})$ that transforms the set of $\mu_i\alpha_i$ into the set of α_i, and hence α^* into $\alpha^{**} = \sum_i \varepsilon_i\mu_i\alpha_{\sigma(i)}$, where $\sigma \in \mathfrak{S}_s$. Applying *a*), show that $\alpha^{**} = \alpha$, so $\mu_i\varepsilon_i = 1$.)

10) Let α be the highest root of an irreducible reduced root system R relative to some basis. Then, $\alpha^\vee$ is the highest root of $R^\vee$ if and only if all the roots are of the same length.

11) With the notation of Prop. 33 of no. 11, show that $\theta_i + \theta_j$ is not a root for any pair (i, j).

12) Let R be a root system in V of rank $\geqslant 3$, $(\alpha_1, \dots, \alpha_l)$ a basis of R, V′ (resp. V″) the subspace of V generated by the α_i for $i \geqslant 2$ (resp. $i \geqslant 3$), $R' = R \cap V'$, $R'' = R \cap V''$. Let d (resp. d', d'') be the determinant of the Cartan matrix of R (resp. R′, R″). Assume that α_1 is orthogonal to all the α_i except α_2, and that $\| \alpha_1 \| = \| \alpha_2 \|$. Show that $d = 2d' - d''$.

13) Let R be a reduced root system, $(\alpha_1, \dots, \alpha_l)$ a basis of R and $\alpha = c_1\alpha_1 + \cdots + c_l\alpha_l$ a root. Then, $c_i(\alpha_i|\alpha_i)/(\alpha|\alpha) \in \mathbf{Z}$ for all i. (Consider the inverse system.)

14) Let R be an irreducible root system, λ the greatest root length, S the set of subsets of R consisting of pairwise orthogonal roots of length λ. Then, any two maximal elements of S are transformed into each other by W(R). (Use Prop. 11, and Prop. 1 of Chap. V, § 3, no. 3.)

15) Let R be a root system of rank l.

a) $-1 \in W(R)$ if and only if R contains l roots that are pairwise strongly orthogonal. (To show that the condition is necessary, argue by induction on l using Prop. 1 of Chap. V, § 3, no. 3.)

b) If $w \in W(R)$ is of order 2, there exists a set S of pairwise strongly orthogonal roots such that w is the product of the s_α ($\alpha \in S$).

16) Let R be a root system, B a basis of R, and R_+ the set of positive roots relative to this basis. For $w \in W(R)$, put $F_w = R_+ \cap w(-R_+)$. Show that the map $w \mapsto F_w$ is a bijection from W(R) to the set of subsets F of R_+ such that F and $R_+ - F$ are closed. (Apply Cor. 1 of Prop. 20 to the subset $P = (R_+ - F) \cup (-F)$.)

¶ 17) Let R be a reduced root system and B a basis of R. For any susbet J of B, let W_J be the subgroup of W(R) generated by the reflections s_α for $\alpha \in J$, and let w_J be the longest element of W_J. Let Φ be the set of w_J.

a) Show that an element $w \in W(R)$ belongs to Φ if and only if

$$W(B) \subseteq R_+(B) \cup (-B).$$

(To show that the condition is sufficient, denote by J_1 the set of $\alpha \in B$ such that $w(\alpha) \in -B$ and put $J = -w(J_1)$. If $\alpha \in J_1$, $w(\alpha) \in -J$ and $w_J w(\alpha) \in B$;

if $\alpha \in B - J_1$, $w_J w(\alpha) \in R_+$: otherwise $w(\alpha)$ would be positive and $w_J w(\alpha)$ negative, which would imply that $w(\alpha)$ belongs to the subsystem generated by the $\beta \in J$ and that α belongs to the subsystem generated by the $\beta \in J_1$, which is absurd. Deduce that $w_J w = 1$.)

18) Let R be a root system and let P be a parabolic subset of R. Show that the complement of P in R is closed.

19) Let R be a root system, and let x be a non-zero element of Q(R) of minimal length. Show that $x \in R$.

¶ 20) Let $(\alpha_1, \dots, \alpha_l)$ be a basis of an irreducible reduced root system R. Let r and p be two integers, with $p \geqslant 2$, such that:

$$(\alpha_1|\alpha_1) = \cdots = (\alpha_r|\alpha_r) = p.(\alpha_{r+1}|\alpha_{r+1}) = \cdots = p.(\alpha_l|\alpha_l).$$

a) Let $\alpha = c_1\alpha_1 + \cdots + c_l\alpha_l$ be a root. Show that $(\alpha|\alpha) = (\alpha_1|\alpha_1)$ (in other words, that α is a long root) if and only if p divides $c_{r+1}, \dots, c_l$.

b) Let h be the Coxeter number of W(R). Show that the number of longest (resp. shortest) roots of R is equal to hr (resp. $h(l-r)$).

21) Let R be a root system and B a basis of R. Let $\alpha, \beta \in B$ and $w \in W(R)$ be such that $\beta = w(\alpha)$. Show that there exists a sequence $\alpha_1, \dots, \alpha_n$ of elements of R and a sequence $w_1, \dots, w_{n-1}$ of elements of W(R) such that

(i) $\alpha_1 = \alpha, \quad \alpha_n = \beta$.

(ii) $w = w_{n-1} \dots w_1$.

(iii) $w_i(\alpha_i) = a_{i+1}$ for $1 \leqslant i \leqslant n-1$.

(iv) For all $i \in [1, n-1]$, there exist $\beta_i \in B$ such that w_i belongs to the subgroup of W(R) generated by the reflections s_{α_i} and s_{β_i}.

¶ 22) With the assumptions and notations of Prop. 33 of no. 11, denote by $\omega_1, \dots, \omega_l$ the fundamental weights of R.

a) Show that $c^{-1}(\omega_i) = \omega_i - \theta_i$. Deduce that $1 - c$ maps P(R) to Q(R).

b) Let f be the connection index of R, and let $m_1, \dots, m_l$ be the exponents of W(R). Show that

$$f = \det(1-c) = \prod_{j=1}^{l} (1 - w^{m_j}) = 2^l \prod_{j=1}^{l} \sin(m_j\pi/h)$$

with $w = e^{2\pi i/h}$.

c) Let p be a prime number. Write h in the form $h = p^a\mathrm{H}$, with H not divisible by p. Show that p divides f if and only if H divides one of the m_j. [2]

23) Let R be a reduced root system, and let X be a subset of P(R). Say that X is *saturated* if the following condition is satisfied:

(S) For all $p \in \mathrm{X}, \alpha \in \mathrm{R}$ and $i \in \mathbf{Z}$ such that i is between 0 and $\langle p, \alpha\check{}\rangle$, $p - i\alpha \in \mathrm{X}$.

a) Show that every saturated subset is stable under the Weyl group W of R.

b) Show that, for any subset A of P(R), there exists a smallest saturated subset S(A) of P(R) containing A.

c) Let C be a chamber of R, and let $p \in \mathrm{P(R)} \cap \overline{\mathrm{C}}$ be a dominant weight. Let S(p) be the smallest saturated subset of P(R) containing p. Let $\Sigma(p)$ be the set of elements $p' \in \mathrm{P(R)}$ such that

(i) $p \equiv p'$ mod. Q(R).

(ii) For all $w \in \mathrm{W}$, $w(p') \leqslant w$ (with respect to the order relation defined by C).

Show that $\Sigma(p)$ is finite, contains p, and is saturated. Conclude that S(p) is contained in $\Sigma(p)$.

d) Show that, if α is a longest element of R, $\mathrm{S}(\alpha) = \mathrm{R} \cup \{0\}$.

24) We retain the notation and assumptions of the preceding exercise.

a) Let $p \in \mathrm{P(R)}$, and let W.p be the orbit of p under W. Show that the following conditions are equivalent:

(i) $\mathrm{S}(p) = \mathrm{W}.p$.

(ii) $\langle p, \alpha\check{}\rangle = 0, 1$ or -1 for all $\alpha \in \mathrm{R}$.

(If (ii) is not satisfied, construct an element $q \in \mathrm{S}(p)$ such that $(q|q) < (p|p)$, and hence $q \notin \mathrm{W}.p$.)

b) Let X be a non-empty saturated subset of P(R). Show that X contains an element p satisfying conditions (i) and (ii) above. (Take p to be an element of X of minimal length.)

c) Assume that R is irreducible. Let C be a chamber of R, let $\mathrm{B} = \{\alpha_i\}_{i\in\mathrm{I}}$ be the corresponding basis, and let

$$\gamma^* = \sum_i n_i\alpha_i\check{}$$

be the highest root of R$\check{}$. Let J be the set of $i \in \mathrm{I}$ such that $n_i = 1$. Let $p \neq 0$ be a dominant weight. Show that conditions (i) and (ii) of *a*) are equivalent to each of the following conditions:

[2] This exercise, hitherto unpublished, was communicated to us by R. Steinberg.

(iii) $\langle p, \gamma^* \rangle = 1$.

(iv) There exists $i \in \mathrm{J}$ such that p is equal to the corresponding fundamental weight.

A weight p satisfying these conditions is called *minuscule.* Show that every non-empty saturated subset of P(R) contains 0 or a minuscule weight.

§ **2.**

We denote by R a reduced root system in a real vector space V.

1) Let $x \in \mathrm{V}$ and let $\mathrm{W}(x)$ be the subgroup of W(R) consisting of the elements w such that

$$w(x) - x \in \mathrm{Q(R)}.$$

Show that $\mathrm{W}(x)$ is generated by reflections. (Use the affine Weyl group of $\mathrm{R}^{\vee}$.)

2) Assume that R is irreducible. Let $\{\alpha_1, \ldots, \alpha_l\}$ be a basis of R, let $\tilde{\alpha} = \sum_i n_i \alpha_i$ be the highest root of R and let f be the connection index of R. Show that $f - 1$ is equal to the number of indices i such that $n_i = 1$.

3) With the notation and assumptions of no. 3, let u be an automorphism of the affine space E that permutes the hyperplanes $\mathrm{L}_{\alpha,k}$ $(\alpha \in \mathrm{R}, k \in \mathbf{Z})$. Show that u is a displacement. (If u_0 is the linear map associated to u, show that the transpose of u leaves R stable, and hence belongs to the group A(R).) Deduce that G is the normaliser of W_a in the group of automorphisms of the affine space E.

4) Let C′ be a chamber relative to W(R) in V^*, and let C be the alcove with vertex 0 contained in C′. Let S_a (resp. S) be the set of reflections in the walls of C (resp. C′). The pairs $(\mathrm{W}_a, \mathrm{S}_a)$ and (W, S) are Coxeter systems, and $\mathrm{S} \subseteq \mathrm{S}_a$. Show that an element $w \in \mathrm{W}_a$ is $(\mathrm{S}, \varnothing)$-reduced (Chap. IV, § 3, Exerc. 3) if and only if $w(\mathrm{C}) \subseteq \mathrm{C}'$.

¶ 5) Assume that R is irreducible, and choose a chamber C of R in V; denote by B the corresponding basis of R.

a) Show that the minuscule weights (§ 1, Exerc. 24) of R form a system of representatives in P(R) of the non-zero elements of P(R)/Q(R). (Apply to $\mathrm{R}^{\vee}$ the corollary of Prop. 6.)

b) Let X be a saturated subset of Q(R) (§ 1, Exerc. 23). Assume that X is non-empty and not reduced to {0}. Let p be a non-zero element of X of minimal length. Show that $p \in \mathrm{R}$. (In view of *a*), p does not satisfy condition (ii) of Exerc. 24 of § 1; hence, there exists $\alpha \in \mathrm{R}$ such that $\langle p, \alpha^{\vee} \rangle \geqslant 2$, so

$p - \alpha \in X$. Since the length of $p - \alpha$ is strictly less than that of p, $p - \alpha = 0$ so $p \in R$.)

c) Let p be a dominant weight not belonging to Q(R). Show that the saturated subset S(p) generated by p (cf. § 1, Exerc. 23) contains a unique minuscule weight. (Remark that S(p) is contained in a non-trivial class mod. Q(R); conclude by applying *a*) and Exerc. 24 *c*) of § 1.)

d) Let p be a dominant weight not belonging to Q(R). Prove that the following two properties are equivalent:

(i) p is minuscule.

(v) There is no dominant weight $q \neq p$ such that $p - q$ is a linear combination of elements of B with non-negative integer coefficients.

(If q satisfies the conditions of (v), let p_1 be a minuscule weight belonging to S(q). Then, $p_1 \equiv p$ mod. Q(R), $p_1 < p$, and *a*) shows that p is not minuscule. Hence, (i) $\Longrightarrow$ (v). Conversely, if p is not minuscule, let $q \in S(p) - W.p$; transforming q by an element of W if necessary, we can assume that $q \in \overline{C}$; by Exerc. 23 of § 1, $q < p$, $q \neq p$, and $q \equiv p$ mod. Q(R). Hence, (v) $\Longrightarrow$ (i).)

§ 3.

The notations and assumptions are those of nos. 2, 3, 4.

1) *a*) Show that, for all i between 1 and l, there exists a unique derivation D_i of A[P] satisfying the following conditions:

a_1) D_i is A-linear.

a_2) $D_i(e^{\omega_j}) = \delta_{ij} e^{\omega_j}$ (δ_{ij} being the Kronecker symbol).

b) Let $(x_i)_{1 \leqslant i \leqslant l}$ be a family of elements of $A[P]^W$ satisfying the condition of Theorem 1. Show that

$$\det(D_i(x_j)) = d.$$

(Show that $\det(D_i(x_j))$ is anti-invariant and has maximal term e^{ρ}, hence the result if 2 is not a zero divisor in A. Treat the general case by using the principle of permanence of algebraic identities.) [3]

2) Let P′ be a subgroup of P(R) containing Q(R). Show that P′ is stable under W. Construct an example where the algebra $A[P]^W$ is not isomorphic to a polynomial algebra (take for R the product of two systems of rank 1).

[3] This exercise, hitherto unpublished, was communicated to us by R. Steinberg.

§ **4.**

If R is a root system, denote by $W^+(R)$ the set of elements of W(R) of determinant 1.

¶ 1) Let R be a root system of type E_8.

a) Show that if $\alpha, \beta \in R$ are congruent modulo 2Q(R), then $\beta = \pm\alpha$.

b) Deduce from *a*) that, if $w \in W(R)$ acts trivially on Q(R)/2Q(R), then $w = \pm 1$.

c) With the notation of no. 10, show that the quadratic form $\frac{1}{2}(x|x)$ on Q(R) defines by passage to the quotient a non-degenerate quadratic form q_8 on the $\mathbf{F}_2$-vector space Q(R)/2Q(R). Show that the pseudo-discriminant of q_8 (cf. *Algebra*, Chap. IX, § 9, Exerc. 9) is zero, and that q_8 is of index 4.

d) Let $\mathbf{O}(q_8)$ be the orthogonal group of Q(R)/2Q(R) for this form. Define, by passing to the quotient, a homomorphism

$$h : W(R) \to \mathbf{O}(q_8).$$

Show (by comparing orders) that the sequence

$$1 \to \{1, -1\} \to W(R) \xrightarrow{h} \mathbf{O}(q_8) \to 1$$

is exact.

e) Show that the image of $W^+(R)$ under h is the subgroup $\mathbf{O}^+(q_8)$ of $\mathbf{O}(q_8)$ defined in *Algebra*, Chap. IX, § 9, no. 5. Deduce that $W^+(R)/\{1, -1\}$ is a simple non-abelian group.

¶ 2) Let R be a root system of type E_6.

a) Put E = Q(R)/3P(R). This is an $\mathbf{F}_3$-vector space of dimension 5. With the notation of no. 12, show that the scalar product $(x|y)$ defines on E a non-degenerate symmetric bilinear form φ. Show that any two distinct elements of R have distinct images in E.

b) Let $\mathbf{O}(\varphi)$ be the orthogonal group of φ. Then, $\mathbf{O}(\varphi) = \{1, -1\} \times \mathbf{SO}(\varphi)$. The spinor norm defines a surjective homomorphism from $\mathbf{SO}(\varphi)$ to $\{1, -1\}$ whose kernel is denoted by $\mathbf{SO}^+(\varphi)$. The group $\mathbf{SO}^+(\varphi)$ is simple of order 25920. The quotient $\mathbf{O}(\varphi)/\mathbf{SO}^+(\varphi)$ is of type (2, 2). Deduce that $\mathbf{O}(\varphi)$ contains a unique subgroup $\Omega(\varphi)$ of index 2, distinct from $\mathbf{SO}(\varphi)$ and not containing -1.

c) Every element of A(R) defines by passage to the quotient an element of $\mathbf{O}(\varphi)$. Show (by comparing orders) that this gives a homomorphism from A(R) to $\mathbf{O}(\varphi)$. The image of W(R) under this homomorphism is $\Omega(\varphi)$, and that of $W^+(R)$ is $\mathbf{SO}^+(\varphi)$. Hence, W(R) is an extension of $\mathbf{Z}/2\mathbf{Z}$ by a simple group of order 25920.

d) Let $F = Q(R)/2Q(R)$. This is an $\mathbf{F}_2$-vector space of dimension 6. Show that the quadratic form $\frac{1}{2}(x|x)$ defines by passage to the quotient a non-degenerate quadratic form q_6 on $\mathbf{F}$, of pseudo-discriminant equal to 1. If $\mathbf{O}(q_6)$ denotes the corresponding orthogonal group, define, by passing to the quotient, a homomorphism

$$h : W(R) \to \mathbf{O}(q_6).$$

Show that h is injective (note that $-1 \notin W(R)$), and then that it is an isomorphism (compare orders). Deduce that there is an isomorphism from $W^+(R)$ to $\mathbf{O}^+(q_6)$ (cf. *Algebra*, Chap. IX, § 9, no. 5).

e) By comparing *c*) and *d*), show[4] that $\mathbf{SO}^+(\varphi)$ is isomorphic to $\mathbf{O}^+(q_6)$.

¶ 3) Let R be a root system of type E_7.

a) Put $E = Q(R)/2P(R)$. This is an $\mathbf{F}_2$-vector space of dimension 6. With the notation in no. 11, show that the scalar product $(x|y)$ defines a non-degenerate alternating bilinear form on E.

b) Deduce from *a*) the existence of an exact sequence

$$1 \to \{1, -1\} \to W(R) \xrightarrow{h} \mathbf{Sp}(6, \mathbf{F}_2) \to 1.$$

(Use the fact that $\mathbf{Sp}(6, \mathbf{F}_2)$ is of order $2^9.3^4.5.7$.)

c) Show that the restriction of h to $W^+(R)$ is an isomorphism from $W^+(R)$ to $\mathbf{Sp}(6, \mathbf{F}_2)$.

d) Give a second proof of *b*) by using the quadratic form q_7 on the $\mathbf{F}_2$-vector space $Q(R)/2Q(R)$ induced by $\frac{1}{2}(x|x)$, as well as the isomorphism

$$\mathbf{O}(q_7) \to \mathbf{Sp}(6, \mathbf{F}_2).$$

¶ 4) Let R be an irreducible reduced root system in V, $(\alpha_1, \dots, \alpha_l)$ a basis of R, $\tilde{\alpha}$ the highest root. Put $\tilde{\alpha} = n_1\alpha_1 + \dots + n_l\alpha_l$. We are going to determine the maximal closed, symmetric subsets of R, distinct from R.

a) Let $i \in \{1, 2, \dots, l\}$. Let R_i be the set of $\alpha \in R$ which are linear combinations of the α_j for $j \neq i$. Show that R_i is maximal if and only if $n_i = 1$.

[4] M. KNESER has shown that all the "exceptional isomorphisms" between the finite classical groups can be obtained by using an analogous method. Cf. Über die Ausnahme-Isomorphismen zwischen klassischen Gruppen, *Hamburger Abh.*, Vol. XXXI (1967), p. 136-140.

b) Let $i \in \{1, 2, \ldots, l\}$ and assume that $n_i > 1$. Let S_i be the set of roots $\sum_{j=1}^{l} m_j \alpha_j$ with $m_i \equiv 0$ (mod. n_i). Show that S_i is maximal if and only if n_i is prime. (If $n_i = ab$ with $a > 1, b > 1$, consider the subset S' of R consisting of the roots $\sum_j m_j \alpha_j$ with $m_i \equiv 0$ (mod. a), and show that S' strictly contains S_i.) Show that the roots $-\tilde{\alpha}, \alpha_j$ $(j \neq i)$ form a basis of S_i (which is of rank l). Deduce the Dynkin graph of S_i.

c) Every maximal closed, symmetric subset of R is transformed by an element of W(R) into one of the subsets described in *a*) or *b*). (Let Σ be such a subset. Then $\Sigma = R \cap H$, where H is a subgroup of Q(R) of finite index (§ 1, Exerc. 6 *b*)); we can assume that Q(R)/H is cyclic. Then there exists $u^* \in V^*$ such that Σ is the set of $\alpha \in R$ such that $\langle u^*, \alpha \rangle \in \mathbf{Z}$.

d) List the maximal, closed, symmetric subsets of R for the different types of irreducible reduced root systems.

5) Let R be a root system, and P′(R) the subgroup of P(R) introduced in § 1, Exerc. 8. Show that P′(R) = P(R) if R is of type A_l with l even, or B_l with $l \equiv 0, 3$ (mod. 4), or D_l with $l \equiv 0, 1$ (mod. 4), or G_2, or F_4, or E_6, or E_8. Show that P′(R) = Q(R) if R is of type C_l, or B_l with $l \equiv 1, 2$ (mod. 4), or E_7, or A_1. If R is of type A_l with l odd and > 1, P′(R)/Q(R) is the unique subgroup of index 2 in the cyclic group P(R)/Q(R). If R is of type D_l with $l \equiv 2, 3$ (mod. 4), P′(R)/Q(R) is the unique subgroup of order 2 of P(R)/Q(R) stable under A(R).

¶ 6) Let R be an irreducible reduced root system, $(\alpha_1, \ldots, \alpha_l)$ a basis of R, $p_1\alpha_1 + \cdots + p_l\alpha_l$ the highest root, $a_1\alpha_1 + \cdots + a_l\alpha_l$ the sum of the positive roots, $m_1, \ldots, m_l$ the exponents of W(R), g its order, f the connection index.

a) Verify that, in each case,

$$l! p_1 p_2 \ldots p_l m_1 m_2 \ldots m_l = a_1 a_2 \ldots a_l.$$

b) Show that

$$g m_1 m_2 \ldots m_l = f a_1 a_2 \ldots a_l.$$

(Use *a*) and Prop. 7 of § 2, no. 4.)

c) For any positive root $\alpha = \sum_i c_i \alpha_i$, let $e(\alpha) = \sum_i c_i$. Calculate in each case the polynomial

$$P(t) = \sum_{\alpha > 0} t^{e(\alpha)}.$$

Verify[5] that $P(t) = t \sum_{i=1}^{l} (1 + t + \cdots + t^{m_i - 1})$.

---

[5] For a proof that does not use the classification, see: B. KOSTANT, The principal three-dimensional subgroup and the Betti numbers of a complex simple Lie group, *Amer. J. of Maths.*, Vol. LXXXI (1959), p. 973-1032.

7) Let R be an irreducible reduced root system.

a) Verify that the canonical homomorphism from A(R)/W(R) to the group of automorphisms of P(R)/Q(R) is injective.

b) Deduce that -1 belongs to W(R) if and only if $Q(R) \supseteq 2P(R)$.

8) Let R_1 and R_2 be two irreducible reduced root systems. Show that if $W(R_1)$ and $W(R_2)$ have the same order, R_1 is isomorphic to R_2 or $R_2\check{}$. (Use the classification.) Does this result still hold without the assumption that R_1 is irreducible?

9) Let R be a root system of rank l, and let p be a prime number dividing the order of A(R). Show that $p \leqslant l+1$. (Reduce to the irreducible case, and use the classification.)

10) *a*) Let (W, S) be an irreducible, finite Coxeter system. Put

$$W(t) = \sum_{w \in W} t^{l(w)} \quad \text{(cf. Chap. IV, § 1, Exerc. 26.)}$$

Let $m_1, \ldots, m_l$ be the exponents of W (Chap. V, § 6, no. 2). Verify the formula

$$W(t) = \prod_{i=1}^{l} (1 + t + \cdots + t^{m_i})$$

for small values of l (use Th. 1 and Exerc. 26 of Chap. IV, § 1)[6].

b) Let R be a reduced, irreducible root system and W (resp. (W_a) the Weyl group (resp. the affine Weyl group) of R, equipped with the Coxeter group structure determined by the choice of an alcove. Define $W(t)$ and the exponents m_i as above and put

$$W_a(t) = \sum_{w \in W_a} t^{l(w)}.$$

Verify the formula

$$W_a(t) = W(t) \prod_{i=1}^{l} \frac{1}{1 - t^{m_i}} = \prod_{i=1}^{l} \frac{1 + t + \cdots + t^{m_i}}{1 - t^{m_i}}$$

for small values of l (use Th. 2 and Exerc. 26 of Chap. IV, § 1)[7].

---

[6] For a proof of this formula that does not use the classification and is valid for all values of l, see: L. SOLOMON, The orders of the finite Chevalley groups, *Journal of Algebra*, Vol. III (1966), p. 376-393.

[7] For a proof of this formula that does not use the classification and is valid for all values of l, see: R. BOTT, An application of the Morse theory to the topology of Lie groups, *Bull. Soc. Math. France*, Vol. LXXXIV (1956), p. 251-281; N. IWAHORI and H. MATSUMOTO, On some Bruhat decomposition and the structure of the Hecke rings of p-adic Chevalley groups, *Publ. Math. Inst. Hautes Et. Sci.*, no. 25 (1965), p. 5-48.

¶ 11) Let (W, S) be a Coxeter system of type H_3 (cf. Th. 1).

a) With the notation of Chap. V, § 6, no. 2, Proof of Lemma 2, show that $\widehat{(z', z'')} = \pi/5$; deduce that the Coxeter number h of W is equal to 10, and that the exponents of W are 1, 5 and 9.

b) Show, by using *a*), that Card(W) = 120, and that the number of reflections in W is 15.

c) Recover the formula Card(W) = 120 by applying Exerc. 5 of Chap. V, § 3.

d) Let $\mathcal{A}_5$ be the alternating group of $\{1, \ldots, 5\}$; if a, b, c, d are distinct elements of $\{1, \ldots, 5\}$, denote by (ab) the transposition of a and b, and $(ab)(cd)$ the product of the transpositions (ab) and (cd). Let

$$r_1 = (14)(23), \quad r_2 = (12)(45), \quad r_3 = (12)(34).$$

Show that $(r_1 r_2)^5 = (r_2 r_3)^3 = (r_1 r_3)^2 = 1$. Deduce the existence of a homomorphism $f : \mathrm{W} \to \mathcal{A}_5$ that takes S to $\{r_1, r_2, r_3\}$; show that f is surjective.

e) Let $\varepsilon : \mathrm{W} \to \{\pm 1\}$ be the homomorphism $w \mapsto (-1)^{l(w)}$. Show that

$$(f, \varepsilon) : \mathrm{W} \to \mathcal{A}_5 \times \{\pm 1\}$$

is an isomorphism. (Use the fact that the two groups being considered have the same order.)

¶ 12) Let $(1, i, j, k)$ be the canonical basis of the field **H** of quaternions, by means of which **H** is identified with $\mathbf{R}^4$. Equip **H** with the scalar product $\frac{1}{2}(x\bar{y} + y\bar{x})$. Let Γ be the multiplicative group of quaternions of norm 1.

a) If $a \in \Gamma$, the orthogonal reflection s_a in **H** which transforms a to $-a$ is the map $x \mapsto -a\bar{x}a$.

b) Let $q = \cos\frac{\pi}{5} - \frac{1}{2}i + (\cos\frac{3\pi}{5})j \in \Gamma$, and $r = \frac{1}{2}(1 + i + j + k) \in \Gamma$. Let Q be the set of quaternions obtained from $1, q, r$ by arbitrary even permutations and sign changes of the coordinates. Then Q is a subgroup of Γ of order 120.

c) Let W be the subgroup of $\mathbf{GL}(\mathbf{H})$ generated by the s_a for $a \in \mathrm{Q}$. Show that W leaves Q stable, is finite, irreducible, and non-crystallographic; deduce that W is of type H_4 (cf. Theorem 1).

d) Show that W acts transitively on Q (use Prop. 3 of Chap. IV, § 1).

e) Let $a_0 \in \mathrm{Q}$, let V be the vector subspace of **H** orthogonal to a_0, and let W_0 be the stabiliser of a_0 in W. Show that the restriction of W_0 to V is an irreducible group generated by reflections (Chap. V, § 3, no. 3) and that it is non-crystallographic. Deduce that W_0 is a Coxeter group of type H_3.

f) Show that $\mathrm{Card(W)} = 2^6 3^2 5^2$ (use *d*), *e*) and Exerc. 11).

g) Show that the Coxeter number of W is equal to 30, and that its exponents are 1, 11, 19, 29.

13) Let V be the hyperplane in $\mathbf{R}^9$ with equation $x_1 + \cdots + x_9 = 0$. Let R be the subset of V consisting of the points

$$(2,2,2,-1,-1,-1,-1,-1,-1), \quad (-2,-2,-2,1,1,1,1,1,1),$$
$$(3,-3,0,0,0,0,0,0,0)$$

together with the points obtained from these by permuting the coordinates. Show that R is a root system in V of type E_8.

14) With the notation in no. 7, show that the automorphism of $\mathbf{R}^{l+1}$ which transforms ε_1 to ε_2, ε_2 to $\varepsilon_3, \ldots, \varepsilon_l$ to ε_{l+1} and ε_{l+1} to ε_1 induces a Coxeter transformation of the system R of type A_l.

15) Determine the minuscule weights (§ 1, Exerc. 24) for each type of reduced, irreducible root system. (One finds the fundamental weights $\omega_1, \ldots, \omega_l$ for A_l, the weight ω_l for B_l, the weight ω_1 for C_l, the weights $\omega_1, \omega_{l-1}, \omega_l$ for D_l, the weights ω_1 and ω_6 for E_6, the weight ω_7 for E_7, and none for E_8, F_4 and G_2.)

¶ 16) Let (W, S) be an irreducible, finite Coxeter system, and let $n = \mathrm{Card}(S)$.

a) If (W, S) is not of type F_4, show that there exists a subset X of S with $n-1$ elements such that (W_X, X) is of type A_{n-1}.

b) Identify W with a subgroup of $\mathbf{GL}(\mathbf{R}^S)$ by means of the canonical representation (Chap. V, § 4). Show that there exists a basis $(e_1, \ldots, e_n)$ of $\mathbf{R}^S$ such that, for every permutation $\sigma \in \mathfrak{S}_n$, the automorphism of $\mathbf{R}^S$ that transforms e_i to $e_{\sigma(i)}$ for $1 \leqslant i \leqslant n$ belongs to W ("Burnside's Theorem"). (When (W, S) is not of type F_4, use *a*); when it is of type F_4, remark that W contains a subgroup of type D_4 (cf. no. 9), which reduces the problem to the preceding case.)

c) Let E be a subgroup of the group of automorphisms of (W, S). Show that the semi-direct product E.W of E by W embeds in a canonical way in $\mathbf{GL}(\mathbf{R}^S)$. Show that the subgroup of $\mathbf{GL}(\mathbf{R}^S)$ thus defined is generated by reflections, except in the following four cases:

(i) (W, S) is of type A_n, $n \geqslant 4$; the group E is of order 2.

(ii) (W, S) is of type D_4; the group E is of order 3.

(iii) (W, S) is of type F_4; the group E is of order 2.

(iv) (W, S) is of type E_6; the group E is of order 2.

Show that, in cases (i) and (iv), $E.W = \{\pm 1\} \times W$. Show that, in case (iii), the group E.W does not leave stable any lattice in $\mathbf{R}^S$.

d) Let W_1 be a finite subgroup of $\mathbf{GL}_n(\mathbf{R})$ generated by reflections, and assume that W_1 is irreducible and essential. Let G be a finite subgroup of $\mathbf{GL}_n(\mathbf{R})$ containing W_1. Show that either G is generated by reflections or is of the form E.W, where E and W are one of the types (i), (ii), (iii), (iv) of *c*).

(Let W be the group generated by the reflections belonging to G. The group G permutes the chambers relative to W. Deduce, as in § 2, no. 3, that G is of the form E.W as above.)

HISTORICAL NOTE (CHAPTERS IV, V AND VI)

(N.B. - The roman numerals in parentheses refer to the bibliography at the end of this note.)

The groups considered in these chapters appeared in connection with various questions of Geometry, Analysis and the Theory of Lie groups, sometimes in the form of permutation groups and sometimes in the form of groups of displacements in euclidean or hyperbolic geometry, and these various points of view have been unified only recently.

The historical roots of the theory are substantially earlier than the introduction of the concept of a group: indeed, they are found in the studies of the "regularity" or "symmetries" of geometrical figures, and notably in the determination of the regular polygons and polyhedra (which certainly goes back to the Pythagoreans), which constitutes the crowning achievement of the *Elements* of Euclid and one of the most admirable creations of the Greek genius. Later, notably with the Arab authors of the high Middle Ages, and then with Kepler, the beginnings of the mathematical theory of regular "tilings" of the plane or the sphere by (not necessarily regular) congruent polygons appear; this is undoubtedly related to the various types of decoration devised by the ancient and Arab civilisations (which can properly be considered as an authentic part of the mathematics developed by these civilisations (XII)).

Around 1830-1840, studies in crystallography (Hessel, Bravais, Möbius) lead to the consideration of a problem that is actually the determination of the finite groups of displacements in euclidean space of 3 dimensions, although the authors quoted above do not yet use the language of group theory; that does not really come into use until about 1860, and it is in the context of the classification of groups that Jordan, in 1869 (VI), determines the discrete groups of orientation-preserving displacements of $\mathbf{R}^3$ (and, more generally, the *closed* subgroups of the group of orientation-preserving displacements).

This stream of ideas develops in many directions until the final years of the 19th century. The most significant of these developments are the following:

1. Continuing a trend that appears very early in the theory of finite groups, "presentations" of finite groups of displacements by generators and relations

of a simple type are sought. Thus, Hamilton, in 1856 (V), proves that the finite groups of rotations of euclidean space $\mathbf{R}^3$ are generated by two generators S, T satisfying the relations $S^p = T^q = (ST)^3 = 1$ for appropriate values of p and q.

2. Discrete groups of displacements may or may not contain reflections. In 1852, Möbius essentially determines the finite groups of displacements in spherical geometry *generated by reflections* (which is equivalent to the same problem for finite groups of euclidean displacements of $\mathbf{R}^3$); he finds that, with the exception of the cyclic groups, such a group has as fundamental domain a spherical triangle with sides of the form $\pi/p, \pi/q, \pi/r$, where p, q, r are three integers > 1 such that $\frac{1}{p} + \frac{1}{q} + \frac{1}{r} > 1$ (III) (cf. Chap. V, § 4, Exerc. 4). He also notices that these groups contain all the finite groups of displacements as subgroups.

3. The latter developments are extended into a new area when the study of "tilings" of the complex plane or of the half-plane by means of figures bounded by circular arcs begins, following the work of Riemann and Schwarz on hypergeometric functions and conformal representations; Klein and Poincaré make it the foundation of the theory of "automorphic functions" and recognise in it (for the case of circular arcs orthogonal to a fixed straight line) a problem equivalent to the determination of the discrete groups of displacements of the non-euclidean hyperbolic plane (identified with the "Poincaré half-plane") (X).

4. The notions of regular polyhedron and of the tiling of $\mathbf{R}^3$ by such polyhedra are extended to all the euclidean spaces $\mathbf{R}^n$ by Schläfli, in work that goes back to about 1850, but which was only published much later and which was ignored for a long time (IV); he determines completely the regular "polytopes" in each $\mathbf{R}^n$, the group of displacements leaving invariant such a polytope, and a fundamental domain of this group which, as in the case $n = 3$ studied by Möbius, is a "chamber" whose projection on the sphere $\mathbf{S}_{n-1}$ is a spherical simplex. However, he does not take up the inverse problem of determining the finite groups of displacements generated by reflections in $\mathbf{R}^n$; this problem will only be solved much later, by Goursat for $n = 4$ (VII), and for arbitrary n in the work of E. Cartan (IX f)) and Coxeter (XIV), to which we shall return later.

With the work of Killing and of E. Cartan on Lie groups, a new stream of ideas begins around 1890 that will develop for a long period without links to the preceding work. In the study of Killing (VIII) and Cartan (IX a)) of the structure of complex semisimple Lie algebras, certain linear forms ω_α on a "Cartan subalgebra" $\mathfrak{h}$ of such a Lie algebra $\mathfrak{g}$ immediately play a basic role; they are the "roots" relative to $\mathfrak{h}$, so called because they appear as the roots of the characteristic equation $\det(\mathrm{ad}_{\mathfrak{g}}(x) - \mathrm{T}) = 0$, considered as functions of $x \in \mathfrak{h}$. The properties of these "roots" established by Killing and Cartan amount to the assertion that, in the language of Chap. VI, they form a "reduced root system" (cf. Chap. VI, § 1, no. 4); they then show that the classification of the complex semisimple Lie algebras reduces to that of the associated "root systems", which itself reduces to the determination of certain matrices with integer coefficients (later called "Cartan matrices"; cf. Chap. VI, § 1, no. 5). Killing and Cartan also show the existence, for every root ω_α, of an involutive permutation S_α of the set of roots[8]; they use in an essential way the transformation $C = S_{\alpha_1} S_{\alpha_2} \dots S_{\alpha_l}$, the product of the permutations associated with l roots forming a fundamental system (a transformation today called a "Coxeter transformation"); they even extend this permutation to a linear transformation of the vector space generated by the fundamental roots ω_{α_i} $(1 \leqslant i \leqslant l)$, and study its eigenvalues ((VIII, II), p. 20; (IX a)), p. 58). But neither Killing, nor Cartan initially, seem to have thought of considering the group $\mathcal{G}'$ generated by the S_α; and when Cartan, a little later (IX b)), determines the Galois group $\mathcal{G}$ of the characteristic equation

$$\det(\mathrm{ad}_{\mathfrak{g}}(x) - T) = 0$$

of a "general element" $x \in \mathfrak{h}$, he studies it initially without bringing in the S_α; thirty years later, under the influence of H. Weyl, he proves (IX c)) that $\mathcal{G}'$ is a normal subgroup of $\mathcal{G}$ and determines in all cases the structure of the quotient group $\mathcal{G}/\mathcal{G}'$ which (for a simple Lie algebra $\mathfrak{g}$) is of order 1 or 2, except for type D_4 where it is isomorphic to $\mathfrak{S}_3$; at the same time he interprets $\mathcal{G}'$ as the group induced by the inner automorphisms of a complex semisimple Lie algebra leaving fixed a Cartan subalgebra[9].

The work of H. Weyl, to which we have just alluded, inaugurated the geometric interpretation of the group $\mathcal{G}'$ (since called the "Weyl group" of $\mathfrak{g}$); he had the idea of considering the S_α as reflections in the vector space of linear forms on $\mathfrak{h}$, in the same way as Killing and Cartan had done for the transformation C. It is also in the memoir (XIII) of H. Weyl that the fundamental domain of the "affine Weyl group" appears (but without the link to the "Weyl group" $\mathcal{G}'$ being clearly indicated); Weyl uses it to to prove that the fundamental group of a compact semisimple group is finite, a crucial point in his proof of the complete reducibility of the linear representations of a complex semisimple Lie algebra. A little later, E. Cartan completes the synthesis of the global points of view of H. Weyl, of his own theory of real or complex semisimple Lie algebras, and of the theory of riemannian symmetric spaces that he was then constructing. In the memoir (IX d)), he completes the determination of the fundamental polytopes of the Weyl group and of the affine Weyl group, and introduces the systems of weights and radical weights (Chap. VI, § 1, no. 9); in (IX e)) he extends this discussion to symmetric spaces, and notably encounters the first examples of non-reduced root systems (Chap. VI, § 4, no. 1). Finally, the article (IX f)) gives the first

[8] The notations ω_α and S_α correspond respectively to the notations α and s_α of Chap. VI, § 1.

[9] The notations $\mathcal{G}$ and $\mathcal{G}'$ correspond respectively to the notations A(R) and W(R) of Chap. VI, § 1, no. 1.

proof that every irreducible finite group generated by reflections in $\mathbf{R}^n$ has a fundamental domain whose projection onto $\mathbf{S}_{n-1}$ is a spherical simplex; it is also in this work that he proves the uniqueness of the highest root (for an arbitrary lexicographic ordering on the root system) by geometrical considerations.

A little later, van der Waerden (XVI), starting from the memoir of H. Weyl, shows that the classification of the complex semisimple Lie algebras is equivalent to that of the reduced root systems, which he carries out by elementary geometric considerations (whereas, with Killing and Cartan, this classification is a result of complicated calculations with determinants). At about the same time, Coxeter determines explicitly all the irreducible finite groups of Euclidean displacements which are generated by reflections (XIV *c*)); this completes the memoir (IX *d*)) of Cartan, which had only determined the "crystallographic" groups (i.e. those associated to a root system, or having an embedding in an infinite discrete group of displacements). The following year (XIV *d*)), Coxeter shows that the finite groups generated by reflections are the only finite groups (up to isomorphism) admitting a presentation by generators R_i subject to relations of the form $(R_iR_j)^{m_{ij}} = 1$ (m_{ij} integers), hence the name "Coxeter" groups since given to groups (finite or not) admitting such a presentation.

The first link between the two streams of research that we have described above seems to have been established by Coxeter (XIV *bis*), and then by Witt (XVII). They observe that the irreducible infinite groups of Euclidean displacements generated by reflections correspond bijectively (up to isomorphism) to complex simple Lie algebras. Witt gives a new determination of discrete groups of this type, and also extends the theorem of Coxeter (XIV *d*)) referred to above by characterising the Coxeter groups isomorphic to infinite discrete groups of Euclidean displacements. This result, and the fact that the analogous groups in hyperbolic geometry are also Coxeter groups[10], has led to the latter groups being studied directly, initially emphasising the geometric realisation ((XV), (XXV)), and then, following J. Tits (XXV), in a purely algebraic framework.

Starting with the work of Witt, the theory of semisimple Lie groups and that of discrete groups generated by reflections continue to interact extremely fruitfully with each other. In 1941, Stifel (XVIII) remarks that the Weyl groups are exactly the finite groups generated by reflections that leave a lattice invariant. Chevalley (XIX *a*)) and Harish-Chandra (XX *a*)) give, in 1948-51, *a priori* proofs of the bijective correspondence between "crystallographic" groups and complex semisimple Lie algebras; until then, it had only been possible to verify this correspondence separately for each type of simple Lie algebra.

[10]These groups, studied in depth in the case of dimension 2, have so far only been considered incidentally in dimensions $\geqslant 3$.

On the other hand, it is observed around 1950 that the polynomials invariant under the Weyl group play an important role in two areas, the theory of infinite-dimensional linear representations (XX *a*)) and in the topology of Lie groups. Coxeter (XIV *f*)) again takes up the study of the transformation C formed by taking the product of the fundamental reflections of a finite group W generated by reflections. He observes (by means of a separate examination of each type) that the algebra of polynomials invariant under W is generated by algebraically independent elements whose degrees are related in a simple way to the eigenvalues of C. A *priori* proofs of these results were given by Chevalley (XIX *b*)) in the first area, and by Coleman (XXIII) and Steinberg (XXIV) in the second.

With the work of A. Borel on linear algebraic groups (XXII), new developments begin which are to lead to a notable enlargement of the theory of Lie groups. A. Borel emphasises the importance of the maximal connected soluble subgroups (since called "Borel subgroups") of a Lie group, and makes them the principal tool for transporting a large part of the classical theory to algebraic groups over an algebraically closed field (but without obtaining a classification of the simple algebraic groups[11]). The Borel subgroups (in the case of real or complex classical groups) had already arisen some years earlier in the work of Gelfand and Neumark on inifinite-dimensional representations; and in 1954, F. Bruhat had discovered the remarkable fact that, for the classical simple groups, the decomposition of the group into double cosets over a Borel subgroup is indexed in a canonical way by the Weyl group (XXI). This result was subsequently extended to all real and complex semisimple groups by Harish-Chandra (XX *b*)). On the other hand, in 1955, Chevalley (XIX *c*)) had succeeded in associating to every complex semisimple Lie algebra $\mathfrak{g}$ and to *every* commutative field k, a group of matrices with coefficients in k having a Bruhat decomposition; and he used this last fact to show, with a small number of exceptions, that the group thus defined was *simple* (in the sense of the theory of abstract groups). He thus "explained" the coincidence, already noticed by Jordan and Lie, between the simple Lie groups (in the sense of the theory of Lie groups) of type A, B, C, D and the classical simple groups defined in a purely algebraic manner over an arbitrary field (a coincidence which had until then only been extended to the exceptional types G_2 and F_4 by Dickson (XI *b*) and *c*))). In particular, by taking a *finite* field k, the construction of Chevalley provided, for each type of complex simple Lie algebra, a family of *finite* simple groups, containing a large number of the then known finite simple groups as well as three new series (corresponding to the simple Lie algebras of types F_4, E_7 and E_8). A little later, by various methods, and using modifications of those of Chevalley, several authors (Herzig, Suzuki,

[11]An algebraic group of dimension > 0 is said to be *simple* (in the sense of algebraic geometry) if it does not contain any normal algebraic subgroup of dimension > 0 other than itself. It is said to be *semisimple* if it is isogenous to a product of simple non-abelian groups.

Ree, Steinberg and Tits) showed on the one hand that the other finite simple groups known at the time could be obtained in an analogous way, with the exception of the alternating groups and the Mathieu groups, and on the other hand constructed other series of new finite simple groups (cf. (XXIX)).

At about the same time, Chevalley (XIX *d*)) again took up the study of linear algebraic groups and showed, using the technique of Bruhat decompositions together with a key result on the normaliser of a Borel subgroup, that the theory of semisimple linear algebraic groups over an *algebraically closed* field k of *arbitrary* characteristic[12] leads to essentially the same types as in the Killing-Cartan classification for $k = \mathbf{C}$. After this, J. Tits (XXV *a*) and *b*)), analysing Chevalley's methods, is led to an axiomatised version of the Bruhat decomposition (the "BN-pairs"), in a remarkably versatile form which involves only the group structure; it is this notion that is now known as a "Tits system". All the simple groups (with the various meanings of the term) we have discussed above are canonically equipped with Tits systems, and Tits himself (XXV *c*)) has proved that the existence of such a system in an abstract group G, together with a few additional properties from pure group theory, allows one to prove that G is *simple*, a theorem which covers the majority of the proofs given until then for these groups (cf. Chap. IV, § 2, no. 6). On the other hand, in collaboration with A. Borel, he has generalised the results of Chevalley in (XIX *d*)) by showing the existence of Tits systems in the group of rational points of a semisimple linear algebraic group over an *arbitrary* field (XXVII).

All the Tits systems encountered in these questions have a finite Weyl group. Another category of examples was discovered by Iwahori and Matsumoto (XXVI); they have shown that if, in Chevalley's construction of (XIX *c*)), k is a p-adic field, the group obtained has a Tits system whose Weyl group is the *affine* Weyl group of the complex semisimple Lie algebra with which one started. This result has been extended by Bruhat and Tits (XXVIII) to all semisimple algebraic groups over a local field.

---

[12]The existence of numerous "pathological" simple Lie algebras over a field of characteristic $p > 0$ could have led some to doubt the universal character of the Killing-Cartan classification.

BIBLIOGRAPHY

(I) J. HESSEL, *Krysallometrie oder Krystallonomie und Krystallographie* (1830, repr. in *Ostwald's Klassiker*, nos. 88 and 89, Leipzig (Teubner), 1897)

(II) A. Bravais, Mémoires sur les polyèdres de forme symétrique, *Journal de Math.*, (1), v. XIV (1849), p. 141-180.

(III) A. MÖBIUS: *a*) Ueber das Gesetz der Symmetrie der Krystalle und die Anwendung dieses Gesetze auf die Eintheilung der Krystalle in Systeme, *J. für die reine und angewandte Math.*, v. XLIII (1852), p. 365-374 (= *Gesammelte Werke*, v. II, Leipzig (Hirzel), 1886, p. 349-360); *b*) Theorie der symmetrischen Figuren, *Gesammelte Werke*, v. II, Leipzig (Hirzel), 1886, p. 561-708.

(IV) L. SCHLÄFLI, Theorie der vielfachen Kontinuität, *Denkschr. der Schweiz. naturforsch. Gesellschaft*, v. XXXVIII (1901), p. 1-237 (= *Ges. math. Abhandlungen*, v. I, Basel (Birkhäuser), 1950, p. 167-387).

(V) W. R. HAMILTON, Memorandum respecting a new system of roots of unity, *Phil. Mag.*, (4), v. XII (1856), p. 446.

(VI) C. JORDAN, Mémoire sur les groupes de mouvements, *Ann. di Mat.*, v. II (1868-69), p. 167-215 and 322-345 (= *Oeuvres*, v. IV, Paris (Gauthier-Villars), 1964, p. 231-302).

(VII) E. GOURSAT, Sur les substitutions orthogonales et les divisions régulières de l'espace, *Ann. Ec. Norm. Sup.*, (3), v. VI (1889), p. 9-102.

(VIII) W. KILLING, Die Zusammensetzung der stetigen endlichen Transformationsgruppen: I) *Math. Ann.*, v. XXXI (1888), p. 252-290; II) *ibid.*, v. XXXIII (1889), p. 1-48; III) *ibid.*, v. XXXIV (1889), p. 57-122; IV) *ibid.*, v. XXXVI (1890), p. 161-189.

(IX) E. CARTAN: *a*) Sur la structure des groupes de transformations finis et continus (Thesis), Paris (Nony), 1894 (= *Oeuvres complètes*, Paris (Gauthier-Villars), 1952, v. I_1, p. 137-287); *b*) Sur la réduction à sa forme canonique de la structure d'un groupe de transformations fini et continu, *Amer. Journ. of Math.*, v. XVIII (1896), p. 1-46 (= *Oeuvres complètes*, Paris (Gauthier-Villars), 1952, v. I_1, p. 293-353); *c*) Le principe de dualité et la théorie des groupes simples et semi-simples, *Bull. Sci. Math.*, v. XLIX (1925), p. 361-374 (= *Oeuvres complètes*, Paris (Gauthier-Villars), 1952, v. I_1, p. 555-568); *d*) La géométrie des groupes simples, *Ann. di Mat.*, (4), v. IV (1927), p. 209-256 (= *Oeuvres complètes*, Paris (Gauthier-Villars), 1952, v. I_2, p. 793-840); *e*) Sur certaines formes riemanniennes remarquables des géométries à groupe fondamental simple, *Ann. Ec. Norm. Sup.*, (3), v. XLIV (1927), p. 345-467 (= *Oeuvres complètes*, Paris (Gauthier-Villars), 1952, v. I_2, p. 867-989); *f*) Complément au mémoire "Sur la géométrie des groupes simples", *Ann. di Mat.*, v, V (1928), p.

253-260 (= *Oeuvres complètes*, Paris (Gauthier-Villars), 1952, v. I_2, p. 1003-1010).

(X) R. FRICKE and F. KLEIN, *Theorie der automorphen Funktionen*, Leipzig (Teubner), 1897.

(XI) L. E. DICKSON: *a*) Theory of linear groups in an arbitrary field, *Trans. Amer. Math. Soc.*, v. II (1901), p. 363-394; *b*) A new system of simple groups, *Math. Ann.*, t. LX (1905), p. 137-150; *c*) A class of groups in an arbitrary realm connected with the configuration of the 27 lines on a cubic surface, *Quart. Journ. of Math.*, v. XXXIII (1901), p. 145-173 and v. XXXIX (1908), p. 205-209.

(XII) A. SPEISER, *Theorie der Gruppen von endlicher Ordnung*, Berlin (Springer), 1924.

(XIII) H. WEYL, Theorie der Darstellung kontinuerlicher halb-einfacher Gruppen durch lineare Transformationen, *Math. Zeitschr.*, v. XXIII (1925), p. 271-309, v. XXIV (1926), p. 328-395 and 789-791 (= *Selecta*, Basel-Stuttgart (Birkhäuser), 1956, p. 262-366).

(XIV) H. S. M. COXETER: *a*) Groups whose fundamental regions are simplexes, *Journ. Lond. Math. Soc.*, v. VI (1931), p. 132-136; *b*) The polytopes with regular prismatic figures, *Proc. Lond. Math. Soc.*, (2), v. XXXIV (1932), p. 126-189; *c*) Discrete groups generated by reflections, *Ann. of Math.*, (2), v. XXXV (1934), p. 588-621; *d*) The complete enumeration of finite groups of the form $R_i^2 = (R_i.R_j)^{k_{ij}} = 1$, *Journ. Lond. Math. Soc.*, v. X (1935), p. 21-25; *e*) *Regular polytopes*, New York (Macmillan), 1948 (2nd ed., 1963); *f*) The product of generators of a finite group generated by reflections, *Duke Math. Journ.*, v. XVIII (1951), p. 765-782.

(XIV *bis*) H. S. M. COXETER and H. WEYL, *The structure and representations of continuous groups* (Inst. for Adv. Study, mimeographed notes by N. Jacobson and R. Brauer, 1934-35): *Appendix*.

(XV) H. S. M. COXETER and W. O. J. MOSER, *Generators and relations for discrete groups*, Ergeb. der Math., Neue Folge, Bd. 14, Berlin (Springer), 1957 (2nd ed., 1963).

(XVI) B. L. van der WAERDEN, Die Klassification der einfachen Lieschen Gruppen, *Math. Zeitschr.*, v. XXXVII (1933), p. 446-462.

(XVII) E. WITT, Spiegelungsgruppen und Aufzählung halbeinfacher Lieschen Ringe, *Abh. Math. Sem. Hamb. Univ.*, v. XIV (1941), p. 289-322.

(XVIII) E. STIFEL, Ueber eine Beziehung zwischen geschlossenen Lie'sche Gruppen und diskontinuierlichen Bewegungsgruppen euklidischer Räume und ihre Anwendung auf die Aufzählung der einfachen Lie'schen Gruppen, *Comm. Math. Helv.*, v. XIV (1941-42), p. 350-380.

(XIX) C. CHEVALLEY: *a*) Sur la classification des algèbres de Lie simples et de leurs représentations, *C. R. Acad. Sci.*, v. CCXXVII (1948), p. 1136-1138; *b*) Invariants of finite groups generated by reflections, *Amer. Journ. of Math.*, v. LXXVII (1955), p. 778-782; *c*) Sur certains groupes simples, *Tohôku Math. Journ.*, (2), v. VII (1955), p. 14-66; *d*) *Classification des groupes de Lie algébriques*, 2 vols., Paris (Inst. H. Poincaré), 1956-58.

(XX) HARISH CHANDRA: *a*) On some applications of the universal enveloping algebra of a semi-simple Lie algebra, *Trans. Amer. Math. Soc.*, v. LXX (1951), p. 28-96; *b*) On a lemma of Bruhat, *Journ. de Math.*, (9), v. XXXV (1956), p. 203-210.

(XXI) F. BRUHAT, Représentations induites des groupes de Lie semi-simples complexes, *C. R. Acad. Sci.*, v. CCXXXVIII (1954), p. 437-439.

(XXII) A. BOREL, Groupes linéaires algébriques, *Ann. of Math.*, (2), v. LXIV (1956), p. 20-80.

(XXIII) A. J. COLEMAN, The Betti numbers of the simple groups, *Can. Journ. of Math.*, v. X (1958), p. 349-356.

(XXIV) R. STEINBERG, Finite reflection groups, *Trans. Amer. Math. Soc.*, v. XCI (1959), p. 493-504.

(XXV) J. TITS: *a*) Groupes simples et géométries associées, *Proc. Int. Congress Math.*, Stockholm, 1962, p. 197-221; *b*) Théorème de Bruhat et sous-groupes paraboliques, *C. R. Acad. Sci.*, v. CCLIV (1962), p. 2910-2912; *c*) Algebraic and abstract simple groups, *Ann. of Math.*, (2), v. LXXX (1964), p. 313-329.

(XXVI) N. IWAHORI and H. MATSUMOTO, On some Bruhat decomposition and the structure of the Hecke rings of p-adic Chevalley groups, *Publ. Math. I.H.E.S.*, no. 25 (1965), p. 5-48.

(XXVII) A. BOREL and J. TITS, Groupes réductifs, *Publ. Math. I.H.E.S.*, no. 27 (1965), p. 55-150.

(XXVIII) F. BRUHAT and J. TITS, Groupes algébriques simples sur un corps local, *Proc. Conf. on local Fields*, p. 23-36, Berlin (Springer), 1967.

(XXIX) R. CARTER, Simple groups and simple Lie algebras, *Journ. Lond. Math. Soc.*, v. XL (1965), p. 193-240.

INDEX OF NOTATION

The reference numbers indicate the chapter, paragraph and number, respectively.

INDEX OF TERMINOLOGY

The reference numbers indicate the chapter, paragraph and number (or, exceptionally, exercise), respectively.

PLATE I

SYSTEMS OF TYPE A_l ($l \geqslant 1$)

(I) V is the hyperplane of $E = \mathbf{R}^{l+1}$ consisting of the points the sum of whose coordinates is zero.
Roots: $\varepsilon_i - \varepsilon_j$ ($i \neq j, 1 \leqslant i \leqslant l+1, 1 \leqslant j \leqslant l+1$).
Number of roots: $n = l(l+1)$.

(II) Basis: $\alpha_1 = \varepsilon_1 - \varepsilon_2, \alpha_2 = \varepsilon_2 - \varepsilon_3, \ldots, \alpha_l = \varepsilon_l - \varepsilon_{l+1}$.
Positive roots: $\varepsilon_i - \varepsilon_j = \sum_{i \leqslant k < j} \alpha_k$ ($1 \leqslant i < j \leqslant l+1$).

(III) Coxeter number: $h = l + 1$.

(IV) Highest root: $\tilde{\alpha} = \varepsilon_1 - \varepsilon_{l+1} = \alpha_1 + \alpha_2 + \cdots + \alpha_l = \omega_1 + \omega_l$.
Completed Dynkin graph ($l \geqslant 2$):

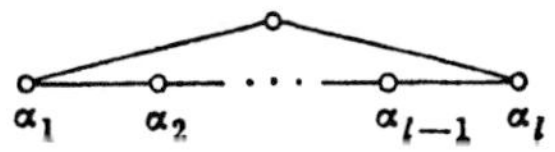

For $l = 1$, the Coxeter graph of the affine Weyl group is

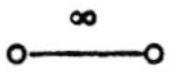

(V) $R^\vee = R$,

$$\Phi_R(x, y) = \frac{(x|y)}{2(l+1)}, \quad \gamma(R) = (l+1)^2.$$

(VI) Fundamental weights:

$$\begin{aligned}
\omega_i &= \varepsilon_1 + \cdots + \varepsilon_i - \frac{i}{l+1} \sum_{j=1}^{l+1} \varepsilon_j \\
&= \frac{1}{l+1} [(l - i + 1)(\alpha_1 + 2\alpha_2 + \cdots + (i-1)\alpha_{i-1}) \\
&\qquad + i((l - i + 1)\alpha_i + (l - i)\alpha_{i+1} + \cdots + \alpha_l)].
\end{aligned}$$

(VII) Sum of the positive roots:

$$\begin{aligned}2\rho &= l\varepsilon_1 + (l-2)\varepsilon_2 + (l-4)\varepsilon_3 + \cdots - (l-2)\varepsilon_l - l\varepsilon_{l+1}\\ &= l\alpha_1 + 2(l-1)\alpha_2 + \cdots + i(l-i+1)\alpha_i + \cdots + l\alpha_l.\end{aligned}$$

(VIII) Q(R): the set of vectors whose coordinates are integers with sum zero.
P(R): generated by Q(R) and $\varepsilon_1 - (l+1)^{-1}(\varepsilon_1 + \varepsilon_2 + \cdots + \varepsilon_{l+1})$.
P(R)/Q(R) is isomorphic to $\mathbf{Z}/(l+1)\mathbf{Z}$.
Connection index: $l+1$.

(IX) Exponents: $1, 2, \ldots, l$.

(X) $W(R) = \mathfrak{S}_{l+1}$, identified with the group of permutations of the ε_i. Order of W(R): $(l+1)!$

(XI) $l = 1$: $A(R) = W(R)$; $w_0 = -1$.
$l \geqslant 2$: $A(R) = W(R) \times \{1, -1\}$ and w_0 transforms α_i to $-\alpha_{l+1-i}$.

(XII) The group $P(R^\vee)/Q(R^\vee)$ is cyclic of order $(l+1)$; it acts on the completed Dynkin graph by circular permutations. If $l \geqslant 2$, the unique non-identity element of A(R)/W(R) acts on P(R)/Q(R) by the automorphism $x \mapsto -x$.

(XIII) Cartan matrix ($l \times l$):

$$\begin{pmatrix} 2 & -1 & 0 & 0 & \cdots & 0 & 0\\ -1 & 2 & -1 & 0 & \cdots & 0 & 0\\ 0 & -1 & 2 & -1 & \cdots & 0 & 0\\ 0 & 0 & -1 & 2 & \cdots & 0 & 0\\ \vdots & \vdots & \vdots & \vdots & \ddots & \vdots & \vdots\\ 0 & 0 & 0 & 0 & \cdots & -1 & 2 \end{pmatrix}$$

PLATE II

SYSTEMS OF TYPE B_l ($l \geqslant 2$)

(I) $V = E = \mathbf{R}^l$.
Roots: $\pm\varepsilon_i$, $(1 \leqslant i \leqslant l)$, $\pm\varepsilon_i \pm \varepsilon_j$ $(1 \leqslant i < j \leqslant l)$.
Number of roots: $n = 2l^2$.

(II) Basis: $\alpha_1 = \varepsilon_1 - \varepsilon_2, \alpha_2 = \varepsilon_2 - \varepsilon_3, \ldots, \alpha_{l-1} = \varepsilon_{l-1} - \varepsilon_l, \alpha_l = \varepsilon_l$.
Positive roots:

$$\varepsilon_i = \sum_{i \leqslant k \leqslant l} \alpha_k \quad (1 \leqslant i \leqslant l),$$

$$\varepsilon_i - \varepsilon_j = \sum_{i \leqslant k < j} \alpha_k \quad (1 \leqslant i < j \leqslant l),$$

$$\varepsilon_i + \varepsilon_j = \sum_{i \leqslant k < j} \alpha_k + 2 \sum_{j \leqslant k \leqslant l} \alpha_k \quad (1 \leqslant i < j \leqslant l),$$

(III) Coxeter number: $h = 2l$.

(IV) Highest root:

$$\tilde{\alpha} = \varepsilon_1 + \varepsilon_2 = \alpha_1 + 2\alpha_2 + 2\alpha_3 + \cdots + 2\alpha_l.$$

We have $\tilde{\alpha} = 2\omega_2$ if $l = 2$, $\tilde{\alpha} = \omega_2$ if $l \geqslant 3$.
Completed Dynkin graph:

for $l = 2$: 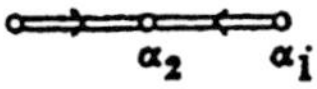

for $l \geqslant 3$: 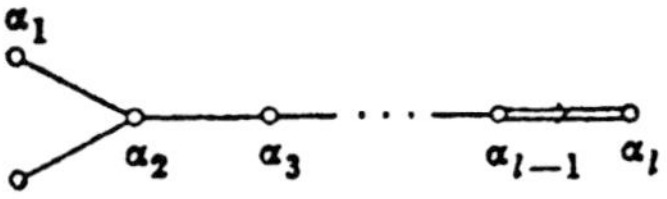

(V) $R^\vee$ is the set of vectors

$$\pm 2\varepsilon_i \ \ (1 \leqslant i \leqslant l), \ \ \pm\varepsilon_i \pm \varepsilon_j \ (1 \leqslant i < j \leqslant l).$$

$$\Phi_R(x, y) = \frac{(x|y)}{4l - 2}, \quad \gamma(R) = (l + 1)(4l - 2).$$

(VI) Fundamental weights:

$$\begin{aligned}\omega_i &= \varepsilon_1 + \varepsilon_2 + \cdots + \varepsilon_i \ (1 \leqslant i < l)\\ &= \alpha_1 + 2\alpha_2 + \cdots + (i-1)\alpha_{i-1} + i(\alpha_i + \alpha_{i+1} + \cdots + \alpha_l)\\ \omega_l &= \frac{1}{2}(\varepsilon_1 + \varepsilon_2 + \cdots + \varepsilon_l)\\ &= \frac{1}{2}(\alpha_1 + 2\alpha_2 + \cdots + l\alpha_l).\end{aligned}$$

(VII) Sum of the positive roots:

$$\begin{aligned}2\rho &= (2l-1)\varepsilon_1 + (2l-3)\varepsilon_2 + \cdots + 3\varepsilon_{l-1} + \varepsilon_l\\ &= (2l-1)\alpha_1 + 2(2l-2)\alpha_2 + \cdots + i(2l-i)\alpha_i + \cdots + l^2\alpha_l.\end{aligned}$$

(VIII) $Q(R) = \bigoplus_{i=1}^{l} \mathbf{Z}\varepsilon_i$, $P(R) = \bigoplus_{i=1}^{l} \mathbf{Z}\varepsilon_i + \mathbf{Z}(\frac{1}{2}\sum_{i=1}^{l} \varepsilon_i)$.
P(R)/Q(R) is isomorphic to $\mathbf{Z}/2\mathbf{Z}$, generated by the image of ω_l.
Connection index: 2.

(IX) Exponents: $1, 3, 5, \ldots, 2l-1$.

(X) W(R) is the semi-direct product of the group $\mathfrak{S}_l$, acting by permutations of the ε_i, by the group $(\mathbf{Z}/2\mathbf{Z})^l$, acting by $\varepsilon_i \mapsto (\pm 1)_i\varepsilon_i$. Its order is $2^l.l!$

(XI) $A(R) = W(R)$; $w_0 = -1$.

(XII) The unique non-trivial element of $P(R^\vee)/Q(R^\vee)$ defines the unique non-trivial automorphism of the completed Dynkin graph.

(XIII) Cartan matrix ($l \times l$):

$$\begin{pmatrix} 2 & -1 & 0 & 0 & \cdots & 0 & 0\\ -1 & 2 & -1 & 0 & \cdots & 0 & 0\\ 0 & -1 & 2 & -1 & \cdots & 0 & 0\\ 0 & 0 & -1 & 2 & \cdots & 0 & 0\\ \vdots & \vdots & \vdots & \vdots & \ddots & \vdots & \vdots\\ 0 & 0 & 0 & 0 & \cdots & 2 & -2\\ 0 & 0 & 0 & 0 & \cdots & -1 & 2 \end{pmatrix}$$

PLATE III

SYSTEMS OF TYPE C_l $(l \geqslant 2)$

(I) $\mathrm{V} = \mathrm{E} = \mathbf{R}^l$.
Roots: $\pm 2\varepsilon_i$, $(1 \leqslant i \leqslant l)$, $\pm\varepsilon_i \pm \varepsilon_j$ $(1 \leqslant i < j \leqslant l)$.
Number of roots: $n = 2l^2$.

(II) Basis: $\alpha_1 = \varepsilon_1 - \varepsilon_2, \alpha_2 = \varepsilon_2 - \varepsilon_3, \dots, \alpha_{l-1} = \varepsilon_{l-1} - \varepsilon_l, \alpha_l = 2\varepsilon_l$.
Positive roots:

$$\varepsilon_i = \varepsilon_i - \varepsilon_j = \sum_{i \leqslant k < j} \alpha_k \quad (1 \leqslant i < j \leqslant l),$$

$$\varepsilon_i + \varepsilon_j = \sum_{i \leqslant k < j} \alpha_k + 2 \sum_{j \leqslant k < l} \alpha_k + \alpha_l \quad (1 \leqslant i < j \leqslant l),$$

$$2\varepsilon_i = \sum_{i \leqslant k < l} \alpha_k + \alpha_l \quad (1 \leqslant i \leqslant l).$$

(III) Coxeter number: $h = 2l$.

(IV) Highest root:

$$\tilde{\alpha} = 2\varepsilon_1 = 2\alpha_1 + 2\alpha_2 + \cdots + 2\alpha_{l-1} + \alpha_l.$$

Completed Dynkin graph:

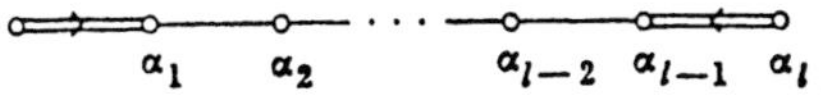

(V) $\mathrm{R}^\vee$ is the set of vectors $\pm\varepsilon_i$, $\pm\varepsilon_i \pm \varepsilon_j$.

$$\Phi_{\mathrm{R}}(x, y) = \frac{(x|y)}{4(l+1)}, \quad \gamma(\mathrm{R}) = (l+1)(4l-2).$$

(VI) Fundamental weights:

$$\begin{aligned} \omega_i &= \varepsilon_1 + \varepsilon_2 + \cdots + \varepsilon_i \ (1 \leqslant i \leqslant l) \\ &= \alpha_1 + 2\alpha_2 + \cdots + (i-1)\alpha_{i-1} \\ &\qquad + i(\alpha_i + \alpha_{i+1} + \cdots + \alpha_{l-1} + \frac{1}{2}\alpha_l). \end{aligned}$$

(VII) Sum of the positive roots:

$$\begin{aligned}2\rho &= 2l\varepsilon_1 + (2l-2)\varepsilon_2 + \cdots + 4\varepsilon_{l-1} + 2\varepsilon_l \\ &= 2l\alpha_1 + 2(2l-1)\alpha_2 + \cdots + i(2l-i+1)\alpha_i + \cdots \\ &\qquad \cdots + (l-1)(l+2)\alpha_{l-1} + \frac{1}{2}l(l+1)\alpha_l.\end{aligned}$$

(VIII) Q(R): the set of points whose coordinates are integers with even sum.
$\mathrm{P(R)} = \bigoplus_{i=1}^{l} \mathbf{Z}\varepsilon_i$.
P(R)/Q(R) is isomorphic to $\mathbf{Z}/2\mathbf{Z}$, generated by the image of ω_1.
Connection index: 2.

(IX) Exponents: $1, 3, 5, \ldots, 2l-1$.

(X) W(R) is the semi-direct product of the group $\mathfrak{S}_l$, acting by permutations of the ε_i, by the group $(\mathbf{Z}/2\mathbf{Z})^l$, acting by $\varepsilon_i \mapsto (\pm 1)_i\varepsilon_i$. Its order is $2^l.l!$

(XI) $\mathrm{A(R)} = \mathrm{W(R)}$; $w_0 = -1$.

(XII) The unique non-trivial element of $\mathrm{P(R^\vee)/Q(R^\vee)}$ defines the unique non-trivial automorphism of the completed Dynkin graph.

(XIII) Cartan matrix ($l \times l$):

$$\begin{pmatrix} 2 & -1 & 0 & 0 & \cdots & 0 & 0 \\ -1 & 2 & -1 & 0 & \cdots & 0 & 0 \\ 0 & -1 & 2 & -1 & \cdots & 0 & 0 \\ 0 & 0 & -1 & 2 & \cdots & 0 & 0 \\ \vdots & \vdots & \vdots & \vdots & \ddots & \vdots & \vdots \\ 0 & 0 & 0 & 0 & \cdots & 2 & -1 \\ 0 & 0 & 0 & 0 & \cdots & -2 & 2 \end{pmatrix}$$

PLATE IV

SYSTEMS OF TYPE D_l ($l \geqslant 3$)

(I) $V = E = \mathbf{R}^l$.
Roots: $\pm\varepsilon_i \pm \varepsilon_j$ $(1 \leqslant i < j \leqslant l)$; (ε_i) the canonical basis of $\mathbf{R}^l$.
Number of roots: $n = 2l(l-1)$.

(II) Basis: $\alpha_1 = \varepsilon_1 - \varepsilon_2, \alpha_2 = \varepsilon_2 - \varepsilon_3, \ldots, \alpha_{l-1} = \varepsilon_{l-1} - \varepsilon_l, \alpha_l = \varepsilon_{l-1} + \varepsilon_l$.
Positive roots:

$$\varepsilon_i - \varepsilon_j = \sum_{i<k<j} \alpha_k \quad (1 \leqslant i < j \leqslant l),$$

$$\varepsilon_i + \varepsilon_l = \sum_{i \leqslant k \leqslant l-2} \alpha_k + \alpha_l \quad (1 \leqslant i < l),$$

$$\varepsilon_i + \varepsilon_j = \sum_{i \leqslant k < j} \alpha_k + 2 \sum_{j \leqslant k < l-1} \alpha_k + \alpha_{l-1} + \alpha_l \quad (1 \leqslant i < j < l).$$

(III) Coxeter number: $h = 2l - 2$.

(IV) Highest root:

$$\tilde{\alpha} = \varepsilon_1 + \varepsilon_2 = \alpha_1 + 2\alpha_2 + \cdots + 2\alpha_{l-2} + \alpha_{l-1} + \alpha_l.$$

We have $\tilde{\alpha} = \omega_2 + \omega_3$ if $l = 3$ and $\tilde{\alpha} = \omega_2$ if $l \geqslant 4$.
Completed Dynkin graph ($l \geqslant 4$):

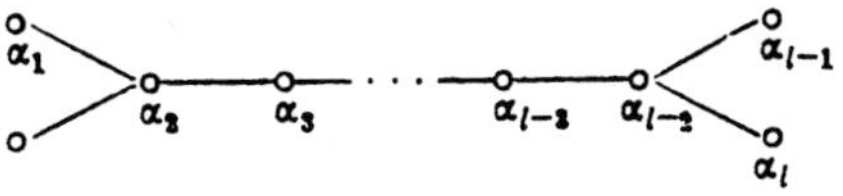

(V) $R^\vee = R$,

$$\Phi_R(x, y) = \frac{(x|y)}{4(l-1)}, \quad \gamma(R) = 4(l-1)^2.$$

(VI) Fundamental weights:

$$\begin{aligned}\omega_i &= \varepsilon_1 + \varepsilon_2 + \cdots + \varepsilon_i \ (1 \leqslant i \leqslant l-2)\\ &= \alpha_1 + 2\alpha_2 + \cdots + (i-1)\alpha_{i-1} + i(\alpha_1 + \alpha_{i+1} + \cdots + \alpha_{l-2})\\ &\qquad + \frac{1}{2}i(\alpha_{l-1} + \alpha_l)\\ \omega_{l-1} &= \frac{1}{2}(\varepsilon_1 + \varepsilon_2 + \cdots + \varepsilon_{l-2} + \varepsilon_{l-1} - \varepsilon_l)\\ &= \frac{1}{2}(\alpha_1 + 2\alpha_2 + \cdots + (l-2)\alpha_{l-2} + \frac{1}{2}l\alpha_{l-1} + \frac{1}{2}(l-2)\alpha_l)\\ \omega_l &= \frac{1}{2}(\varepsilon_1 + \varepsilon_2 + \cdots + \varepsilon_{l-2} + \varepsilon_{l-1} + \varepsilon_l)\\ &= \frac{1}{2}(\alpha_1 + 2\alpha_2 + \cdots + (l-2)\alpha_{l-2} + \frac{1}{2}(l-2)\alpha_{l-1} + \frac{1}{2}l\alpha_l).\end{aligned}$$

(VII) Sum of the positive roots:

$$\begin{aligned}2\rho &= 2(l-1)\varepsilon_1 + 2(l-2)\varepsilon_2 + \cdots + 2\varepsilon_{l-1}\\ &= 2(l-1)\alpha_1 + 2(2l-3)\alpha_2 + \cdots + 2(il - \frac{i(i+1)}{2})\alpha_i + \cdots\\ &\qquad \cdots + \frac{l(l-1)}{2}(\alpha_{l-1} + \alpha_l).\end{aligned}$$

(VIII) Q(R): the set of points whose coordinates are integers with even sum.

$$\mathrm{P(R)} = \bigoplus_{i=1}^{l} \mathbf{Z}\varepsilon_i + \mathbf{Z}(\frac{1}{2}\sum_{i=1}^{l}\varepsilon_i).$$

l odd: P(R)/Q(R) is isomorphic to $\mathbf{Z}/4\mathbf{Z}$, generated by the image of ω_l; we have $\omega_1 \equiv 2\omega_l$ and $\omega_{l-1} \equiv 3\omega_l$ mod. Q(R).
l even: P(R)/Q(R) is isomorphic to $(\mathbf{Z}/2\mathbf{Z}) \times (\mathbf{Z}/2\mathbf{Z})$; the three elements of order 2 are the images of ω_1, ω_{l-1} and ω_l.
Connection index: 4.

(IX) Exponents: $1, 3, 5, \ldots, 2l-5, 2l-3, l-1$ (the last appearing twice if l is even and once if l is odd).

(X) W(R) is the semi-direct product of the group $\mathfrak{S}_l$, acting by permutations of the ε_i, by the group $(\mathbf{Z}/2\mathbf{Z})^{l-1}$, acting by $\varepsilon_i \mapsto (\pm 1)_i\varepsilon_i$ with $\prod_i (\pm 1)_i = 1$. Its order is $2^{l-1}.l!$

(XI) $l \neq 4$: A(R)/W(R) $= \mathbf{Z}/2\mathbf{Z}$ acting on the Dynkin graph by transposition of the nodes α_{l-1} and α_l.
$l = 4$: A(R)/W(R) $= \mathfrak{S}_3$, acting on the Dynkin graph by permuting the nodes α_1, α_3 and α_4.
$w_0 = -1$ if l is even; $w_0 = -\varepsilon$ if l is odd, where ε is the automorphism that interchanges α_{l-1} and α_l and leaves the other α_i fixed.

(XII) Action of $P(R^\vee)/Q(R^\vee) = P(R)/Q(R)$ on the completed Dynkin graph:
l odd: ω_l transforms α_0 into α_1, α_l into α_1, α_1 into α_{l-1} and α_{l-1} into α_0; it interchanges α_j and α_{l-j} for $2 \leqslant j \leqslant l-2$.
l even: ω_l (resp. ω_{l-1}) interchanges α_0 and α_l (resp. α_0 and α_{l-1}), α_1 and α_{l-1} (resp. α_1 and α_l) and interchanges α_j and α_{l-j} for $2 \leqslant j \leqslant l-2$.

(XIII) Cartan matrix ($l \times l$):

$$\begin{pmatrix} 2 & -1 & \cdots & 0 & 0 & 0 & 0 \\ -1 & 2 & \cdots & 0 & 0 & 0 & 0 \\ \vdots & \vdots & \ddots & \vdots & \vdots & \vdots & \vdots \\ 0 & 0 & \cdots & 2 & -1 & 0 & 0 \\ 0 & 0 & \cdots & -1 & 2 & -1 & -1 \\ 0 & 0 & \cdots & 0 & -1 & 2 & 0 \\ 0 & 0 & \cdots & 0 & -1 & 0 & 2 \end{pmatrix}$$

PLATE V

SYSTEM OF TYPE E_6

(I) V is the subspace of $E = \mathbf{R}^8$ consisting of the points whose coordinates (ξ_i) are such that $\xi_6 = \xi_7 = -\xi_8$.
Roots: $\pm\varepsilon_i \pm \varepsilon_j$ $(1 \leqslant i < j \leqslant 5)$,

$$\pm\frac{1}{2}(\varepsilon_8 - \varepsilon_7 - \varepsilon_6 + \sum_{i=1}^{5}(-1)^{\nu(i)}\varepsilon_i) \text{ with } \sum_{i=1}^{5}\nu(i) \text{ even.}$$

Number of roots: $n = 72$.

(II) Basis: $\alpha_1 = \frac{1}{2}(\varepsilon_1+\varepsilon_8)-\frac{1}{2}(\varepsilon_2+\varepsilon_3+\varepsilon_4+\varepsilon_5+\varepsilon_6+\varepsilon_7)$, $\alpha_2 = \varepsilon_1+\varepsilon_2$, $\alpha_3 = \varepsilon_2 - \varepsilon_1$, $\alpha_4 = \varepsilon_3 - \varepsilon_2$, $\alpha_5 = \varepsilon_4 - \varepsilon_3$, $\alpha_6 = \varepsilon_5 - \varepsilon_4$.
Positive roots: $\pm\varepsilon_i + \varepsilon_j$ $(1 \leqslant i < j \leqslant 5)$,

$$\frac{1}{2}(\varepsilon_8 - \varepsilon_7 - \varepsilon_6 + \sum_{i=1}^{5}(-1)^{\nu(i)}\varepsilon_i) \text{ with } \sum_{i=1}^{5}\nu(i) \text{ even.}$$

Positive roots with at least one coefficient $\geqslant 2$ (we denote the root $a\alpha_1 + b\alpha_2 + c\alpha_3 + d\alpha_4 + e\alpha_5 + f\alpha_6$) by $\begin{smallmatrix} a & c & d & e & f \\ & & b & & \end{smallmatrix}$)[13]:

$$\begin{matrix} 01210 & 11210 & 01211 & 12210 & 11211 & 01221 \\ 1 & 1 & 1 & 1 & 1 & 1 \end{matrix}$$

$$\begin{matrix} 12211 & 11221 & 12221 & 12321 & 12321 \\ 1 & 1 & 1 & 1 & 2 \end{matrix}$$

(III) Coxeter number: $h = 12$.

(IV) Highest root:

$$\tilde{\alpha} = \frac{1}{2}(\varepsilon_1 + \varepsilon_2 + \varepsilon_3 + \varepsilon_4 + \varepsilon_5 - \varepsilon_6 - \varepsilon_7 + \varepsilon_8)$$
$$= \alpha_1 + 2\alpha_2 + 2\alpha_3 + 3\alpha_4 + 2\alpha_5 + \alpha_6 = \omega_2.$$

---

[13] The other positive roots can be obtained by applying Cor. 3 of Prop. 19 of Chap. VI, § 1, no. 6.

Completed Dynkin graph:

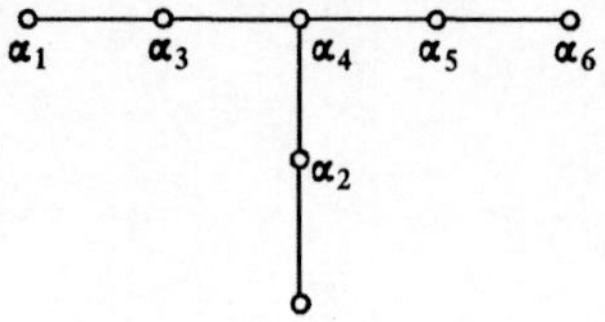

(V) $R = R^{\check{}}$,

$$\Phi_R(x, y) = (x|y)/24, \qquad \gamma(R) = 144.$$

(VI) Fundamental weights:

$$\omega_1 = \frac{2}{3}(\varepsilon_8 - \varepsilon_7 - \varepsilon_6) = \frac{1}{3}(4\alpha_1 + 3\alpha_2 + 5\alpha_3 + 6\alpha_4 + 4\alpha_5 + 2\alpha_6)$$

$$\omega_2 = \frac{1}{2}(\varepsilon_1 + \varepsilon_2 + \varepsilon_3 + \varepsilon_4 + \varepsilon_5 - \varepsilon_6 - \varepsilon_7 + \varepsilon_8)$$
$$= \alpha_1 + 2\alpha_2 + 2\alpha_3 + 3\alpha_4 + 2\alpha_5 + \alpha_6 = \tilde{\alpha}$$

$$\omega_3 = \frac{5}{6}(\varepsilon_8 - \varepsilon_7 - \varepsilon_6) + \frac{1}{2}(-\varepsilon_1 + \varepsilon_2 + \varepsilon_3 + \varepsilon_4 + \varepsilon_5)$$
$$= \frac{1}{3}(5\alpha_1 + 6\alpha_2 + 10\alpha_3 + 12\alpha_4 + 8\alpha_5 + 4\alpha_6)$$

$$\omega_4 = \varepsilon_3 + \varepsilon_4 + \varepsilon_5 - \varepsilon_6 - \varepsilon_7 + \varepsilon_8$$
$$= 2\alpha_1 + 3\alpha_2 + 4\alpha_3 + 6\alpha_4 + 4\alpha_5 + 2\alpha_6$$

$$\omega_5 = \frac{2}{3}(\varepsilon_8 - \varepsilon_7 - \varepsilon_6) + \varepsilon_4 + \varepsilon_5$$
$$= \frac{1}{3}(4\alpha_1 + 6\alpha_2 + 8\alpha_3 + 12\alpha_4 + 10\alpha_5 + 5\alpha_6)$$

$$\omega_6 = \frac{1}{3}(\varepsilon_8 - \varepsilon_7 - \varepsilon_6) + \varepsilon_5$$
$$= \frac{1}{3}(2\alpha_1 + 3\alpha_2 + 4\alpha_3 + 6\alpha_4 + 5\alpha_5 + 4\alpha_6).$$

(VII) Sum of the positive roots:

$$2\rho = 2(\varepsilon_2 + 2\varepsilon_3 + 3\varepsilon_4 + 4\varepsilon_5 + 4(\varepsilon_8 - \varepsilon_7 - \varepsilon_6))$$
$$= 2(8\alpha_1 + 11\alpha_2 + 15\alpha_3 + 21\alpha_4 + 15\alpha_5 + 8\alpha_6).$$

(VIII) $P(R)/Q(R)$ is isomorphic to $\mathbf{Z}/3\mathbf{Z}$.
Connection index: 3.

(IX) Exponents: $1, 4, 5, 7, 8, 11$.

(X) Order of $W(R)$: $2^7.3^4.5$.

(XI) $A(R) = W(R) \times \{1, -1\}$; w_0 transforms $\alpha_1, \alpha_2, \alpha_3, \alpha_4, \alpha_5, \alpha_6$, respectively, into $-\alpha_6, -\alpha_2, -\alpha_5, -\alpha_4, -\alpha_3, -\alpha_1$.

(XII) The non-identity element of A(R)/W(R) defines the automorphism $x \mapsto -x$ of P(R)/Q(R).
The group of automorphisms of the completed Dynkin diagram is isomorphic to $\mathfrak{S}_3$; its elements of order 3 are induced by the two non-trivial elements of $P(R^\vee)/Q(R^\vee)$.

(XIII) Cartan matrix:

$$\begin{pmatrix} 2 & 0 & -1 & 0 & 0 & 0 \\ 0 & 2 & 0 & -1 & 0 & 0 \\ -1 & 0 & 2 & -1 & 0 & 0 \\ 0 & -1 & -1 & 2 & -1 & 0 \\ 0 & 0 & 0 & -1 & 2 & -1 \\ 0 & 0 & 0 & 0 & -1 & 2 \end{pmatrix}$$

PLATE VI

SYSTEM OF TYPE E_7

(I) V is the hyperplane in $E = \mathbf{R}^8$ orthogonal to $\varepsilon_7 + \varepsilon_8$.
Roots: $\pm\varepsilon_i \pm \varepsilon_j$ $(1 \leqslant i \leqslant j \leqslant 6)$, $\pm(\varepsilon_7 - \varepsilon_8)$,

$$\pm\frac{1}{2}(\varepsilon_7 - \varepsilon_8 + \sum_{i=1}^{6}(-1)^{\nu(\mathrm{i})}\varepsilon_i) \quad \text{with } \sum_{i=1}^{8}\nu(i) \text{ odd.}$$

Number of roots: $n = 126$.

(II) Basis:

$$\alpha_1 = \frac{1}{2}(\varepsilon_1 + \varepsilon_8) - \frac{1}{2}(\varepsilon_2 + \varepsilon_3 + \varepsilon_4 + \varepsilon_5 + \varepsilon_6 + \varepsilon_7),$$

$$\alpha_2 = \varepsilon_1 + \varepsilon_2,\ \alpha_3 = \varepsilon_2 - \varepsilon_1,\ \alpha_4 = \varepsilon_3 - \varepsilon_2,\ \alpha_5 = \varepsilon_4 - \varepsilon_3,$$

$$\alpha_6 = \varepsilon_5 - \varepsilon_4,\ \alpha_7 = \varepsilon_6 - \varepsilon_5.$$

Positive roots:

$$\pm\varepsilon_i + \varepsilon_j \quad (1 \leqslant i < j \leqslant 6), \quad -\varepsilon_7 + \varepsilon_8,$$

$$\frac{1}{2}(-\varepsilon_7 + \varepsilon_8 + \sum_{i=1}^{6}(-1)^{\nu(\mathrm{i})}\varepsilon_i) \quad \text{with } \sum_{i=1}^{6}\nu(i) \text{ odd.}$$

Positive roots containing α_7 and having at least one coefficient $\geqslant 2$ (we denote the root $a\alpha_1 + b\alpha_2 + c\alpha_3 + d\alpha_4 + e\alpha_5 + f\alpha_6 + g\alpha_7$ by $\begin{smallmatrix} a\,c\,d\,e\,f\,g \\ b \end{smallmatrix}$)[14]:

012111	112111	012211	122111	112211
1	1	1	1	1
012221	122211	112221	122221	123211
1	1	1	1	1
123221	123211	123321	123221	123321
1	2	1	2	2

[14] The positive roots not containing α_7 come from E_6. The positive roots all of whose coefficients are $\leqslant 1$ can be obtained by applying Cor. 3 of Prop. 19 of Chap. VI, § 1, no. 6.

1 2 4 3 2 1   1 3 4 3 2 1   2 3 4 3 2 1
    2   2   2

(III) Coxeter number: $h = 18$.

(IV) Highest root:

$$\tilde{\alpha} = \varepsilon_8 - \varepsilon_7 = 2\alpha_1 + 2\alpha_2 + 3\alpha_3 + 4\alpha_4 + 3\alpha_5 + 2\alpha_6 + \alpha_7 = \omega_1.$$

Completed Dynkin graph:

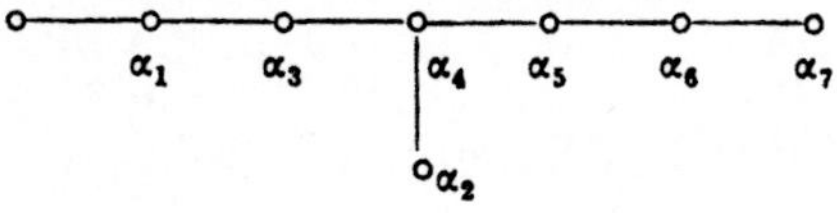

(V) $R^\vee = R$.

$$\Phi_R(x, y) = (x|y)/36, \qquad \gamma(R) = 2^2.3^4.$$

(VI) Fundamental weights:

$$\begin{aligned}
\omega_1 &= \varepsilon_8 - \varepsilon_7 = 2\alpha_1 + 2\alpha_2 + 3\alpha_3 + 4\alpha_4 + 3\alpha_5 + 2\alpha_6 + \alpha_7\\
\omega_2 &= \frac{1}{2}(\varepsilon_1 + \varepsilon_2 + \varepsilon_3 + \varepsilon_4 + \varepsilon_5 + \varepsilon_6 - 2\varepsilon_7 + 2\varepsilon_8)\\
&= \frac{1}{2}(4\alpha_1 + 7\alpha_2 + 8\alpha_3 + 12\alpha_4 + 9\alpha_5 + 8\alpha_6 + 3\alpha_7)\\
\omega_3 &= \frac{1}{2}(-\varepsilon_1 + \varepsilon_2 + \varepsilon_3 + \varepsilon_4 + \varepsilon_5 + \varepsilon_6 - 3\varepsilon_7 + 3\varepsilon_8)\\
&= 3\alpha_1 + 4\alpha_2 + 6\alpha_3 + 8\alpha_4 + 6\alpha_5 + 4\alpha_6 + 2\alpha_7\\
\omega_4 &= \varepsilon_3 + \varepsilon_4 + \varepsilon_5 + \varepsilon_6 + 2(\varepsilon_8 - \varepsilon_7)\\
&= 4\alpha_1 + 6\alpha_2 + 8\alpha_3 + 12\alpha_4 + 9\alpha_5 + 6\alpha_6 + 3\alpha_7\\
\omega_5 &= \varepsilon_4 + \varepsilon_5 + \varepsilon_6 + \frac{3}{2}(\varepsilon_8 - \varepsilon_7)\\
&= \frac{1}{2}(6\alpha_1 + 9\alpha_2 + 12\alpha_3 + 18\alpha_4 + 15\alpha_5 + 10\alpha_6 + 5\alpha_7)\\
\omega_6 &= \varepsilon_5 + \varepsilon_6 - \varepsilon_7 + \varepsilon_8\\
&= 2\alpha_1 + 3\alpha_2 + 4\alpha_3 + 6\alpha_4 + 5\alpha_5 + 4\alpha_6 + 2\alpha_7\\
\omega_7 &= \varepsilon_6 + \frac{1}{2}(\varepsilon_8 - \varepsilon_7)\\
&= \frac{1}{2}(2\alpha_1 + 3\alpha_2 + 4\alpha_3 + 6\alpha_4 + 5\alpha_5 + 4\alpha_6 + 3\alpha_7).
\end{aligned}$$

(VII) Sum of the positive roots:

$$\begin{aligned}
2\rho &= 2\varepsilon_2 + 4\varepsilon_3 + 6\varepsilon_4 + 8\varepsilon_5 + 10\varepsilon_6 - 17\varepsilon_7 + 17\varepsilon_8\\
&= 34\alpha_1 + 49\alpha_2 + 66\alpha_3 + 96\alpha_4 + 75\alpha_5 + 52\alpha_6 + 27\alpha_7.
\end{aligned}$$

(VIII) P(R)/Q(R) is isomorphic to $\mathbf{Z}/2\mathbf{Z}$.
Connection index: 2.

(IX) Exponents: $1, 5, 7, 9, 11, 13, 17$.

(X) Order of W(R): $2^{10}.3^4.5.7$.

(XI) $A(R) = W(R)$, $w_0 = -1$.

(XII) $P(R\check{})/Q(R\check{})$ has only one non-identity element; it defines the unique non-trivial automorphism of the Dynkin graph.

(XIII) Cartan matrix:

$$\begin{pmatrix} 2 & 0 & -1 & 0 & 0 & 0 & 0 \\ 0 & 2 & 0 & -1 & 0 & 0 & 0 \\ -1 & 0 & 2 & -1 & 0 & 0 & 0 \\ 0 & -1 & -1 & 2 & -1 & 0 & 0 \\ 0 & 0 & 0 & -1 & 2 & -1 & 0 \\ 0 & 0 & 0 & 0 & -1 & 2 & -1 \\ 0 & 0 & 0 & 0 & 0 & -1 & 2 \end{pmatrix}$$

PLATE VII

SYSTEM OF TYPE E_8

(I) $V = E = \mathbf{R}^8$.

Roots: $\pm\varepsilon_i \pm \varepsilon_j$ $(i < j)$, $\frac{1}{2}\sum_{i=1}^{8}(-1)^{\nu(i)}\varepsilon_i$ with $\sum_{i=1}^{8}\nu(i)$ even.

Number of roots: $n = 240$.

(II) Basis:

$$\alpha_1 = \frac{1}{2}(\varepsilon_1 + \varepsilon_8) - \frac{1}{2}(\varepsilon_2 + \varepsilon_3 + \varepsilon_4 + \varepsilon_5 + \varepsilon_6 + \varepsilon_7),$$

$$\alpha_2 = \varepsilon_1 + \varepsilon_2,\ \alpha_3 = \varepsilon_2 - \varepsilon_1,\ \alpha_4 = \varepsilon_3 - \varepsilon_2,\ \alpha_5 = \varepsilon_4 - \varepsilon_3,$$

$$\alpha_6 = \varepsilon_5 - \varepsilon_4,\ \alpha_7 = \varepsilon_6 - \varepsilon_5,\ \alpha_8 = \varepsilon_7 - \varepsilon_6.$$

Positive roots:

$$\pm\varepsilon_i + \varepsilon_j\ (i < j),\ \frac{1}{2}(\varepsilon_8 + \sum_{i=1}^{7}(-1)^{\nu(i)}\varepsilon_i) \text{ with } \sum_{i=1}^{7}\nu(i) \text{ even.}$$

Positive roots containing α_8 and having at least one coefficient $\geqslant 2$(we denote the root $a\alpha_1 + b\alpha_2 + c\alpha_3 + d\alpha_4 + e\alpha_5 + f\alpha_6 + g\alpha_7 + h\alpha_8$ by $\begin{smallmatrix} a\,c\,d\,e\,f\,g\,h \\ b \end{smallmatrix}$)[15]:

0121111	0122111	1121111	0122211	1221111
1	1	1	1	1
1122111	1222111	1122211	0122221	1232111
1	1	1	1	1
1222211	1122221	1232211	1232211	1222221
1	1	2	1	1
1232211	1233211	1232221	1233211	1232221
2	1	1	2	2

[15] The positive roots not containing α_8 come from E_7. The positive roots all of whose coefficients are $\leqslant 1$ can be obtained by applying Cor. 3 of Prop. 19 of Chap. VI, § 1, no. 6.

1233321	1243211	1233221	1233321	1343211
1	2	2	1	2
1243221	1233321	2343211	1343221	1243321
2	2	2	2	2
2343221	1343321	1244321	2343321	1344321
2	2	2	2	2
1354321	2344321	1354321	2354321	2354321
2	2	3	2	3
2454321	2454321	2464321	2465321	2465421
2	3	3	3	3
	2465431	2465432		
	3	3		

(III) Coxeter number: $h = 30$.

(IV) Highest root:

$$\tilde{\alpha} = \varepsilon_7 + \varepsilon_8 = 2\alpha_1 + 3\alpha_2 + 4\alpha_3 + 6\alpha_4 + 5\alpha_5 + 4\alpha_6 + 3\alpha_7 + 2\alpha_8$$
$$= \omega_8.$$

Completed Dynkin graph is:

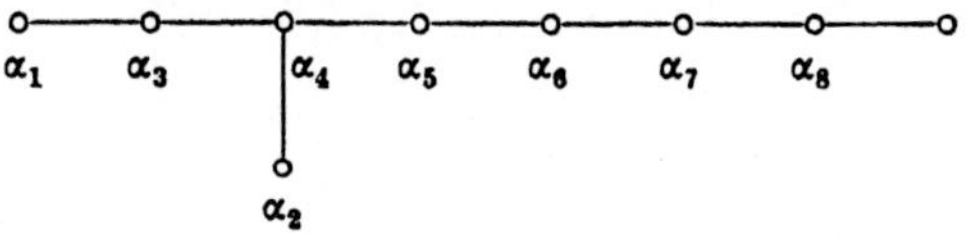

(V) $\mathrm{R}^{\check{}} = \mathrm{R}$.

$$\Phi_{\mathrm{R}}(x, y) = (x|y)/60, \qquad \gamma(\mathrm{R}) = 900.$$

(VI) Fundamental weights:

$$\omega_1 = 2\varepsilon_8 = 4\alpha_1 + 5\alpha_2 + 7\alpha_3 + 10\alpha_4 + 8\alpha_5 + 6\alpha_6 + 4\alpha_7 + 2\alpha_8$$
$$\omega_2 = \frac{1}{2}(\varepsilon_1 + \varepsilon_2 + \varepsilon_3 + \varepsilon_4 + \varepsilon_5 + \varepsilon_6 + \varepsilon_7 + 5\varepsilon_8)$$
$$= 5\alpha_1 + 8\alpha_2 + 10\alpha_3 + 15\alpha_4 + 12\alpha_5 + 9\alpha_6 + 6\alpha_7 + 3\alpha_8$$
$$\omega_3 = \frac{1}{2}(-\varepsilon_1 + \varepsilon_2 + \varepsilon_3 + \varepsilon_4 + \varepsilon_5 + \varepsilon_6 + \varepsilon_7 + 7\varepsilon_8)$$
$$= 7\alpha_1 + 10\alpha_2 + 14\alpha_3 + 20\alpha_4 + 16\alpha_5 + 12\alpha_6 + 8\alpha_7 + 4\alpha_8$$
$$\omega_4 = \varepsilon_3 + \varepsilon_4 + \varepsilon_5 + \varepsilon_6 + \varepsilon_7 + 5\varepsilon_8$$
$$= 10\alpha_1 + 15\alpha_2 + 20\alpha_3 + 30\alpha_4 + 24\alpha_5 + 18\alpha_6 + 12\alpha_7 + 6\alpha_8$$

$$\begin{aligned}
\omega_5 &= \varepsilon_4 + \varepsilon_5 + \varepsilon_6 + \varepsilon_7 + 4\varepsilon_8 \\
&= 8\alpha_1 + 12\alpha_2 + 16\alpha_3 + 24\alpha_4 + 20\alpha_5 + 15\alpha_6 + 10\alpha_7 + 5\alpha_8 \\
\omega_6 &= \varepsilon_5 + \varepsilon_6 + \varepsilon_7 + 3\varepsilon_8 \\
&= 6\alpha_1 + 9\alpha_2 + 12\alpha_3 + 18\alpha_4 + 15\alpha_5 + 12\alpha_6 + 8\alpha_7 + 4\alpha_8 \\
\omega_7 &= \varepsilon_6 + \varepsilon_7 + 2\varepsilon_8 \\
&= 4\alpha_1 + 6\alpha_2 + 8\alpha_3 + 12\alpha_4 + 10\alpha_5 + 8\alpha_6 + 6\alpha_7 + 3\alpha_8 \\
\omega_8 &= \varepsilon_7 + \varepsilon_8 \\
&= 5\alpha_1 + 8\alpha_2 + 10\alpha_3 + 15\alpha_4 + 12\alpha_5 + 9\alpha_6 + 6\alpha_7 + 3\alpha_8 = \tilde{\alpha}.
\end{aligned}$$

(VII) Sum of the positive roots:

$$\begin{aligned}
2\rho &= 2(\varepsilon_2 + 2\varepsilon_3 + 3\varepsilon_4 + 4\varepsilon_5 + 5\varepsilon_6 + 6\varepsilon_7 + 23\varepsilon_8) \\
&= 2(46\alpha_1 + 68\alpha_2 + 91\alpha_3 + 135\alpha_4 + 110\alpha_5 + 84\alpha_6 + 57\alpha_7 + 29\alpha_8).
\end{aligned}$$

(VIII) Q(R): the set of points with coordinates ξ_i such that $2\xi_i \in \mathbf{Z}$, $\xi_i - \xi_j \in \mathbf{Z}$, $\sum_{i=1}^{8} \xi_i \in 2\mathbf{Z}$.

Connection index: 1.

(IX) Exponents: $1, 7, 11, 13, 17, 19, 23, 29$.

(X) Order of W(R): $2^{14}.3^5.5^2.7$.

(XI) and (XII) $A(R) = W(R)$, $w_0 = -1$.

(XIII) Cartan matrix:

$$\begin{pmatrix}
2 & 0 & -1 & 0 & 0 & 0 & 0 & 0 \\
0 & 2 & 0 & -1 & 0 & 0 & 0 & 0 \\
-1 & 0 & 2 & -1 & 0 & 0 & 0 & 0 \\
0 & -1 & -1 & 2 & -1 & 0 & 0 & 0 \\
0 & 0 & 0 & -1 & 2 & -1 & 0 & 0 \\
0 & 0 & 0 & 0 & -1 & 2 & -1 & 0 \\
0 & 0 & 0 & 0 & 0 & -1 & 2 & -1 \\
0 & 0 & 0 & 0 & 0 & 0 & -1 & 2
\end{pmatrix}$$

PLATE VIII

SYSTEM OF TYPE F_4

(I) $V = E = \mathbf{R}^4$.

Roots:

$$\pm\varepsilon_i,\ (1 \leqslant i \leqslant 4), \qquad \pm\,\varepsilon_i \pm \varepsilon_j\ (1 \leqslant i < j \leqslant 4),$$
$$\frac{1}{2}(\pm\varepsilon_1 \pm\varepsilon_2 \pm \varepsilon_3 \pm \varepsilon_4).$$

Number of roots: $n = 48$.

(II) Basis:

$$\alpha_1 = \varepsilon_2 - \varepsilon_3,\ \alpha_2 = \varepsilon_3 - \varepsilon_4,\ \alpha_3 = \varepsilon_4,\ \alpha_4 = \frac{1}{2}(\varepsilon_1 - \varepsilon_2 - \varepsilon_3 - \varepsilon_4).$$

Positive roots:

$$\varepsilon_i\ \ (1 \leqslant i \leqslant 4), \quad \varepsilon_i \pm \varepsilon_j\ \ (1 \leqslant i < j \leqslant 4),\ \ \frac{1}{2}(\varepsilon_1 \pm \varepsilon_2 \pm \varepsilon_3 \pm \varepsilon_4).$$

Positive roots having at least one coefficient $\geqslant 2$ (we denote the root $a\alpha_1 + b\alpha_2 + c\alpha_3 + d\alpha_4$ by $a\,b\,c\,d$)[16]:

0120 1120 0121 1220 1121 0122 1221 1122
1231 1222 1232 1242 1342 2342

(III) Number of roots: $h = 12$.

(IV) Highest root: $\tilde{\alpha} = \varepsilon_1 + \varepsilon_2 = 2\alpha_1 + 3\alpha_2 + 4\alpha_3 + 2\alpha_4 = \omega_1$.

Completed Dynkin graph:

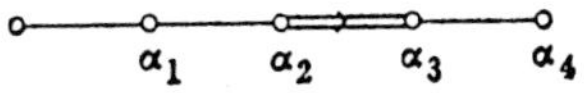

[16]The other positive roots can be obtained by applying Cor. 3 of Prop. 19 of Chap. VI, § 1, no. 6.

(V) R˘ the set of vectors $\pm 2\varepsilon_i, \pm\varepsilon_i \pm \varepsilon_j, \pm\varepsilon_1 \pm \varepsilon_2 \pm \varepsilon_3 \pm \varepsilon_4$.

$$\Phi_{\mathrm{R}}(x, y) = \frac{(x|y)}{18}, \quad \gamma(\mathrm{R}) = 2.3^4.$$

(VI) Fundamental weights:

$$\begin{aligned}
\omega_1 &= \varepsilon_1 + \varepsilon_2 = 2\alpha_1 + 3\alpha_2 + 4\alpha_3 + 2\alpha_4 \\
\omega_2 &= 2\varepsilon_1 + \varepsilon_2 + \varepsilon_3 = 3\alpha_1 + 6\alpha_2 + 8\alpha_3 + 4\alpha_4 \\
\omega_3 &= \frac{1}{2}(3\varepsilon_1 + \varepsilon_2 + \varepsilon_3 + \varepsilon_4) = 2\alpha_1 + 4\alpha_2 + 6\alpha_3 + 3\alpha_4 \\
\omega_4 &= \varepsilon_1 = \alpha_1 + 2\alpha_2 + 3\alpha_3 + 2\alpha_4.
\end{aligned}$$

(VII) Sum of the positive roots:

$$2\rho = 11\varepsilon_1 + 5\varepsilon_2 + 3\varepsilon_3 + \varepsilon_4 = 16\alpha_1 + 30\alpha_2 + 42\alpha_3 + 22\alpha_4.$$

(VIII) $\mathrm{Q}(\mathrm{R}) = \bigoplus_{i=1}^{4} \mathbf{Z}\varepsilon_i + \mathbf{Z}(\frac{1}{2}\sum_{i=1}^{4} \varepsilon_i)$.
$\mathrm{P}(\mathrm{R}) = \mathrm{Q}(\mathrm{R})$.
Connection index: 1.

(IX) Exponents: $1, 5, 7, 11$.

(X) and (XI) $\mathrm{A}(\mathrm{R}) = \mathrm{W}(\mathrm{R})$, $w_0 = -1$.

(XIII) Cartan matrix:

$$\begin{pmatrix} 2 & -1 & 0 & 0 \\ -1 & 2 & -2 & 0 \\ 0 & -1 & 2 & -1 \\ 0 & 0 & -1 & 2 \end{pmatrix}$$

PLATE IX

SYSTEM OF TYPE G_2

(I) V is the hyperplane in $E = \mathbf{R}^3$ with equation $\xi_1 + \xi_2 + \xi_3 = 0$.
Roots:

$$\pm(\varepsilon_1 - \varepsilon_2),\quad \pm(\varepsilon_1 - \varepsilon_3),\quad \pm(\varepsilon_2 - \varepsilon_3),\quad \pm(2\varepsilon_1 - \varepsilon_2 - \varepsilon_3),$$
$$\pm(2\varepsilon_2 - \varepsilon_1 - \varepsilon_3),\quad \pm(2\varepsilon_3 - \varepsilon_1 - \varepsilon_2).$$

Number of roots: $n = 12$.

(II) Basis: $\alpha_1 = \varepsilon_1 - \varepsilon_2, \alpha_2 = -2\varepsilon_1 + \varepsilon_2 + \varepsilon_3$.
Positive roots: $\alpha_1, \alpha_1 + \alpha_2, 2\alpha_1 + \alpha_2, 3\alpha_1 + \alpha_2, 3\alpha_1 + 2\alpha_2$.

(III) Coxeter number: $h = 6$.

(IV) Highest root: $\tilde{\alpha} = -\varepsilon_1 - \varepsilon_2 + 2\varepsilon_3 = 3\alpha_1 + 2\alpha_2 = \omega_2$.
Completed Dynkin graph:

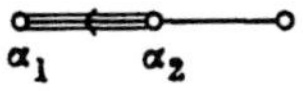

(V) R˘ is the set of vectors

$$\pm\alpha_1,\quad \pm(\alpha_1 + \alpha_2),\quad \pm(2\alpha_1 + \alpha_2),\quad \pm\frac{1}{3}\alpha_2,$$
$$\pm\frac{1}{3}(3\alpha_1 + \alpha_2),\quad \pm\frac{1}{3}(3\alpha_1 + 2\alpha_2).$$
$$\Phi_R(x, y) = \frac{(x|y)}{24},\quad \gamma(R) = 48.$$

(VI) Fundamental weights:

$$\omega_1 = 2\alpha_1 + \alpha_2,\quad \omega_2 = 3\alpha_1 + 2\alpha_2 = \tilde{\alpha}.$$

(VII) Sum of the positive roots:

$$2\rho = 2(5\alpha_1 + 3\alpha_2).$$

(VIII) P(R) = Q(R).
Connection index: 1.

(IX) Exponents: 1, 5.

(X) W(R): the dihedral group of order 12.

(XI) and (XII): A(R) = W(R), $w_0 = -1$.

(XIII) Cartan matrix:

$$\begin{pmatrix} 2 & -1 \\ -3 & 2 \end{pmatrix}$$

PLATE X

IRREDUCIBLE SYSTEMS OF RANK 2

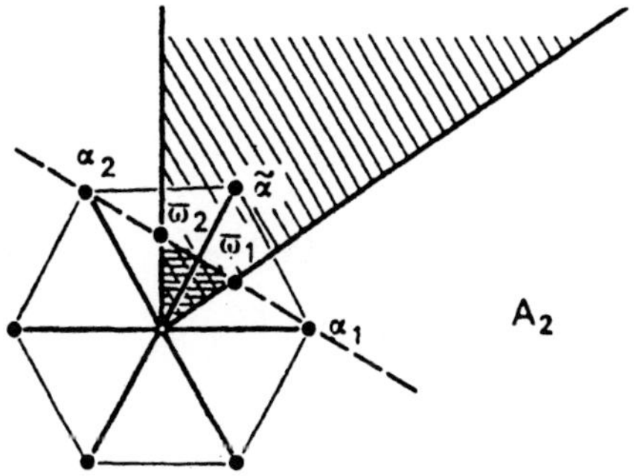

A_2

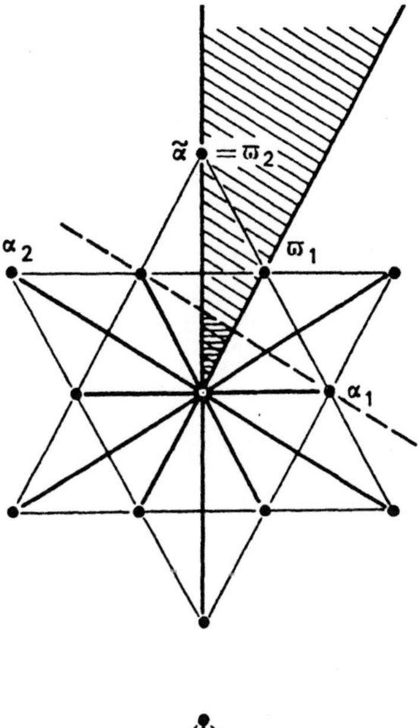

G_2

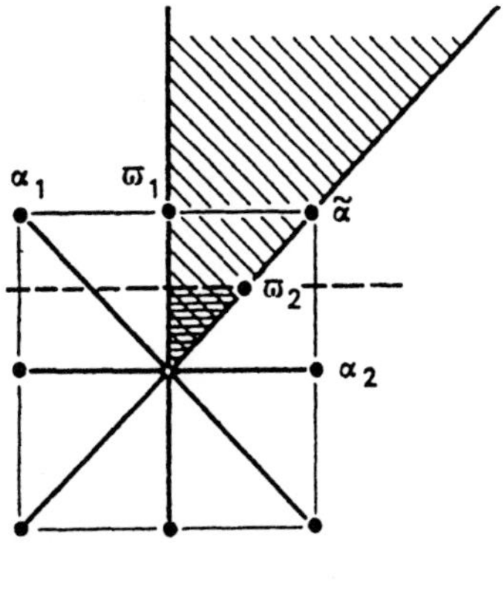

B_2

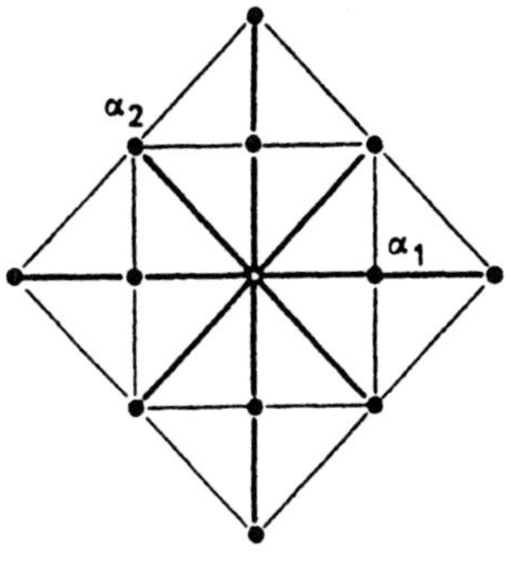

BC_2

The first three diagrams above represent the root systems R of type A_2, B_2 and G_2. The shaded region represents the chamber C corresponding to the basis (α_1, α_2). The line $(x|\beta) = 1$, where β denotes the highest root of the inverse system $R^\vee$, is shown dotted, and the doubly shaded region represents the alcove of $R^\vee$ with vertex 0 contained in C.

The last diagram represents the unique irreducible *non-reduced* root system of rank 2.

SUMMARY OF THE PRINCIPAL PROPERTIES OF ROOT SYSTEMS

(In this summary we restrict ourselves to the case of reduced root systems and work over the field of real numbers.)

1) Let V be a real vector space. A reduced root system in V is a subset R of V with the following properties:

(i) R is finite and generates V.

(ii) For all $\alpha \in \mathrm{R}$, there exists $\alpha\check{} \in \mathrm{V}^*$ such that $\langle \alpha, \alpha\check{} \rangle = 2$, and such that the map

$$s_\alpha : x \mapsto x - \langle x, \alpha\check{} \rangle \alpha$$

from V to V transforms R to R.

(iii) For all $\alpha \in \mathrm{R}$, $\alpha\check{}(\mathrm{R}) \subseteq \mathbf{Z}$.

(iv) If $\alpha \in \mathrm{R}$, then $2\alpha \notin \mathrm{R}$.

In view of (i), the element $\alpha\check{}$, whose existence is guaranteed by (ii), is unique; thus (iii) makes sense. The map s_α is a reflection that leaves fixed the points of $\mathrm{L}_\alpha = \mathrm{Ker}(\alpha\check{})$ and transforms α to $-\alpha$.

The elements of R are called roots. The dimension of V is called the rank of the root system.

2) The group of automorphisms of V that leave R stable is denoted by A(R). The s_α ($\alpha \in \mathrm{R}$) generate a subgroup W(R) of A(R), called the Weyl group of R; this subgroup is normal in A(R). The only reflections belonging to W(R) are the s_α.

3) The set $\mathrm{R}\check{}$ of $\alpha\check{}$ (for $\alpha \in \mathrm{R}$) is a reduced root system in V^*, called the inverse system of R. The map $\alpha \mapsto \alpha\check{}$ is a bijection, called canonical, from R to $\mathrm{R}\check{}$. We have $(\mathrm{R}\check{})\check{} = \mathrm{R}$, and the canonical bijections $\mathrm{R} \to \mathrm{R}\check{}$, $\mathrm{R}\check{} \to \mathrm{R}$ are mutual inverses. The map $u \mapsto {}^t u^{-1}$ defines an isomorphism from W(R) to $\mathrm{W}(\mathrm{R}\check{})$ by means of which we identify these two groups.

4) Let V be a real vector space that is the direct sum of vector subspaces $\mathrm{V}_1, \dots, \mathrm{V}_r$. For all i, let R_i be a reduced root system in V_i. Then the union R of the R_i is a root system in V, called the direct sum of the R_i. The group W(R) can be identified with the product of the $\mathrm{W}(\mathrm{R}_i)$. If $\mathrm{R} \neq \varnothing$ and R is not the direct sum of two non-empty root systems, R is said to be irreducible. This is equivalent to saying that W(R) is irreducible. Every reduced root system

R is a direct sum of irreducible reduced root systems, uniquely determined up to a permutation, and called the irreducible components of R.

5) Let R be a reduced root system in V. There exist scalar products on V invariant under W(R). In the following, we denote by $(x|y)$ such a scalar product. If V and V* are identified using $(x|y)$, we have $\alpha^\vee = \frac{2\alpha}{(\alpha|\alpha)}$. The reflection s_α is the orthogonal reflection which transforms α to $-\alpha$. If R is irreducible, the Weyl group acts transitively on the set of roots of a given length. If R is irreducible, the scalar product $(x|y)$ is unique up to multiplication by a constant.

6) Let R be a reduced root system. For $\alpha, \beta \in \mathrm{R}$, put

$$\langle \alpha, \beta^\vee \rangle = n(\alpha, \beta) \in \mathbf{Z}.$$

We have

$$n(\alpha,\alpha) = 2,$$
$$s_\beta(\alpha) = \alpha - n(\alpha,\beta)\beta,$$
$$n(\alpha,\beta) = \frac{2(\alpha|\beta)}{(\beta|\beta)}.$$

The only possibilities are the following, up to interchanging α and β:

$n(\alpha,\beta) = n(\beta,\alpha) = 0;$	$(\widehat{\alpha,\beta}) = \frac{\pi}{2};$	$s_\alpha s_\beta$ of order 2;
$n(\alpha,\beta) = n(\beta,\alpha) = 1;$	$(\widehat{\alpha,\beta}) = \frac{\pi}{3};$ $\Vert \alpha \Vert = \Vert \beta \Vert;$	$s_\alpha s_\beta$ of order 3;
$n(\alpha,\beta) = n(\beta,\alpha) = -1;$	$(\widehat{\alpha,\beta}) = \frac{2\pi}{3};$ $\Vert \alpha \Vert = \Vert \beta \Vert;$	$s_\alpha s_\beta$ of order 3;
$n(\alpha,\beta) = 1,\ n(\beta,\alpha) = 2;$	$(\widehat{\alpha,\beta}) = \frac{\pi}{4};$ $\Vert \beta \Vert = \sqrt{2} \Vert \alpha \Vert;$	$s_\alpha s_\beta$ of order 4;
$n(\alpha,\beta) = -1,\ n(\beta,\alpha) = -2;$	$(\widehat{\alpha,\beta}) = \frac{3\pi}{4};$ $\Vert \beta \Vert = \sqrt{2} \Vert \alpha \Vert;$	$s_\alpha s_\beta$ of order 4;
$n(\alpha,\beta) = 1,\ n(\beta,\alpha) = 3;$	$(\widehat{\alpha,\beta}) = \frac{\pi}{6};$ $\Vert \beta \Vert = \sqrt{3} \Vert \alpha \Vert;$	$s_\alpha s_\beta$ of order 6;
$n(\alpha,\beta) = -1,\ n(\beta,\alpha) = -3;$	$(\widehat{\alpha,\beta}) = \frac{5\pi}{6};$ $\Vert \beta \Vert = \sqrt{3} \Vert \alpha \Vert;$	$s_\alpha s_\beta$ of order 6;
$n(\alpha,\beta) = n(\beta,\alpha) = 2;$	$\alpha = \beta;$	
$n(\alpha,\beta) = n(\beta,\alpha) = -2;$	$\alpha = -\beta;$	

7) Let $\alpha, \beta \in \mathrm{R}$. If $(\alpha|\beta) > 0$, $\alpha - \beta$ is a root unless $\alpha = \beta$. If $(\alpha|\beta) < 0$, $\alpha + \beta$ is a root unless $\alpha = -\beta$.

8) Let α, β be two non-proportional roots. The set I of $j \in \mathbf{Z}$ such that $\beta + j\alpha \in \mathrm{R}$ is an interval $[-q, p]$ of $\mathbf{Z}$ containing 0. We have

$$p - q = -n(\beta,\alpha), \quad \frac{q+1}{p} = \frac{(\beta+\alpha|\beta+\alpha)}{(\beta|\beta)}.$$

Let S be the set of $\beta + j\alpha$ for $j \in I$. Then $s_\alpha(S) = S$ and $s_\alpha(\beta + p\alpha) = \beta - q\alpha$. We call S the α-chain of roots defined by β, $\beta - q\alpha$ its origin, $\beta + p\alpha$ its end, and $p + q$ its length.

If T is an α-chain with origin γ, the length of T is $-n(\gamma, \alpha)$.

9) Let X be the union of the $\operatorname{Ker} \check{\alpha}$ ($\alpha \in R$). The connected components of $V - X$ are called the chambers of R in V. They are open simplicial cones. The Weyl group acts simply-transitively on the set of chambers. If C is a chamber, $\overline{C}$ is a fundamental domain for W(R). We have $(x|y) > 0$ for $x, y \in C$. The bijection from V to V^* corresponding to $(x|y)$ defines a bijection from the set of chambers of R in V to the set of chambers of $\check{R}$ in V^*; we denote by $\check{C}$ the chamber that is the image of C under this bijection.

10) Let C be a chamber of R. Let $L_1, L_2, \ldots, L_l$ be the walls of C. For all i, there exists a unique root α_i such that $L_i = L_{\alpha_i}$ and α_i is on the same side of L_i as C. The family $(\alpha_1, \ldots, \alpha_l)$ is a basis of V, and C is the set of $x \in V$ such that $\langle \check{\alpha}_i, x \rangle > 0$ for all i, in other words such that $(\alpha_i|x) > 0$ for all i. Then $\{\alpha_1, \ldots, \alpha_l\}$ is called the basis B(C) of R defined by C. We have $(\alpha_i|\alpha_j) \leqslant 0$ when $i \neq j$. The group W(R) acts simply-transitively on the set of bases. Every root is transformed by some element of W(R) to an element of B(C). We have $\{\check{\alpha}_1, \ldots, \check{\alpha}_l\} = B(\check{C})$.

11) Put $s_{\alpha_i} = s_i$, let S be the set of the s_i, and let m_{ij} be the order of $s_i s_j$. The pair (W(R), S) is a Coxeter system with Coxeter matrix (m_{ij}); in other words, W(R) is defined by the family of generators $(s_i)_{1 \leqslant i \leqslant l}$ and the relations $(s_i s_j)^{m_{ij}} = 1$. Two elements s_i and s_j are conjugate in W(R) if and only if there exists a sequence of indices $(i_1, i_2, \ldots, i_q)$ such that $i_1 = i, i_q = j$ and each of the $m_{i_l i_{l+1}}$ is equal to 3.

12) Let $n_{ij} = n(\alpha_i, \alpha_j)$. The matrix $(n_{ij})_{1 \leqslant i,j \leqslant l}$ is called the Cartan matrix of R. It is independent (up to a permutation of $1, 2, \ldots, l$) of the choice of C. We have $n_{ii} = 2, n_{ij} \in \{0, -1, -2, -3\}$ for $i \neq j$. If two root systems have the same Cartan matrix they are isomorphic.

13) Let G be the subgroup of A(R) that leaves B(C) stable. Then A(R) is the semi-direct product of G by W(R).

14) The order relation on V (resp. V^*) defined by C is the order relation, compatible with the vector space structure of V (resp. V^*), for which the elements $\geqslant 0$ are the linear combinations of the α_i (resp. $\check{\alpha}_i$) with coefficients $\geqslant 0$. These elements are called positive for C, or for B(C). These order relations are also defined by $\check{C}$. An element of V is $\geqslant 0$ if and only if its values on $\check{C}$ are $\geqslant 0$. The set of elements $\geqslant 0$ for C contains $\overline{C}$ but is in general distinct from $\overline{C}$. Let $x \in V$. Then $x \in \overline{C}$ if and only if $x \geqslant w(x)$ for all $w \in W(R)$; and $x \in C$ if and only if $x > w(x)$ for all $w \in W(R)$ distinct from 1.

15) Every root is either positive or negative for C. We denote by $R_+(C)$ the set of roots that are positive for C, so that $R = R_+(C) \cup (-R_+(C))$ is

a partition of R. The reflection s_i transforms α_i to $-\alpha_i$ and permutes the elements of $R_+(C)$ distinct from α_i among themselves.

16) Let B be a basis of R. Every positive (resp. negative) root for B is a linear combination of elements of B with coefficients that are integers $\geqslant 0$ (resp. $\leqslant 0$).

17) Let $(\beta_1, \beta_2, \ldots, \beta_n)$ be a sequence of roots that are positive for C and such that $\beta_1 + \cdots + \beta_n$ is a root. There exists a permutation $\pi \in \mathfrak{S}_n$ such that, for all $i \in \{1, 2, \ldots, n\}$, $\beta_{\pi(1)} + \beta_{\pi(2)} + \cdots + \beta_{\pi(i)}$ is a root.

18) Let $\alpha \in R_+(C)$. Then $\alpha \in B(C)$ if and only if α cannot be written as a sum of positive roots.

19) Let C be a chamber, $(\alpha_1, \alpha_2, \ldots, \alpha_l)$ the corresponding basis. For any subset J of $I = \{1, 2, \ldots, l\}$, let W_J be the subgroup of W(R) generated by the s_i such that $i \in J$. Let C_J be the set of linear combinations of the α_j with $j \in J$ and with coefficients > 0, so that C_J is a facet of C.

Let $J \subset I$, $g \in W(R)$. The following conditions are equivalent:

a) g leaves a point of C_J invariant;
b) g leaves every point of C_J invariant;
c) g leaves every point of $\overline{C_J}$ invariant;
d) $g(C_J) = C_J$;
e) $g(\overline{C_J}) = \overline{C_J}$;
f) $g \in W_J$.

Let $J, J' \subset \{1, 2, \ldots, l\}$ and $g, g' \in W(R)$. The following conditions are equivalent:

a) $g(C_J) = g'(C_{J'})$;
b) $g(C_J) \cap g'(C_{J'}) \neq \varnothing$;
c) $gW_J = g'W_{J'}$;
d) $J = J'$ and $g' \in gW_J$.

Let $J_1, J_2, \ldots, J_r \subset I$ and $J = J_1 \cap \cdots \cap J_r$. Then $W_J = W_{J_1} \cap \cdots \cap W_{J_r}$.
For all $g \in W(R)$, there exists $J \subset I$ such that $\overline{C} \cap g(\overline{C}) = \overline{C_J}$ and $g \in W_J$.

20) Let P be a subset of R. Then P is said to be closed if the conditions $\alpha \in P, \beta \in P, \alpha + \beta \in R$ imply $\alpha + \beta \in P$; and P is said to be parabolic if P is closed and $P \cup (-P) = R$. The following conditions are equivalent:

a) P is parabolic;
b) P is closed and there exists a chamber C such that $P \supset R_+(C)$;
c) there exist a chamber C and a subset Σ of B(C) such that P is the union of $R_+(C)$ and the set Q of roots that are linear combinations of elements of Σ with coefficients that are integers $\leqslant 0$.

Assume that these conditions are satisfied and let V_1 be the vector subspace of V generated by Σ. Then

$$P \cap (-P) = Q \cup (-Q) = V_1 \cap R,$$

and $P \cap (-P)$ is a root system in V_1 with basis Σ.

Let P', C', Σ' have analogous properties. If there exists an element of W(R) transforming P to P′, there exists an element of W(R) transforming C to C′, Σ to Σ' and P to P′.

21) Let P be a subset of R. The following conditions are equivalent:

a) there exists a chamber C such that $P = R_+(C)$;

b) P is closed, and $\{P, -P\}$ is a partition of R.

The chamber C is then unique.

Assume that V is equipped with the structure of an ordered vector space such that every root is either positive or negative. Let R_+ be the set of positive roots for this structure. There exists a unique chamber C such that $R_+ = R_+(C)$.

22) A subset B of R is a basis of R if and only if the elements of B are linearly independent and every root is a linear combination of elements of B with coefficients that are all $\geqslant 0$ or all $\leqslant 0$.

23) Let P be a closed subset of R such that $P \cap (-P) = \varnothing$. There exists a chamber C such that $P \subset R_+(C)$.

24) A subset P of R is called symmetric if $P = -P$. Let P be a subset of R, and let V_1 (resp. Γ) be the vector subspace (resp. the additive subgroup) of V generated by P. The following conditions are equivalent:

a) P is closed and symmetric;

b) P is closed and P is a root system in V_1;

c) $\Gamma \cap R = P$.

25) Assume that R is irreducible. Let C be a chamber; put

$$B(C) = \{\alpha_1, \ldots, \alpha_l\}.$$

There exists a highest element of R (for the order defined by C), that is, an element $\tilde{\alpha} = n_1\alpha_1 + \cdots + n_l\alpha_l$ of R such that, for any root

$$p_1\alpha_1 + \cdots + p_l\alpha_l,$$

$n_1 \geqslant p_1, \ldots, n_l \geqslant p_l$. Then $\tilde{\alpha} \in \overline{C}$ and $\| \tilde{\alpha} \| \geqslant \| \alpha \|$ for every root α.

26) The subgroup of V generated by R is denoted by Q(R); the elements of Q(R) are called the radical weights of R. The group Q(R) is a discrete subgroup of V of rank $l = \dim V$. Any basis of R is a basis of Q(R).

The subgroup of V associated to $Q(R^\vee)$ is denoted by P(R); the elements of P(R) are called the weights of R. The group P(R) is a discrete subgroup of V of rank l containing Q(R). The groups $P(R)/Q(R)$, $P(R^\vee)/Q(R^\vee)$ are finite and isomorphic; their order f is called the connection index of R. With the notation of 25), the order of W(R) is $l!n_1n_2\ldots n_lf$.

The group A(R) leaves P(R), Q(R) stable, and hence acts on P(R)/Q(R). The group W(R) acts trivially on P(R)/Q(R), so A(R)/W(R) acts on P(R)/Q(R).

27) Let C be a chamber. Let $B = (\alpha_1, \dots, \alpha_l)$ be the corresponding basis of R. The dual basis $(\omega_1, \dots, \omega_l)$ of $(\check{\alpha_1}, \dots, \check{\alpha_l})$ is a basis of P(R). The ω_i are called the fundamental weights (for C, or for B). The set of linear combinations of the ω_i with coefficients > 0 (resp. $\geqslant 0$) is C (resp. $\overline{C}$). The linear combinations of the ω_i with integer coefficients $\geqslant 0$ are called the dominant weights. Every element of P(R) can be transformed by some element of W(R) to a unique dominant weight. The dominant weights are the elements ω of V such that $\frac{2(\omega|\alpha_i)}{(\alpha_i|\alpha_i)}$ is an integer $\geqslant 0$ for all i.

28) Let $\rho = \frac{1}{2} \sum_{\alpha \in R_+(C)} \alpha$. Then, $\rho = \omega_1 + \cdots + \omega_l \in C$.

29) Let T be the group of translations of V^* whose vectors belong to $Q(R\check{})$. The group of affine tranformations of V^* generated by T and W(R) is the semi-direct product of W(R) by T. This group is called the affine Weyl group of R and is denoted by $W_a(R)$. It acts properly on V^*. For $\alpha \in R$ and $\lambda \in \mathbf{Z}$, let $s_{\alpha,\lambda}$ be the map $x^* \mapsto x^* - \langle x^*, \alpha\rangle \alpha\check{} + \lambda\alpha\check{}$; this is an affine reflection, and the set $L_{\alpha,\lambda}$ of its fixed points is defined by the equation $\langle x^*, \alpha\rangle = \lambda$; we have $L_{\alpha,\lambda} = L_\alpha + \frac{1}{2}\lambda\alpha\check{}$. The $s_{\alpha,\lambda}$ are the affine reflections belonging to $W_a(R)$, and they generate the group $W_a(R)$.

30) Let E be the union of the $L_{\alpha,\lambda}$ for $\alpha \in R$ and $\lambda \in \mathbf{Z}$. The connected components of $V^* - E$ are called the alcoves of R. If R is irreducible, each alcove is an open simplex; in general, an alcove is a product of open simplices. The group $W_a(R)$ acts simply-transitively on the set of alcoves. If C is an alcove, $\overline{C}$ is a fundamental domain for $W_a(R)$. Let $\sigma_1, \dots, \sigma_q$ be the reflections in $W_a(R)$ corresponding to the walls of C; let μ_{ij} be the order of $\sigma_i\sigma_j$. Then $W_a(R)$ is defined by the generators σ_i and the relations $(\sigma_i\sigma_j)^{\mu_{ij}} = 1$.

31) If $p \in P(R\check{})$, there exists an alcove C such that p is an extremal point of $\overline{C}$. If C′ is an alcove, there is a unique radical weight that is an extremal point of $\overline{C'}$.

Let $x^* \in V^*$; the following conditions are equivalent:

a) $x^* \in P(R\check{})$;

b) for all $\alpha \in R$, the hyperplane parallel to L_α and passing through x^* is one of the $L_{\alpha,\lambda}$.

Let C′ be a chamber of $R\check{}$. There exists a unique alcove C contained in C′ and such that $0 \in \overline{C}$. Assume that R is irreducible, and let β be the highest root of R (for C′); then C is the set of $x^* \in C'$ such that $\langle x^*, \beta\rangle < 1$.

32) Let S be the symmetric algebra of V, S^W the subalgebra consisting of the elements invariant under $W = W(R)$, g the order of W, $l = \dim V$. There exist homogeneous, algebraically independent elements $I_1, I_2, \dots, I_l$ that generate S^W. The S^W-module S has a basis consisting of g homogeneous elements. Let $\mathfrak{a}$ be the ideal of S generated by the homogeneous elements of S^W of degree > 0; the representation of W on $S/\mathfrak{a}$, induced by the representation of W

on S by passage to the quotient, is isomorphic to the regular representation of W (over **R**).

33) Let $I_1, I_2, \dots, I_l$ be homogeneous, algebraically independent elements generating S^W. Their degrees $k_1, k_2, \dots, k_l$ are uniquely determined (up to order) by R. We have $g = k_1 k_2 \dots k_l$. The number of roots is $2\sum_{i=1}^{l}(k_i - 1)$.

34) An element A of S is said to be anti-invariant under W if $w(A) = \det(w).A$ for all $w \in W$. Let $R = R_1 \cup (-R_1)$ be a partition of R, and put $\pi = \prod_{\alpha \in R_1} \alpha$. The element π of S is anti-invariant; the anti-invariant elements of S are the elements of the form πI, with $I \in S^W$.

35) Let E be the group algebra **Z**[P] of the group of weights P of R. If $p \in P$, we denote by e^p the corresponding element of E. We have $e^p e^{p'} = e^{p+p'}$ and the e^p form a basis of E. There is an action of the group W on E such that $w(e^p) = e^{w(p)}$ if $w \in W$ and $p \in P$. An element $z \in E$ is said to be anti-invariant if $w(z) = \det(w).z$ for all $w \in W$. For all $z \in E$, put $J(z) = \sum_{w \in W} \det(w).w(z)$. Let C be a chamber. The elements $J(e^p)$, where $p \in P \cap C$, form a basis of the group of anti-invariant elements of E. If ρ is half the sum of the positive roots, we have:

$$J(e^\rho) = e^\rho \prod_{\alpha > 0}(1 - e^{-\alpha}) = \prod_{\alpha > 0}(e^{\alpha/2} - e^{-\alpha/2}),$$

the products being taken over the set of roots > 0.

36) With the notation of 35), put

$$z_p = J(e^{p+\rho})/J(e^\rho) \quad \text{for } p \in P.$$

The z_p, for $p \in P \cap \overline{C}$, form a basis of the group E^W of elements of E invariant under W. If $\omega_1, \dots, \omega_l$ are the fundamental weights of R, the elements z_{ω_i}, $1 \leqslant i \leqslant l$, are algebraically independent and generate the ring E^W.

37) Let C be a chamber of R, $(\alpha_1, \dots, \alpha_l)$ the corresponding basis. The element $c = s_1 s_2 \dots s_l$ of W is called the Coxeter transformation of R. The conjugacy class of c does not depend on C or on the numbering of the α_i. The order h of c is called the Coxeter number of R. The eigenvalues of c are of the form $\exp\frac{2i\pi m_j}{h}$, where the integers $m_1, m_2, \dots, m_l$ (called the exponents of R) are such that $1 \leqslant m_1 \leqslant m_2 \leqslant \dots \leqslant m_l \leqslant h - 1$.

Assume that R is irreducible. Then

$$m_1 = 1, \quad m_l = h - 1.$$

$$m_j + m_{l+1-j} = h \quad (1 \leqslant j \leqslant l).$$

$$m_1 + m_2 + \dots + m_l = \frac{1}{2}lh = \frac{1}{2}\mathrm{Card}(R).$$

Every $m \in \{1, 2, \ldots, h-1\}$ coprime to h is equal to exactly one of the m_j. The numbers $m_1+1, m_2+1, \ldots, m_l+1$ coincide, up to order, with the integers denoted by $k_1, k_2, \ldots, k_l$ in 33). With the notation of 25), $n_1+\cdots+n_l = h-1$. There exist l orbits of $\{1, c, c^2, \ldots, c^{h-1}\}$ on R, each of which has h elements.

If h is even, $c^{h/2}$ transforms C to $-$C. We have $-1 \in$ W if and only if the exponents of W are all odd; in that case, h is even and $c^{h/2} = -1$.